Pathology and Pathobiology
of the
Urinary Bladder and Prostate

UNITED STATES AND CANADIAN ACADEMY OF PATHOLOGY, INC.

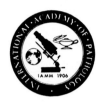

MONOGRAPHS IN PATHOLOGY

SERIES EDITOR, F. Stephen Vogel, M.D.
Secretary-Treasurer

UNITED STATES AND CANADIAN ACADEMY OF PATHOLOGY, INC.

Pathology and Pathobiology
of the
Urinary Bladder and Prostate

EDITED BY

RONALD S. WEINSTEIN, M.D.
Professor and Head
Department of Pathology
University of Arizona College of Medicine
Tucson, Arizona

WILLIAM A. GARDNER, JR., M.D.
Professor and Chairman
Department of Pathology
University of South Alabama
College of Medicine
Mobile, Alabama

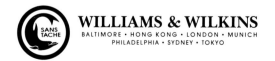

WILLIAMS & WILKINS
BALTIMORE · HONG KONG · LONDON · MUNICH
PHILADELPHIA · SYDNEY · TOKYO

Publisher: Deanna F. Gemmill
Associate Publisher: Carole E. Pippin
Copy Editor: Ann Donaldson, ELS
Designer: Norman Och
Illustration Planner: Lorraine Wrzosek

Printed in the United States of America

Library of Congress Cataloging-in-Publication Data
Pathology and pathobiology of the urinary bladder and prostate / edited by Ronald S. Weinstein, William A. Gardner, Jr.
    p.   cm.—(Monographs in pathology; no. 34)
    At head of title: United States and Canadian Academy of Pathology.
    Includes bibliographical references and index.
    ISBN 0-683-08911-0
    1. Bladder—Pathophysiology. 2. Prostate—Pathophysiology. I. Weinstein, Ronald S. II. Gardner, William A., 1939–   . III. United States and Canadian Academy of Pathology. IV. Series.
    [DNLM: 1. Bladder—pathology—congresses. 2. Bladder Diseases—pathology—congresses. 3. Prostate—pathology—congresses. 4. Prostate Diseases—pathology—congresses. W1 MO568H no. 34]
RC919.P34 1992
616.99′262—dc20
DNLM/DLC
for Library of Congress   92-5499
                                                                                            CIP

Foreword

The co-directors of the Long Course that was presented at the 1991 meeting of the United States and Canadian Academy of Pathology served as co-editors of this 34th issue in the "*Monographs in Pathology*" series. Members of the faculty each authored a Chapter for the text. Although time imposed restraints upon the content of the oral presentations, this fetter was relaxed during the compilation of the monograph. Thus, this volume contains much additional material that has been screened carefully for its practical and scientific value to the conduct of medicine and pathology.

The Academy expresses sincere appreciation to Drs. Ronald Weinstein and William Gardner, and this gratitude extends fully to the many additional contributors. The assistance of Williams & Wilkins and its staff is gratefully acknowledged.

F. STEPHEN VOGEL, M.D.
Series Editor

Preface

This monograph presents, in expanded form, the United States and Canadian Academy of Pathology's Long Course, *Pathology and Pathobiology of the Urinary Bladder and Prostate*. Held at the annual meeting of the Academy on March 20, 1991, in Chicago, this represents the first time that these organs have been the focus of attention in this distinguished series. Any pathologist at all familiar with the concepts and practices of urogenital pathology, is aware of the extraordinary contributions of Dr. Kash Mostofi to the field. In addition to his position as one of the premier urologic pathologists in the world, his historical leadership role in the USCAP and IAP makes it all the more appropriate that Chapter 1 in this volume be a tribute to Dr. Mostofi.

This monograph is by no means intended to be a comprehensive text on the pathology of the bladder and prostate, but rather to bring together recent concepts, techniques, and diagnostic interpretations that are new, perhaps contentious, or even possibly neglected.

In Chapter 2, Dr. Ronald S. Weinstein introduces two themes in molecular genetics that are currently thought to have a bearing on bladder cancer. First is a consideration of some modern concepts regarding tumorigenesis. An examination of ways in which clinical bladder cancer could possibly be explained by some recently introduced concepts of the molecular genetics of neoplasia follows. The point is emphasized that some aspects of bladder tumor progression seem to fit popular concepts of multistep oncogenesis while other clinical presentations could represent variations or exceptions. A second topic, the molecular genetic basis of failures of certain forms of cancer therapies, is surveyed and related to urinary bladder where potentially relevant. An extensive bibliography is included since many of the key references may not be readily available to practicing pathologists who lack easy access to libraries with basic science collections.

Chapter 3 is a review of distinctive and diagnostically troublesome nonmalignant lesions of the urinary bladder. Dr. George M. Farrow draws on his vast experience at the Mayo Clinic to assemble a collection of cases that illustrate the considerable capacity of bladder mucosa to express diverse forms of differentiation of both epithelial and mesenchymal components. His figures provide a mini-atlas of such lesions. This is followed by a thorough presentation, by Dr. William M. Murphy, of the spectrum of bladder cancers, detailing both their tumorigenesis and histopathological varieties. Dr. Murphy critically evaluates the value of tumor markers in the workup of bladder cancer, and scrutinizes popular ideas on tumor progression in the bladder.

In Chapter 5, Drs. Leopold G. Koss and Bogdan Czerniak present an update on the use of image analysis and flow cytometry for studying tumors of prostate and bladder. They attempt to relate the results of studies on DNA content to molecular events and to provide a glimpse of future horizons in urogenital tumor research.

Chapter 6, written by Drs. William A. Gardner, Jr., and Betsy D. Bennett, is an exploration of the extraordinary gaps in knowledge of inflammatory and neoplastic disease of the prostate. Next, Dr. Jonathan I. Epstein focuses attention on an area of frequent quandary for both pathologists and urologists, the atypical proliferations of prostate epithelium. Modern concepts of intraductal dysplasia (PIN) and the relationship of such lesions to various forms of adenocarcinoma are discussed. The author carefully outlines many questions that remain to be answered by additional clinical and pathological studies. Chapter 8, by Drs. Gary J. Miller and James M. Cygan, demonstrates the utility of comprehensive study, using macrosections, of resected prostate glands.

Chapter 9, by Dr. Donald S. Coffey and colleagues, is a summary of the final lecture of the full-day course on the pathobiology of prostate. This turned out to be a *tour de force* by most accounts. Presenting a lecture on basic science and holding the interest of a clinically oriented audience, following 6 hours of formal lectures, can be challenging. Dr. Coffey, a master educator, succeeded in captivating, stimulating, and motivating the large audience made up mostly of clinicians. He provided them with novel and provocative ideas on the laboratory assessment of prostate cancer and left some participants hungering for a sabbatical in a basic science laboratory.

The editors wish to express their sincere gratitude to the Academy for the invitation to organize and chair this Long Course, to the USCAP Education Committee and their liaison, Dr. Authur H. Cohen, for guidance and useful advice; to Dr. Nathan Kaufman, for his encouragement, suggestions, and support; to Mr. James Crimmins and his staff for attending to local arrangements; to Dr. F. Stephen Vogel, for bringing the manuscript to completion; and to the contributors for their outstanding presentations at the Long Course, and their timely submission of completed manuscripts.

RONALD S. WEINSTEIN, M.D.
WILLIAM A. GARDNER, JR., M.D.
Monograph Editors

Contributors

BETSY D. BENNETT, M.D., PH.D.
  Professor and Vice Chair, Department of Pathology, University of Southern Alabama, College of Medicine, Mobile, Alabama
H. BALLENTINE CARTER, M.D.
  Assistant Professor of Urology, Department of Urology, The Johns Hopkins University School of Medicine, Baltimore, Maryland
DONALD S. COFFEY, PH.D.
  Professor of Urology, Oncology, and Pharmacology, Department of Urology, The Johns Hopkins University School of Medicine, Baltimore, Maryland
JAMES M. CYGAN, M.D.
  ACS Summer Fellow, Department of Pathology, University of Colorado Health Sciences Center, Denver, Colorado
BOGDAN CZERNIAK, M.D.
  Assistant Professor, Department of Pathology, Montefiore Medical Center, Albert Einstein College of Medicine, Bronx, New York
JONATHAN I. EPSTEIN, M.D.
  Associate Professor of Pathology and Urology, The Johns Hopkins University Medical Institute, The Johns Hopkins Hospital, Baltimore, Maryland
GEORGE M. FARROW, M.D.
  Professor of Pathology, Department of Pathology, Mayo Clinic, Rochester, Minnesota
WILLIAM A. GARDNER, JR., M.D.
  Professor and Chairman, Department of Pathology, University of Southern Alabama, College of Medicine, Mobile, Alabama
LEOPOLD G. KOSS, M.D.
  Professor and Chairman, Department of Pathology, Montefiore Medical Center, Albert Einstein College of Medicine, Bronx, New York
GARY J. MILLER, M.D.
  Assistant Professor of Pathology, Department of Pathology and Division of Urology, University of Colorado Health Sciences Center, Denver, Colorado
WILLIAM M. MURPHY, M.D.
  Professor of Urology, Nephropathology, Urologic Pathology, and Cytology, Department of Pathology, Baptist Memorial Hospital, Memphis, Tennessee
ALAN W. PARTIN, M.D., PH.D.
  Resident, Department of Urology, The Johns Hopkins University School of Medicine, Baltimore, Maryland
RONALD S. WEINSTEIN, M.D.
  Professor and Head, Department of Pathology, University of Arizona College of Medicine, Tucson, Arizona

Contents

Chapter 1

Kash Mostofi, M.D.: A Tribute

RONALD S. WEINSTEIN AND WILLIAM A. GARDNER, JR.

This monograph, which summarizes the contents of lectures delivered at the 1991 Long Course given at the annual meeting of the United States and Canadian Academy of Pathology (USCAP), covers selected topics on urinary bladder and prostate pathology. It is ironic that this was the first USCAP/International Academy of Pathology Long Course on these urogenital organs even though the father of USCAP Long Courses was Dr. Fathollah Keshvar (Kash) Mostofi, the world's leading urogenital pathologist (Fig. 1.1).

Before these Long Course lectures commenced, Dr. Mostofi was invited to the podium to be acknowledged, both for his role in creating the Long Course series and for his contributions to the field of urogenital pathology. As Dr. Mostofi approached the podium, he was met with the thunderous applause of a thousand grateful pathologists. It was announced that Dr. Mostofi would soon celebrate his 80th birthday. The audience responded by rising and robustly singing, "Happy Birthday—Kash Mostofi!"

A question worthy of consideration is, "what makes Kash Mostofi *unique*?" Several possibilities merit consideration. Dr. Mostofi brings to the fields of pathology and medicine an unusual combination of talents, interests, and perspectives that have provided the foundation for a career of accomplishment that continues to flower. His intelligence, personal commitment to excellence, professionalism, integrity, and humanism are admirable. His willingness to make long-term commitments to organizations and projects is unusual and accounts for many of his successes.

What sets Dr. Mostofi apart from other leaders is his particular talent as a consummate problem-solver. Where others see problems, barriers, and doom-and-gloom, Dr. Mostofi sees solutions, and his visions are clear and often prophetic. For generations, colleagues have followed his inspired leadership, allowing him to add immeasurably to the richness of our field. Not only does Dr. Mostofi envision solutions to challenging problems, he has the capacity to create innovative programs to provide solutions, and to nurture them for years until they mature.

A survey of some of the highlights of Dr. Mostofi's career provides a panoramic view of a life of accomplishment. Dr. Mostofi was born in Teheran, Iran, at the beginning of the second decade of this century. He received his A.B. and B.Sc.

1

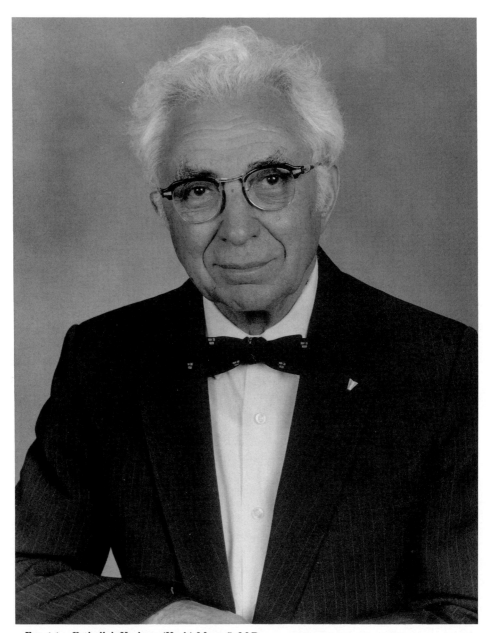

FIG. 1.1.   Fathollah Keshvar (Kash) Mostofi, M.D.

degrees in 1935 at the University of Nebraska and his M.D. from Harvard Medical School in 1939. Following a rotating internship in Bethlehem, Pennsylvania, he returned to Harvard where he trained in pathology at the Peter Bent Brigham Hospital, the Boston Lying-In Hospital & Free Hospital for Women, and the Children's Hospital. Dr. Mostofi accepted a junior faculty position at the Massachusetts General Hospital from 1943 to 1944. He spent the next 4 years on active duty in the military service, and stayed active in the military in subsequent years, retiring as colonel in 1971.

Following active duty, Dr. Mostofi spent a year as Special Research Fellow at the National Cancer Institute in Bethesda, Maryland, and then joined the staff of the Armed Forces Institute of Pathology (AFIP) as Chairman of Genitourinary Pathology in 1948. In addition to his Chair, he was Scientific Director of the American Registry of Pathology, and Chairman, Center for Advanced Pathology, and Associate Director for Consultation, from 1977 to 1986.

Throughout his career at the AFIP, Dr. Mostofi has functioned as one of its most effective section Chairmen. His range of activities, and the standards he set for his section, defined the role of Section Chairman at the AFIP for later generations. He also holds professorships at several medical colleges, including Johns Hopkins, Georgetown, the Uniformed Services University of the Health Sciences, and the University of Maryland. He is currently a member of 35 professional organizations.

Best known of Dr. Mostofi's scientific contributions are his classifications of urogenital tumors. His work on testicular tumors was adopted, with minor modifications, by the World Health Organization (WHO), as have been his classifications of tumors of bladder, prostate, and kidney. WHO publications that he authored are printed in English, French, Spanish, and Russian, and are distributed to all medical schools and all pathology societies. Dr. Mostofi's AFIP fascicle on "Tumors of Male Sex Organs" sold over 25,000 copies and it is now being reprinted.

Dr. Mostofi's contributions have extended far beyond urogenital pathology. For example, he has studied human factors in aircraft accidents since he became interested in the investigation of the crashes of several Comet aircraft in 1954. With Wing Commander Bruce Harvey, RAF (later Air Vice Marshal), Dr. Mostofi helped organize the Joint (American-British-Canadian) Committee on Aviation Pathology, and served as Secretary of this Committee from 1954 to 1960. Among its accomplishments, the Committee developed detailed instructions and procedures for examining and recording findings on the remains of crash victims. These have been widely utilized. On another occasion, the Director of the AFIP asked Dr. Mostofi to organize an international cooperative research program on schistosomiasis, an important military disease. When budgetary limitations prevented the attainment of the goal with in-house funding, Dr. Mostofi arranged for an international symposium and published a book with contributions from 30 world authorities, without any funding from the United States. This is the only book that has been published on the pathology of schistosomiasis.

Dr. Mostofi has been an innovator in the area of continuing medical education. One innovation that has endured for a generation is the "USCAP Long Course."

The lineage of the Long Course recorded in this monograph extends back to the first pathology "Long Course" presented at the annual meeting of the United States-Canadian Division of the International Academy of Pathology (predecessor organization of the USCAP) in 1953, which Dr. Mostofi organized. The Long Course and subsequent monographs have constituted major continuing educational programs at succeeding yearly meetings. Another innovation relevant to this year's Long Course is Dr. Mostofi's annual 5-day course on urologic pathology. In the 17 years that the course has been given, all urologists in the military and more than half of the urologists in this country, including most of the United States professors of urology, have taken the course.

Many important honors have been bestowed on Dr. Mostofi for his outstanding achievements. In 1972, he received the first and only Gold Medallion of the United States-Canadian Division of the International Academy of Pathology (IAP). In 1977, the Division established the F. K. Mostofi Distinguished Service Award, to be presented annually to a person who has contributed significantly to the progress of pathology. At its annual meeting held in mid-March 1977 at Toronto, President Jack Layton presented Dr. Mostofi with a portrait, executed by the renowned photographer, Mr. Yousof Karsh. These honors were in recognition of Dr. Mostofi's long and faithful service to the Academy: as Secretary-Treasurer of both the IAP and the United States-Canadian Division from 1952–1970; and subsequently as Vice President and President of the Division, followed by two terms as President of the international body. As Secretary-Treasurer of the IAP, Dr. Mostofi has been credited with nurturing this society into a dynamic international organization with 23 divisions, world-wide.

As Secretary-Treasurer of the International Council of Societies of Pathology, an office he has held since 1984, Dr. Mostofi assisted the World Health Organization in the selection of members to various WHO Scientific Panels dealing with pathology and/or cancer. The objective has been to develop an internationally accepted histological classification of chronic disease, particularly cancer. Dr. Mostofi has organized the distribution of teaching aids prepared by WHO to many of the 70 national societies belonging to the group, and publicizing the program throughout the world. On many occasions, he has been selected by the National Research Council-National Academy of Science to represent the United States at international congresses and on multinational committees. His broad knowledge of medical issues, his interest in world health care, and his keen analytical skills and sound judgment, have made him a highly respected representative of this country and a credit to the field of pathology.

Whereas Dr. Mostofi's professional contributions are meritorious, it is thoughts of the man behind the curriculum vitae that are treasured by his students, colleagues, and friends. Physicians world-wide know Dr. Mostofi for his gentle manner, his inquiring and creative mind, and his deep commitment to patient care. Unquestionably, he is the most readily recognized pathologist in the world today. A familiar sight at pathology meetings everywhere is the entrance into a lecture hall or reception area of an alert, tall, trim, stylishly dressed, grey-haired gentleman, with an endearing smile, who radiates good will and has the unmistakable presence of a citizen of the world. He is a trusted colleague and a dependable friend. He always seems glad to be wherever he is, and delighted that he might have an opportunity to learn or to add something useful to the proceedings.

The co-directors of this Long Course thank Dr. Mostofi for attending, and for his inspiration.

Chapter 2

Genetics of Tumorigenesis and Multidrug Resistance in Urinary Bladder Cancer

RONALD S. WEINSTEIN

INTRODUCTION

Recent advances in cytogenetics and molecular genetics have provided a framework for studies on the pathogenesis of human cancers[246] and on the rational use of chemotherapy.[216,217,234,308] This presentation addresses two somewhat unrelated genetic themes in cancer research: (1) the roles of oncogenes and suppressor genes in human carcinogenesis; and (2) genetic control mechanisms that modulate tumor sensitivity to certain forms of chemotherapy. Work in each of these areas in recent years has generated information published in many hundreds of papers and numerous monographs. The objective of this presentation is to provide the pathologist with an intellectual framework for dealing with each of these topics. Obviously, this will require including some information that is tangential to studies on the urinary bladder. Although early observations in molecular genetics actually came from studies utilizing bladder cancer cells,[230,277,279] much of the subsequent oncogene and cancer pharmacology research has been performed on cells from other organs and, in certain instances, the relevance of this work to the genitourinary tract is unclear. Nevertheless, general principles that are emerging appear to be relevant to the theme of this monograph on urinary bladder and prostate pathology and therefore merit consideration.

The discovery that genes are involved in multistage tumorigenesis is a major advance in tumor biology, with implications for diagnosis and treatment.[245,310] Many laboratories have identified cellular genes, some of which are oncogenes, whose alterations during tumorigenesis trigger phases in tumor initiation and progression that culminate in the full expression of the malignant phenotype.[311,313] Over the past decade, more than 50 oncogenes have been characterized,[269] their tissue distributions in normal tissues and tumors have been cataloged,[91] and putative roles of oncogenes and suppressor genes in tumorigenesis have been delineated.[304,305] Models of carcinogenesis have been constructed that illustrate the accumulation of various types of sequential events. The variety of features these models portray help to underline the complexity of the process of carcinogenesis and, in some instances, may even suggest that more than one pathway can lead to the eventual development of a malignant tumor.[22,98,215]

For pedagogical purposes, the colorectal adenoma-cancer model developed by Vogelstein and his colleagues[150,304,305] will be described as an example of multistage tumor progression. (Fig. 2.1) While the applicability to bladder malignancies of some of the specific oncogenes and suppressor genes implicated by Vogelstein's group in colorectal carcinogenesis is unclear, it seems likely that the central concept of Vogelstein's work, that multiple oncogenic hits are required for completion of carcinogenesis, is applicable to bladder transitional cell carcinomas. This fits the late onset of transitional cell carcinoma in most bladder cancer patients, suggesting a requirement for multiple events to occur to complete urothelial transformation into the malignant state.[97,223] Another concept, that bladder cancers have a chemical carcinogenic etiology, is also consistent with the Vogelstein scheme. The demonstration, in skin, that *ras* oncogene activation by point mutation can indeed be induced by chemical carcinogens, such as dimethylbenzanthracene, provides evidence for a link between chemical carcinogenesis

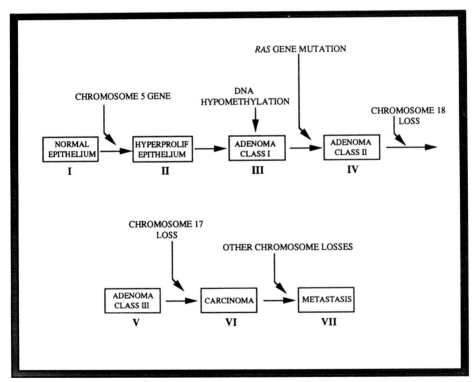

FIG. 2.1. The Vogelstein model for colorectal tumorigenesis. Tumorigenesis proceeds through a series of genetic alterations involving tumor-suppressor genes (particularly those on chromosomes 5, 17, and 18) and oncogenes (*ras*). The tumors continue to progress once carcinomas have formed, and the accumulated loss of suppressor genes on additional chromosomes correlates with the ability of the carcinomas to metastasize. A parallel series of events could be involved in tumorigenesis in the urinary bladder. See text for details.

and oncogenes.[15,131] Activated *ras* genes are found in chemically induced benign and malignant tumors in urinary bladder although, interestingly, not in the hyperplastic or preneoplastic lesions preceding tumor development.[306] Details of the Vogelstein model are still being elaborated so that the analogy between colorectal cancer and bladder cancer is incomplete. Additional time will be required to establish the applicability of some of the specific features of the Vogelstein model to tumors in other organs, including bladder.

Molecular genetics is also playing a central role in the study of cancer pharmacology.[108,109,308] Discovery of genes, unrelated to oncogenes, that endow subpopulations of cancer cells with mechanisms to circumvent the toxic effects of certain anticancer drugs has provided a basis for the development of novel approaches to therapy that are currently being tested in clinical trials.[118,242,290] Thus, genetics in concert with cellular and molecular pharmacology has produced new insights into the development of potentially useful novel treatment strategies.

The topic of genetic modulation of cancer drug sensitivity will be introduced using a truly remarkable gene, the multidrug resistance (*MDR1*) gene, as an example of a gene that profoundly influences the sensitivity of certain tumor cells to drugs.[118,234,242,296] At the outset, it should be stressed that many unrelated mechanisms can confer drug resistance to tumors.[151] These include alterations in drug uptake,[26,107,153] intracellular drug accumulation[41,68,171] and distribution,[104,128,129,324] increased metabolic inactivation of drugs,[120,229,271] decreased drug activation,[6,169,231] altered target proteins[3,39,110,119,147] or levels of normal target proteins,[222,257] and altered DNA repair mechanisms.[42,79] The situation is further complicated by the fact that these mechanisms are not mutually exclusive, and that several interrelated mechanisms can be involved in the resistance process.[18,62,78,198,216] It is possible that several different resistance mechanisms become operative in individual cancer patients over the course of their disease.[198]

Justifications for singling out P-glycoprotein (Pgp, P-170, Mdr1 protein, or Mdr1), the product of the *MDR1* gene, for consideration at this time are that Mdr1 is expressed in some normal transitional epithelia and bladder tumors[318] and is well characterized.[78,101,135,141,238] It serves as an instructive example of a mediator of drug resistance that can be manipulated both experimentally[290] and clinically in a way that reverses drug resistance and reestablishes drug sensitivity.[64,65,193,194,227,236,249] Mdr1 mediates multidrug resistance, a complex phenomenon characterized by a broad cross-resistance of cancer cells to a spectrum of apparently dissimilar natural-product compounds. Mdr1 functions, in cancer cells, as an energy-driven ~170 kDa membrane efflux transporter with unusually broad substrate specificity that decreases the steady state accumulation of drugs.[47,104,117,122,159] This glycoprotein is present in plasma membranes and on the luminal side of the Golgi stacks.[325] It transports an assortment of structurally dissimilar natural-product drugs, including doxorubicin and vinblastine, out of tumor cells directly from the cytosol or may facilitate vectorial transport of drugs sequestered in endocytic vesicles. Functioning as a pump, Mdr1 prevents the accumulation of toxic drugs at their targets.[17,34,117] Many details of this transport process remain to be elucidated.[239]

What caught the attention of oncologists is that the Mdr1 transporter function can be inhibited by structurally unrelated agents such as calcium channel blockers and quinidine. Inhibition of the Mdr1 pump function reverses drug resistance in Mdr1-expressing tumor cells and reestablishes the drug-sensitive phenotype.[233,324] Another type of multidrug resistance, associated with alterations in the essential nuclear enzyme topoisomerase II, has been called "atypical" multidrug resistance.[20,67] It is mentioned so that the reader will be aware of the fact that there are several ways in which cancer cells may achieve a multidrug resistant state, not all of which are amenable to pump inhibition.

Most of the early studies testing Mdr1 inhibitors utilized tissue culture systems[20]; however, a few recent studies on patients indicated that Mdr1 pump inhibition might be useful as a therapeutic strategy in the clinical setting. For example, early clinical trials on a small series of patients with drug-refractory hematological malignancies, using Mdr1 inhibitors as adjuvants to chemotherapy, produced some remissions.[194,249] This raised the possibility that use of intravesical chemotherapy in combination with the administration of intravesical Mdr1 inhibitors might benefit bladder cancer patients,[175] but the results of such clinical trials have not been reported. This approach to bladder chemotherapy would be worth considering for the treatment of superficial disease in which Mdr1 inhibitors could gain direct access to tumor cells via the urinary space.

In summary, this discussion will focus on two major themes in cancer biology that are currently at center stage in the world of cancer molecular genetics, carcinogenesis and drug resistance.

CENTRAL ROLE OF GENETIC ALTERATIONS IN CARCINOGENESIS

Malignant cell populations are characterized by a genetic instability that leads to the spontaneous generation of variant cell forms with different phenotypic and genotypic properties. It is widely held that the origin of human cancer is at least partially explained by the accumulation of such genetic changes within a single cell and its progeny.[212,213,311] These genetic changes have been shown to include the somatic activation of "dominantly acting" protooncogenes through point mutation, rearrangement, or amplification,[27,267] and the germline or somatic inactivation of tumor-suppressor genes through point mutation and/or deletion.[123,158,200] Protooncogenes are normal cellular genes involved in cellular proliferation and differentiation that have the potential of contributing to the development of tumors when their structure or expression is altered.[51,157]

The existence of tumor-suppressor genes was deduced from studies with somatic cell hybrids. When malignant cells were fused with normal cells, the resulting hybrids were nontumorigenic.[124,272] These experiments indicated that a gene (or genes) from a normal cell might replace a defective function in a malignant cell and possibly render it responsive to normal regulators of cell growth.[273] The tumor-suppressor gene may represent the critical target in the allelic loss event. Such genes may encode proteins that regulate normal growth and, thus, indirectly suppress neoplastic development.[28,181,312] For purposes of discussion, specific examples of oncogenes and suppressor genes are introduced.

The discovery that a single point mutation can account for the transforming properties of an oncogene was first reported simultaneously by two groups working with closely related bladder cancer cell lines. Tabin *et al.*[277] studied the EJ bladder carcinoma cell line and detected a mutated p21 protein, discussed below, in the absence of altered expression levels. Reddy *et al.*[230] demonstrated that a single point mutation of guanosine-to-thymidine, resulting in the incorporation of valine instead of glycine at the 12th amino acid residue of the T24 oncogene-encoded p21 protein in the T24 human bladder carcinoma cell line, produced oncogene activation.

The *ras* gene family studied by Tabin and Reddy belongs to a gene family with several members, with varying degrees of homology in their effector regions (Table 2.1). The Ha-, Ki-, and N-*ras* genes are family members and encode for similar proteins known as p21. Normal p21 proteins are probably signal-transducing proteins based on their structural and functional homology with G proteins, which are well-characterized signal transducers. G proteins carry messages from activated cell surface receptors to specific cytoplasmic effectors that generate secondary messengers. Normal p21 proteins have several biochemical properties, including the ability to bind to GTP and to manifest GTPase activity.[16] Phospholipase is the putative effector for *ras* proteins.[25] Phospholipase produces secondary messages involved in the initiation of cell growth. It is known that *ras* genes acquire transforming potential (*e.g.*, become "activated") by single mutations affecting amino acids 12, 13, or 61.[139,230,277,279,326] Activated p21 proteins lack GTPase activity because of a conformational change in the catalytic site of the protein.[185,283] This loss of GTPase activity permits restricted production of secondary message which may, in turn, result in uncontrolled cell growth in tumors. Although p21 may affect cell growth, it should be noted that induction of the metastatic phenotype is not an intrinsic property of *ras* oncogenes. About 15% of all human tumors, including carcinomas, sarcomas, and leukemias, contain mutated c-*ras* oncogenes.[90,268]

Several genes, including *ras*, p53, and nm23 can induce metastatic behavior

TABLE 2.1.   *ras* GENE COMPARISONS[a]

Gene	Size	Chromosomal Location
Ras genes		
c-Ha-*ras*-1	<6 kb	Chromosome 11 (11p15.1-p15.5)
c-Ki-*ras*-2	>40 kb	Chromosome 12 (12p12.2-pter)
N-*ras*	10 kb	Chromosome 1 (1p22-p32)
Ras pseudogenes		
c-Ha-*ras*-2		X Chromosome
c-Ki-*ras*-1		Chromosome 6 (6p12-p32)

[a] From (with permission) Fenoglio-Preiser, C. M., Longacre, T. A., and Linstrom, M. G. Oncogenes and tumor suppressor genes in solid tumors: Breast, gynecologic, and urologic tumors. In *Molecular Diagnostics in Pathology*, edited by C. M. Fenoglio-Preiser and C. L. Willman. Baltimore, Williams & Wilkins, 1991, pp. 219–259.

upon transfection.[74,165,206,225,226,282] The *ras*, described above, is probably not causally related to the generation of metastases. The p53 is a gene on chromosome 17 and codes for nuclear protein p53.[77,205] This protein may participate in triggering of the metastatic cascade. Originally studied as a tumor-associated antigen, p53 encodes a DNA-binding nuclear phosphoprotein. The specific function of p53 is unknown.[163,207] What *is* known is that when p53 is introduced in a mutant form, it is associated with the development of metastases.[13] Classification of p53 as a tumor-suppressor gene has been confirmed by transfecting the wild-type p53 gene into human colorectal carcinoma cells, resulting in suppression of growth.[14]

Recently, another metastasis suppressor gene, nm23, has been found by Steeg and her co-workers[274] to be expressed in benign and malignant nonmetastatic processes and to be downregulated and/or lost in metastatic tumors. The protein product of nm23 has been identified as a nucleoside diphosphate (NDP) kinase. NDP kinases participate in several major functions that could play roles in carcinogenesis, including microtubule assembly-disassembly[205] and signal transduction through G proteins.[154] The nm23-like DNP kinases could function both as dominant oncogenes and as suppressor genes, depending on whether they are normal or defective and which signal transduction pathway is involved.[173] Based on observations on p53 and nm23, as well as other considerations, Liotta *et al.*[173] have proposed that induction of the metastatic phenotype is a complex process that requires a complement of genes.

Vogelstein and his colleagues,[131,303] who have had an interest in bladder cancer in addition to colon cancer, have shown that the most common cancer-related genetic change known at the gene level is p53 mutation. The normal allele of the p53 gene encodes a 53-kDa nuclear phosphoprotein involved in the control of cell proliferation. Several mutant alleles of p53, with single base substitutions, code for proteins that have altered growth regulatory properties.[14,71,75,76,92,130,189] A broad spectrum of alterations in p53, including point mutations, allelic losses, deletions, and rearrangements, have been demonstrated in various human tumors.[1,36,192,278] It has been proposed that these aberrations, together with alterations of oncogenes and additional suppressor genes, constitute the mutational network leading to malignancy.[131]

COLORECTAL CARCINOMA AS A PARADIGM FOR HUMAN TUMORIGENESIS

The most comprehensive studies on the accumulation of sequential genetic changes during human tumorigenesis have been reported for colorectal carcinomas by Vogelstein and his co-workers.[84,304] General aspects of this model may be directly relevant to bladder carcinogenesis, whereas some specific features may not be applicable. Early events preceding the development of malignant colorectal tumors include the loss of alleles representing a gene on 5q21[87] responsible for familial adenomatous polyposis (FAP), followed by *ras* gene activation (Fig. 2.1). Vogelstein *et al.*[304] found that *ras* is the only dominantly acting oncogene involved in carcinogenesis in a large percentage of colorectal tumors. Losses of 5q21 alleles are the earliest genetic alterations identified in sporadic colorectal neoplasms. They have been found in adenomas as small as 5 mm in diameter.

The gene responsible for FAP was recently isolated by two teams of researchers, one led by Vogelstein and Kinszler at Johns Hopkins and Nakamura of the Tokyo Cancer Institute,[155] and the other by White at the University of Utah.[166] This gene has been designated APC, for adenomatous polyposis coli. The APC gene has been found to be mutated in FAP families susceptible to hereditary colorectal cancers as well as in some nonhereditary (sporadic) colon cancers. Another gene, designated MCC for mutated in colon cancer, was also localized to 5q21. MCC has been implicated only in nonhereditary colon cancer. Both of these genes act as tumor-suppressor genes, although their specific functions remain to be elucidated. Neither the APC gene nor the MCC gene show significant resemblances to other genes now in databases, suggesting that they may represent some new kind of gene. Unfortunately, the lack of homology to other genes is likely to increase the work required to delineate their functions.[183]

Activation of a *ras* gene appears to occur next in colorectal carcinogenesis (Fig. 2.1). Vogelstein's group found mutations in the Ki-*ras* gene in approximately 50% of large colorectal adenomas and in a similar percentage in colorectal carcinomas.[31,304] Based on the time of appearance of the *ras* gene mutations, it was deduced that *ras* gene abnormalities probably have a role relatively early in tumorigenesis but following the changes in chromosome 5q.

Continuing with the Vogelstein model, somewhat later events included loss of sequences on 18q and 17p, which are observed in more than 70% of colorectal carcinomas.[86,196,199,305] It is uncertain whether the alterations of 17p and 18q are directly and causally associated with metastatic potential, or only represent markers of generalized chromosomal alterations that are associated with tumor aggressiveness.[149] The target gene on chromosome 18q21, termed "deleted in colorectal carcinomas" (or the DCC gene), is expressed in most normal tissues, including brain tissue where the highest expression is found, and in colonic mucosa. The gene is very large with a mRNA transcript size of 10 to 12 kilobase. Its expression is greatly reduced or absent in most colorectal carcinomas.[84] In addition, somatic mutations within the gene have been discovered in a number of colorectal cancers. These include a homozygous deletion at the 5′ end of the gene, a point mutation within one of the introns, and DNA insertions within a fragment immediately downstream of one of the exons.[84]

Although a full-length cDNA or genomic clone for the DCC gene is not yet available, partial sequencing has produced interesting preliminary conclusions. Several features of the DCC gene may be relevant to its role in tumorigenesis. The predicted amino acid sequence of the cDNA of the DCC gene specifies a protein with a sequence homologous to neural cell adhesion molecules (N-CAMs) and other related cell surface glycoproteins.[84] The DCC gene contains four immunoglobulin-like domains of the C2 class and a fibronectin type III-related domain similar to the domains present in N-CAM and other members of this family of cell adhesion molecules. This suggests that somatic mutations within the DCC gene, which have been observed in colorectal cancers,[84] could play a role in tumor pathogenesis by introducing abnormal cell-cell interactions affecting growth control and differentiation,[73,247] and that these might account for some of the aberrant cell-cell interactions that are characteristic of carcinomas.

The target of chromosome 17p loss in colorectal tumors is the p53 gene, which functions as a suppressor gene in normal tissue.[13,76,92] The p53 protein functions as a homodimer. Complexing of one mutant subunit with a wild-type subunit may be sufficient to subvert normal function.

In summary, Vogelstein's model of colorectal carcinogenesis provides a paradigm for human tumorigenesis in which the development of a malignant tumor proceeds through a series of genetic alterations including *ras* gene activation and the loss of tumor-suppressor genes on chromosomes 5, 17, and 18. The model accommodates the possibility that other chromosomal losses may be required to complete the cascade,[305] and that abnormalities in additional epigenetic processes may play additional roles. For example, DNA hypomethylation is consistently found in colorectal tumors at all stages of development and, therefore, probably represents a relatively early event in neoplasia. The degree of loss in colorectal carcinomas is estimated to be in the range of 10–20 million methyl groups per cell.[88,106] Hypomethylation may contribute to increased "stickiness" of chromatin during mitosis, impairing segregation and promoting aberrant segregation of chromosomal regions.[260] This could explain the loss of wild-type tumor-suppressor genes.[106]

BLADDER CANCER AND THE VOGELSTEIN MODEL

The applicability of the Vogelstein model of colorectal carcinogenesis to bladder carcinogenesis deserves serious consideration for many reasons, including the fact that some bladder transitional cell carcinomas arise as papillary lesions. Furthermore, in bladder there is a correlation between tumor stage and tumor ploidy, which is consistent with the concept of progressive derangements in the tumor cell genome, although alternative interpretations are possible.[211,286] Also, there is some overlap in associated genes (*e.g.*, *ras* and p53) in the two tumor systems. Other gene alterations (*e.g.*, in the APC gene) may be organ-specific and are not expected to be involved in bladder carcinogenesis.

Does the Vogelstein model, showing the accumulation of molecular derangements in the tumor cell genome over time, fit the clinical course of all bladder cancer cases? Are there groups of bladder cancer patients who do not fit this model particularly well? Correlative molecular genetics-histopathology studies on bladder will be required to provide definitive answers to these questions. However, longitudinal clinical studies have included some patients who might be exceptions to the Vogelstein scheme, although the model could be applicable to the majority of cases of bladder cancer.

There is a growing consensus that bladder cancers behave as several different distinct entities when viewed from the perspective of rates of clinical progression.[61,202] At one end of the spectrum are low-grade, superficial transitional cell carcinomas and at the other end of the spectrum are certain high-grade, high-stage transitional cell carcinomas. A long-standing issue is whether the former, low-grade, superficial cancers progress into the latter, high-grade, deeply infiltrating bladder cancers.[7,53,72,164,232]

Historical perspective helps in understanding various perceptions of the natural history of bladder cancer. Concepts of carcinogenesis in human bladder changed significantly in the 1980s. Up to that time, speculations on tumor progression in human bladder were heavily influenced by a belief that the usual fate of patients with superficial tumors, and flat carcinoma *in situ*, was to progress to deeply infiltrating carcinoma. This was broadened in the 1980s to accommodate two additional possibilities: (1) that some cancers can persist for many years without ever progressing to deep invasion or metastasis; and (2) that other cancers actually become deeply invasive very early in their clinical course, skipping a clinically detectable preinvasive phase of development.[35,61,320]

Figure 2.2*A* is a cartoon that portrays the pre-1982 view that bladder cancer progression was inevitable and generally occurred at an accelerating rate.[321] Time courses for clinical progression of bladder tumors are illustrated for three hypothetical patients: curve A portrays a tumor that progressed relatively rapidly; curve B shows a tumor with an intermediate rate of progression; and curve C represents a tumor with a relatively slow rate of progression. Note that all three curves indicate that the development of clinically advanced disease is the expected outcome without treatment, given sufficient time. The "bad actors" among tumors (*e.g.*, curve A) and the "good actors" among tumors (*e.g.*, curve C) are characterized by the slopes of the respective curves, not the end point of the disease. Note that the endpoint, deep invasion, is the same for all three patients. Disease progression, as illustrated by this family of curves, might well be explained by an accumulation of events similar to those represented in the Vogelstein model. Curves such as these provided a strong argument for the development of bladder cancer screening programs since they showed a significant time interval between the development of superficial lesions and deeply invasive bladder cancer.

Two new groups of bladder cancer patients were recognized in the 1980s. The time courses of their diseases necessitated modification of some of the concepts that are illustrated in Figure 2.2*A*. In a large longitudinal study, carried out by the National Bladder Cancer Group in the United States, involving 147 patients with previously untreated TaG1 transitional cell carcinomas, the issue of the inevitability of progression of superficial bladder cancer was examined in detail. Dr. George R. Prout, Jr. and Dr. Gilbert H. Friedell, a urologist and a pathologist, respectively, jointly headed the collaborative. Working with Dr. Bruce Barton, a statistician, and the author, they found that most of the patients who came to urologists with TaG1 papillary transitional cell carcinoma never experienced progression of their disease to either higher grade (not shown) or higher stage disease, contrary to expectation (Table 2.2). Of course, we could not completely exclude the possibility that, given sufficient time, progression to advanced disease would occur in these patients. This was regarded as unlikely since the average follow-up was over 4 years. Many of the National Bladder Cancer Group's patients were followed for over a decade on a surveillance protocol and were found to have recurrent tumors but no evidence of progression in tumor grade or stage. It is now appreciated that these observations are consistent with the notion that papillary transitional cell carcinomas may represent epithelium in which

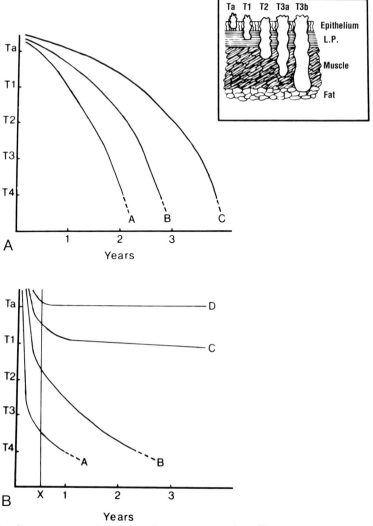

FIG. 2.2. Curves representing rates of tumor progression. Time zero represents the initial appearance of identifiable cancer cells. The inset in the upper right-hand corner illustrates levels of tumor invasion. UICC (Union Internationale Contre le Cancer) nomenclature: Ta = papillary carcinoma, noninvasive; T1 = invasion confined to the lamina propria (L. P.); T2 = tumor invasion of superficial muscle in the bladder wall; T3a = tumor invasion of deep muscle; T3b = tumor invasion of perivesical fat. T4 (not shown) would indicate that the tumor is fixed to the pelvis or invades other pelvic organs. (A) Pre-1982 view of tumor progression is one of gradual acceleration of the invasive process after a relatively long lag period. Curves A, B, and C represent relatively rapid, intermediate, and slow rates of progression, respectively. The *dotted lines* indicate that death accompanies deep invasion. (B) Updated representations of tumor progression in urinary bladder including more recently recognized groups of patients (curves A and D; see text for details). This representation includes highly aggressive tumors (curves A and B) that tend to express their capacity to invade the bladder wall very early in the clinical course. Carcinomas that are minimally invasive at the time of discovery (curves C and D) have a high likelihood of remaining superficial and not life-threatening. The prediction is that, at time point "X" in tumor progression, carcinomas with different aggressive potentials will display markedly different levels of bladder wall penetration. Adapted with permission from Weinstein, R. S., and Pauli, B. U. Cell junctions and the biological behavior of cancer. In *Junctional Complexes in Epithelial Cells*, edited by M. Stoker, J. Bock, and S. Clark. New York, John Wiley & Sons, 1987, pp. 240–260.

TABLE 2.2.   TUMOR PROGRESSION IN LOW-GRADE, LOW-STAGE BLADDER CANCER[a]

	No.	%
Patients[b]	147	100
No subsequent invasion	139	95.0
Lamina propria invasion	6	4.1
Muscle invasion	2	1.4
Metastases	0	0

[a] G. R. Prout, Jr., G. H. Friedell, B. Barton, and R. S. Weinstein, unpublished data, 1985. Average follow-up interval = 49.3 months.

[b] Patients entered into the study with no prior therapy.

the carcinogenic process has been aborted after initiation and promotion are complete.[80,81,224]

Another group of patients who may be at variance with the Vogelstein model are those with bladder cancers that invade deeply into the connective tissue and muscle of the bladder, but who have surprisingly brief histories of symptoms when they are first seen by the urologist. These patients have no prior history of bladder cancer at the time of initial biopsy.[35,61,146] The discovery that the large majority of patients who will develop muscle-invading bladder cancer actually present *initially* with higher grade invasive carcinomas, and not low-grade papillary lesions came as a surprise when it was announced to the urology community in 1982.[35,61,146] The finding provided circumstantial evidence that some deeply invasive cancers of the bladder may evolve very rapidly in the absence of preexisting low-grade, superficial papillary precursor lesions. The Vogelstein model does not specify an actual time line for tumor progression, but it seems to imply a requirement for a substantial time interval for the accumulation of multiple genetic events.

A clinical implication of the rapid progression of this group of bladder cancers is that efforts to screen for the precursor lesions of deeply invasive bladder carcinoma may be thwarted since their precursor lesions may exist briefly, lowering the probability of detection. Ironically, many neoplastic bladder lesions that might be detectable by screening methods are of less concern since they behave as benign tumors despite their malignant histopathological phenotype.

Figure 2.2*B* is an updated representation of tumor progression that incorporates these two additional groups of bladder cancer patients.[321] Many examples of patients fitting each of these curves are in the National Bladder Cancer Group's databank. Curve A represents a patient with an explosive onset of deeply invasive bladder cancer. The evolution of deep invasion and metastasis occurred before clinical detection at time "X." Curve B represents a patient with a scenario in which the disease progressed to an advanced stage, but over a longer time course. Curve C shows minimal progression and curve D shows no progression. Curve C illustrates disease progression in a patient who presents initially with a T1 lesion, that is, with tumor cells in the lamina propria. In these patients, tumor recurrences may have cells invading into the lamina propria, but no progression beyond this level of invasion in the majority of cases. There are exceptions where the tumor does eventually extend to a deeper level in the bladder wall. Curve D represents a patient who presents initially with TaG1 papillary transitional cell carcinoma. Approximately 50% of such patients have recurrences. The National Bladder Cancer Group's databank includes patients with more than a dozen recurrences over a decade, all of which showed the same histopathology as the first tumor. The National Bladder Cancer Group found that the best predictor of the histopathology of a recurrent bladder tumor is the histopathology of the previous surgical specimen.

Based on these considerations, it is hypothesized that many invasive bladder carcinomas do not progress through histopathologically benign developmental stages of carcinogenesis, unlike the typical situation in colon and rectum. Furthermore, most TaG1 papillary transitional cell carcinomas may be *formes frustes* of cancer (Table 2.2). This is also consistent with data showing that progression of papillary transitional cell carcinomas of low cytologic grade is not directly related to the number or frequency of recurrences.[138,168,170,285]

The literature on carcinoma *in situ* in bladder can be interpreted as suggesting that some cases of carcinoma *in situ*, especially in the absence of solid bladder tumors, may also represent *formes frustes* of cancer that do not progress.[228,320] A benign clinical course for carcinoma *in situ* may occur less frequently than for nonprogression of TaG1 papillary lesions, but many such cases are recorded.[4,82,83,228,320] For practical reasons, urologists focus their attention on the potential of carcinoma *in situ* lesions to progress, and often discount cases in which malignant lesions have not fulfilled the prediction of invasion. To some extent, the idea that carcinoma *in situ* inevitably progresses to invasive disease is overemphasized in the literature, although one must be careful not to minimize the importance of this entity. In the author's experience, urologists see carcinoma *in situ* in the bladder as a very threatening lesion, which is true in many cases.[228] On the other hand, there are lessons to be learned from the cases in which the carcinoma *in situ* does not progress to invasive disease, in urinary bladder as in other organs.[53,187,188] Cancer cell biologists are in a different boat than urologists and should consider paying more attention to cytologically malignant lesions that do not progress, since those lesions can provide important insights into triggering mechanisms of the malignant cascade and unique information on host defense mechanisms that provide barriers to invasion.[125,219,322]

Despite these exceptions, some cases of bladder cancer appear to fit the Vogelstein model of progression especially well with respect to their time course. Of course, it is recognized that this could be coincidental. It remains to be determined if sequential genetic events correlate with discrete histopathological phases of bladder tumorigenesis.

GENES INVOLVED IN URINARY BLADDER CARCINOGENESIS

Table 2.3 summarizes the oncogenes that have been associated with bladder cancers.[221,248] Abnormalities in *ras* genes have been found in transitional cell carcinomas, both *in situ* and in tissue culture systems. For brief reviews, see References 248 and 178. A *ras*-related oncogene has been described in the urine of bladder cancer patients.[275]

In early studies, Fujita *et al.*[99,100] evaluated a large series of urinary tract

TABLE 2.3. ALTERATIONS IN GENES IN BLADDER TUMORS

Change	Oncogenes	Source	Reference No.
Mutations	c-Ha-*ras*	Bladder TCC[a]	178
		Urothelial TCC	99, 100
		EJ cell line	277, 279
		T24 cell line	230
		WEB cell line	180
	c-Ki-*ras*	A1688 cell line	254
		A1633 cell line	294
	N-*ras*	HT1197 cell line	32
	p53	Urothelial TCC	131
Amplifications	c-Ha-*ras*	T24 (MGH-U1) line	160
	c-Ki-*ras*	Bladder TCC	100
Translocations	NR[b]		
Deletion	RB gene	Bladder cancer	172
	c-Ha-*ras*	T24 cell line	52
Over-expression	Ha-*ras*	Bladder TCC	302
	c-*erb* B-1	Bladder TCC	24, 203

[a] TCC, transitional cell carcinoma.
[b] NR, not reported.

tumors, and cell lines derived from urinary tract tumors, for *ras* oncogenes by molecular genetic analysis. Ha-*ras* genes were detected in 2 of 38 tumors and found to contain a single base mutation at codon 61, leading to substitutions of arginine and leucine for glutamine at that position. An additional Ha-*ras* oncogene mutation was identified in a bladder carcinoma at codon 12. In 1 of 21 tumors, they found a 40-fold amplification of the Ki-*ras* gene. Bos[30] showed a detection rate of mutated *ras* genes at a frequency of less than 10% in primary bladder tumors. Thus, while codons 12 and 61 appear as hotspots of *ras* oncogene activation in bladder cancers, the prevalence of these mutations is probably low.[89,139]

Different results were reported in an immunohistochemical study. Viola *et al.*[302] described increased expression of *ras* p21 in all of their cases of high-grade bladder carcinomas and proposed that increased p21 could be an indicator of malignant potential in premalignant lesions of the bladder. The association of p21 expression with tumor grade and stage was not confirmed by Malone *et al.*[178] Fenoglio-Preiser *et al.*[91] suggest that the discrepancy might be explained by the use of antibody RAP-5 in the study of Viola *et al.* This antibody lacks specificity and, in addition, may not detect *ras* protein in bladder tumors.[251,307,323]

Deletion of Ha-*ras* in urological tumors is a more common event. Fearon *et al.*[85] found chromosomal deletion of 11p, the region coding for Ha-*ras*, in 5 of 11 bladder transitional cell carcinomas. Ishikawa *et al.*[136] studied transitional cell carcinomas from heterozygous individuals and found deletions of one allele in 38% of the tumors.

Another gene associated with colorectal carcinogenesis is p53. There have been p53 gene base substitution mutations detected in many other human malignancies including bladder cancers.[131] Hollstein *et al.*[131] found that 98% of mutations in various tumors occurred within a 600-base pair region of the p53 gene, between codons 110 and 307, thus defining the regions of the p53 protein that are probably essential for its biological activities. They also found that different tumor types exhibited different mutational spectra. Fifteen cases of bladder cancer were described with p53 mutations, of which seven were G:C to A:T transitions. Three mutations occurred at CpG dinucleotides.

One of the genes associated with colorectal carcinogenesis, the APC gene, is less likely to have a role in bladder carcinogenesis than *ras* or p53. On the other hand, the history of the discovery of the APC gene, which is associated with familial adenomatous polyposis, is instructive. It is conceivable that parallel discoveries could shed light on the bladder cancer tumorigenesis. The first clue to the location of the gene responsible for FAP came from the work of Herrera *et al.,*[126] who demonstrated a constitutional deletion of chromosomal band 5q21 in an FAP patient. This cytogenetic finding stimulated performance of linkage analyses that demonstrated that 5q21 chromosome markers were tightly linked to the development of polyps in numerous FAP kindred.[29,167] Other studies suggested that genes from the same region may participate in tumorigenesis in kindred as well as in patients with sporadic colorectal cancer.[156,166] Thus, the stage was set for subsequent cytogenetic studies.

It remains to be seen if cytogenetic analysis of bladder tumors will provide comparable clues to the locations of genes critical to bladder carcinogenesis. Table 2.4 summarizes chromosomal changes found in bladder, prostate, and renal tumors. The lack of consistent changes from organ to organ reflects a degree of organ specificity for some of the chromosomal changes.

To date, a broad spectrum of chromosomal alterations have been associated with transitional cell carcinoma of the bladder.[253,309] Primary chromosomal changes include structural alterations of chromosome 5, such as i(5p) and the deletion of the long arm,[11,105,252] monosomy of chromosome 9,[23,270,299] and trisomy of chromosome 7 (Fig. 2.3).[11,23,105,300] One case has been described with del(5)(q13q22) as the only karyotypic abnormality.[8] Other single cases have been reported with del(10) (q24),[23] trisomy of chromosome 20,[270] or del(21)(q22.1q22.3)[12] as sole karyotypic changes. Loss of a Y chromosome is the only chromosomal change in several transitional cell carcinomas. Possible secondary events are seen as occasional changes in chromosomes 1, 3, 6, 8, 10, 11, 13, and 17. In bladder cancer, 5q- and 11p- are generally associated with a poor prognosis, and +7 and 9q- are associated with an improved prognosis.[253]

Fearon *et al.*[85] used molecular probes to study transitional cell carcinomas. The

TABLE 2.4. CHROMOSOMAL CHANGES IN GENITOURINARY TUMORS

Tumor Type	Chromosomal Change	Loss of Heterozygosity
Bladder	5p, −9, +7, +21	11p, 9q, 17p
	del 21 (q22;23)	
	del 10 (q24)	
Prostate	2p, 7q, 10q	
Renal	3p, 11–23 deletions	3p, 6 pericentric
	+7, t(5;14)	
	−4, −14, +20	

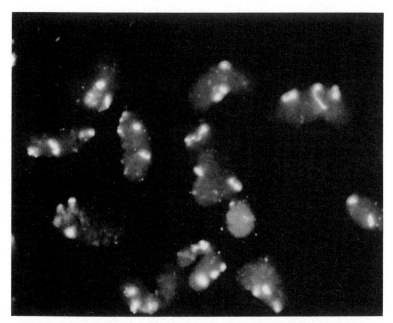

FIG. 2.3.   Cytogenetic analysis using fluorescence *in situ* hybridization (FISH). The patient, a 76-year-old female, had a moderately well-differentiated transitional cell carcinoma in the left renal pelvis, with areas of squamous cell carcinoma. There was a previous Grade II transitional cell carcinoma of the right renal pelvis treated with a right nephrectomy. This preparation demonstrated normal results for all probes except chromosome 7, which showed 9% of cells with three spots indicating trisomy of 7. (Courtesy of C. S. Berger and A. A. Sandberg, Scottsdale, AZ.)

region containing the c-Ha-*ras*-1 gene on 11p was lost, as evidenced by loss of constitutional heterozygosity for this locus, as well as the locus for the insulin gene, in 5 of 12 tumors. Transitional cell carcinomas were also screened for loss of constitutional heterozygosity with probes for chromosomes 1–3, 12–15, 17, 18, and 20. They found two tumors with triploidy of loci on chromosomes 13 and 20 and one tumor with triploidy of a chromosome 15 locus. Loss of heterozygosity was also seen for 2p and 14q. Tsi *et al.*[288] confirmed and extended the findings of Fearon *et al.* They screened 25 tumors with DNA probes derived from loci on 6p, 9q, 11p, 14q, and 17p. Tsi *et al.* found loss of heterozygosity for 11p sequences in approximately 40% of tumors. Even higher frequencies of reduction to homozygosity or hemizygosity were seen with alleles from loci on chromosome 9p and chromosome 17p. Fearon *et al.* did not detect a loss of heterozygosity for 17q and suggested that the loss of 17p alleles is a subchromosomal event. They proposed that the loss of 17p alleles may involve the p53 suppressor gene.[13,14,86]

Studies based on karyotypes have important limitations. Until recently, detection of cytogenetic abnormalities was limited to those that were visible with the light microscope and occurred in mitotically active cells that could be recovered from the tumor. Some DNA lesions detectable by molecular genetic techniques in nearly all tumors of a given type may not be detected by cytogenetics.[309] A limitation of molecular genetic analysis techniques has been that they have not been amenable to the analysis of clonal heterogeneity in a tumor. The application of interphase fluorescent *in situ* hybridization,[133] the use of polymerase chain reaction (PCR) for small numbers of cells or single cells,[182] and the characterization of DNA polymorphisms detectable by PCR amplification should result in the answering of critical questions pertaining to tumor clonality.

MOLECULAR GENETICS AND MECHANISMS OF CANCER DRUG RESISTANCE

The second topic to be considered is the genetic basis of clinical failures of cancer therapy.[308] Recently, the literature on various types of drug resistance has been discussed in several excellent monographs.[70,151,240] There is an urgent need to understand the mechanisms of drug resistance, since this information could potentially be used to develop novel strategies to reverse drug resistance.[65]

A goal of the clinical laboratory is to develop, and ultimately offer, chemosensitivity tests that will enable the clinician to tailor therapy to the biology of cancers in individual patients. Currently, therapeutic decisions are based in large measure on conventional tumor histology, although tumor markers are useful for the evaluation of some types of tumors. Pathologists recognize that few of the existing transitional epithelial cell biochemical markers are clinically useful for predicting the future biological behavior of individual bladder tumors or their responses to therapy. The expression of markers, such as the tissue ABO(H) blood group antigens or EGF receptors, is not known to correlate with responses to therapy, although these therapy issues have not been systematically examined.[54,232]

Of the forms of cancer drug resistance described to date, the best characterized is so-called "classic multidrug resistance," a genetically controlled form of resistance to chemotherapy. Studies on Mdr1 have provided important insights into one of the mechanisms by which cells may circumvent the toxic effects of drugs and have suggested novel therapeutic strategies.[44] They also illustrate some of the complexities encountered in attempting to assess drug resistance in clinical specimens.[314,316] There is some evidence that increased expression of the *MDR1* gene *in vivo* may be only one manifestation of a coordinated cellular defense mechanism.[112,198] This could further complicate the analysis of drug resistant tumors.

Cancers exhibiting *intrinsic* classic multidrug resistance do not respond to chemotherapy upon primary exposure to "natural-product" cytotoxic drugs. Some cancers that do respond initially to standard chemotherapy regimens, employing natural-product drugs, subsequently become resistant to these drugs and, simultaneously, to many other drugs to which the patient has had no previous exposure. This represents multidrug resistance in an *acquired* form.[216,234] Tumors displaying either the intrinsic or acquired form of multidrug resistance are usually not cross-resistant to alkylating agents, most antimetabolites, or heavy metals.[33] While many cancer cells exhibiting the multidrug resistance phenotype have elevated levels of *MDR1* gene expression, drug resistance mechanisms unrelated to drug transport and Mdr1 protein have been implicated in conferring multidrug resistance as well.[67,195] It has also been shown experimentally that acquired multidrug resistance mediated by several different mechanisms, one of which is *MDR*1 gene hyperexpression, can be produced by chemically related compounds in the same cancer cell line.[280] Fractionated irradiation has been shown to induce overexpression of Mdr1 protein in mammalian tumor cell lines and lung carcinoma xenographs, raising the possibility that treatment modalities other than chemotherapy may account for the acquired multidrug resistance phenotype in some instances.[127,184]

The genetic basis of classic multidrug resistance has been elucidated.[296] The *MDR*1 gene, which is responsible for classic multidrug resistance, has been cloned and classified as a member of the *MDR* gene superfamily.[49,103,141,295] Its encoded pleiotropic protein, an isoform in the P-glycoprotein family of proteins, is called Mdr1.[140,293,316] Mdr1 overexpression has been implicated in multidrug resistance in human tumors arising at many different sites.[94,111,142]

Resistance to natural-product drugs is conferred by Mdr1 by preventing the intracellular accumulation of the agents, thus rendering the drugs unable to reach critical cellular targets.[104,129,289,324] Drugs implicated in multidrug resistance have various intracellular targets including DNA, topoisomerase II, ribosomes, and microtubules.[17] This spectrum of intracellular targets drew the attention of early investigators to a potential role of the plasma membrane in mediating multidrug resistance.[140] It turned out that Mdr1-mediated efflux transport at the plasma membrane provides protection against these drugs in the following manner: lipophilic drugs cross the cell membrane by Fickian diffusion or by carrier-mediated passive transport (Fig. 2.4); the transporter then ejects the drug from the cell in a process energized by the hydrolysis of ATP at a nucleotide binding site on the Mdr1 polypeptide.[59,135] The discovery that Mdr1 is a transporter led to the conceptualization of novel strategies to overcome this type of drug resistance. It was shown that chemosensitivity to various drugs can be reestablished by blocking efflux transporter activity. Pump inhibitors, such as the calcium channel blocker verapamil or other classes of compounds that can function as effector-inhibitors of Mdr1, have been effective in reversing drug resistance in tumors (Table 2.5).[292,324,327] Results of early clinical trials on lymphoma and multiple myeloma patients, using pump inhibitors as therapeutic adjuvants, appear to justify expanding such studies to urinary bladder.[194,249]

THE MULTIDRUG RESISTANCE GENE FAMILY

The so-called multidrug resistance genes, referred to as *MDR* genes in humans and *mdr* genes in rodents (see Tables 2.6 and 2.7), belong to a superfamily of genes found in both prokaryotes and eukaryotes and include the human cystic fibrosis transmembrane regulator.[141,235] Recent genetic evidence suggests that the transport of antigens or peptide fragments across membranes, for presentation by the MHC-Class I molecules, may also be mediated by a related molecular pump.[69,287] Mammalian *MDR* genes are related to an evolutionarily conserved family of *MDR*-like genes in nonmammalian species.[96,141,186,214,238] Many members of this superfamily have been implicated in the ATP-dependent transport of a remarkably broad spectrum of substances across membranes.[5,141]

Analysis of hybridization patterns and sequencing of cDNA and genomic clones

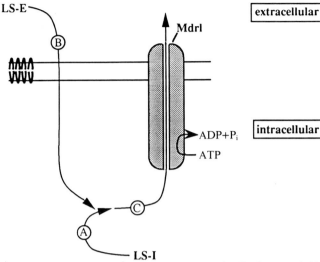

FIG. 2.4.   Pathways of lipophilic substance (LS) efflux via Mdr1 (P-glycoprotein) in normal tissues and tumors. It is proposed that lipophilic substances may be synthesized within the intracellular compartment (*LS-I*) or come to the cell via the extracellular space (*LS-E*). Theoretically, substances arriving via the extracellular route could include xenobiotic lipophilic substances, such as drugs or foster lipophilic substances, such as endogenous substances synthesized by other cells and recirculated through the cell. Transport process is energized by the hydrolysis of adenosine triphosphate (*ATP*) to adenosine diphosphate plus inorganic phosphate (*ADP* + P_i). (*A*) Intracellular pathway. (*B*) Extracellular pathway. (*C*) Common pathway. With permission from Weinstein, R. S., Kuszak, J. R., Kluskens, L. F., and Coon, J. S. P-glycoproteins in pathology: The multidrug resistance gene family in humans. *Hum. Pathol. 21:* 949–958, 1990.

TABLE 2.5.   AGENTS THAT REVERSE MULTIDRUG RESISTANCE[a]

Calcium channel blockers and their analogs, *e.g.*, R- and L-verapamil
Analogs of cytotoxic drugs, *i.e.*, vinca alkaloids
Quinidine and its optical isomer, quinine
Cyclosporine and its analogs
Phenothiazines
Reserpine analogs
Hydrophobic cephalosporins
Steroids, *i.e.*, deoxycorticosterone
Surfactants, *i.e.*, Solutol-HS-15
Other nontoxic natural products

[a] Modified with permission, from Pastan, I., and Gottesman, M. M. Drug resistance: Biological warfare at the cellular level. In *Molecular Foundations of Oncology*, edited by S. Broder. Baltimore, Williams & Wilkins, 1991, pp. 83–93.

have shown that human cells contain two, and rodent cells three, *mdr* genes (Table 2.6).[49,60,134,204] The two human genes, *MDR*1 and *MDR*2, encode for highly homologous integral membrane proteins in humans.[49,103,295] Historically, both of these genes have been called multidrug-resistance genes based on structural similarities. To date, only *MDR*1 has been linked to the multidrug resistance phenomenon in humans. The product of the *MDR*2 gene, the Mdr2 protein, has not been shown to be a transporter or to make any contribution to the drug

TABLE 2.6.   NOMENCLATURE FOR MULTIDRUG RESISTANCE GENES[a]

Gene	Designation		
	Class I	Class II	Class III
Human	*MDR*1		*MDR*2[b]
Mouse	*Mdr*3	*Mdr*1	*Mdr*2
Hamster	*Pgp*1	*Pgp*2	*Pgp*3

[a] Adapted from Juranka, P. F., Zastawny, R. L., and Ling, V. P-glycoprotein: Multidrug-resistance and a super family of membrane-associated transport proteins. *FASEB J. 3:* 2583–2592, 1989, and Kanamar, H., Kakehi, Y., Yoshida, O., Nakaniski, S., Pastan, I., and Gottesman, M. M. MDR1 RNA levels in human renal cell carcinomas: Correlation with grade and prediction of reversal of doxorubicin resistance by quinidine in tumor explants. *J. Natl. Cancer Inst. 81:* 844–849, 1989.

[b] Also known as *MDR*3.

TABLE 2.7.   NOMENCLATURE FOR HUMAN *MDR* GENE PRODUCTS

Gene	Message	Protein[a]
*MDR*1	*MDR*1 mRNA	Mdr1
*MDR*2	*MDR*2 mRNA	Mdr2

[a] Also called P-glycoprotein, Pgp, and P-170.

resistance phenotype. Although Mdr2 is unrelated to multidrug resistance, it continues to be called an multidrug resistance protein. Another complexity of nomenclature is that the products of both the *MDR*1 and *MDR*2 genes are commonly called P-glycoprotein, Pgp, or P-170, reflecting the molecular weight of the first P-glycoprotein to be identified (molecular weight = 170kDa).[9,10] For the sake of precision, we prefer to distinguish between the two gene products and to refer to the isoforms encoded by human *MDR*1 and *MDR*2 genes as Mdr1 and Mdr2, respectively (Table 2.7).[319] Relationships and the current nomenclature of the *MDR* genes in several species are summarized in Table 2.6. This information is useful as a guide to the literature on *MDR* reagents derived from various species.

Human Mdr1 is a 1280-residue protein and consists of two halves, the N-terminal and C-terminal halves, that share a high degree of sequence similarity (Fig. 2.5).[33,234] Each half-molecule consists of an extensive hydrophobic region containing six putative transmembrane domains arranged in pairs, followed by a hydrophilic cytoplasmic region containing the consensus sequence for potential nucleotide-binding sites.[47,117] Multiple linking polypeptides join the transmembrane segments together at both the cytoplasmic and extracellular surfaces of the plasma membrane.[47] The polypeptide component of the Mdr1 monomer has a molecular weight of 120–140 kDa. There is a single glycosylation locus in the extracellular region of the N-terminal half of the molecule. Variability in glycosylation can give rise to Mdr1 proteins of molecular weights ranging from 135 to 180 kDa.[78,115]

On the basis of sequence homology between the N-terminal and C-terminal halves of Mdr1 and Mdr2, it was initially suggested that the gene arose by duplication of a primordial gene.[47] If this is the case, it would be predicted that

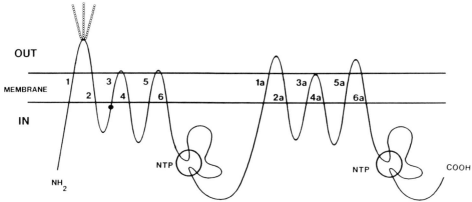

FIG. 2.5.   Schematic model of Mdr1, the human multidrug transporter. The predicted glycosylation sites are marked by chains, and the predicted nucleotide-binding folds are circled. Positions of introns are marked by arrows and intron types. NTP, nucleoside triphosphate-binding sites. With permission from Roninson, I. B. Structures and evolution of P-glycoproteins. In *Molecular and Cellular Biology of Multidrug Resistance in Tumor Cells*, edited by I. B. Roninson. New York, Plenum Press, 1991, pp. 395–402.

introns would be found in similar positions in the two halves of the protein-coding sequence, since intron positions are conserved in almost all cases of internal duplication.[284] Roninson's group[48] has reevaluated this question and proposed the alternative hypothesis that primordial proteins corresponding to the left and the right halves of Mdr1 were formed independently by fusion of closely related genes.

Mdr2, the other human P-glycoprotein, and its gene, *MDR2*, also have been characterized.[297] Both the *MDR1* and *MDR2* genes have been localized to human chromosome 7, band q21.1.[40] They are linked within 330 kilobase pairs of DNA.[50] Mdr2 shares a high level of sequence homology with Mdr1 in human, and its analogous isoforms in mouse, with greater than 75% identical amino acid residues.[49,60,297] The more conserved regions are those including or adjacent to the nucleotide-binding sites within the cytoplasmic domains of P-glycoproteins. Generally, nucleic acid probes that distinguish *MDR1* and *MDR2* mRNAs are targeted to highly divergent sequences corresponding to amino acid sequences at the exterior surface of the membrane.

LABORATORY ASSESSMENT OF *MDR*1 GENE EXPRESSION

Mdr1 expression can be quantitated by: (1) measuring protein levels, (2) measuring *MDR* mRNA levels, and (3) assessing *MDR1* gene amplification. Quantification of the protein by immunoblotting or immunocytochemistry is often less sensitive than measuring *MDR* message.[113,237] Since the human *MDR1* gene does not generally require gene amplification and *MDR1* gene amplification may not occur *in vivo*, measurement of *MDR1* gene amplification is not of value as a clinical test.[265] Mdr1 pump function and inhibition can be evaluated by flow cytometry and nonflow cytometry.[104,152,176,197,324]

TISSUE SAMPLING ISSUES

Sampling issues are complex due to the heterogeneity of expression of Mdr1 in normal tissues and tumors and the fact that Mdr1 is expressed in some nonepithelial cells, including lymphocytes and macrophages as well as in endothelial cells in some organs.[58,259] In the bulk tissue samples required for analysis of *MDR*1 mRNA by slot blot analysis or quantitative PCR, the relative contributions of various irrelevant cellular components are generally unknown. If present, stromal cells, inflammatory cells, or endothelial cells expressing Mdr1 will result in an overestimate of the Mdr1 content of tumor cells.[259] Thresholds for monoclonal antibody detection systems used in immunohistochemistry are also a matter of concern.[37,45]

Sample preservation methods also need to be systematically evaluated. Potentially adverse effects of ischemia at surgery and time-related postoperative or postmortem degradation on *MDR*1 mRNA levels have not been explored. Levels of expression of Mdr1 and *MDR*1 mRNA have not been compared in surgical specimens and autopsy specimens. The effects of carrier fluids, length of storage, storage temperatures, chemical preservatives, and freezing will need to be determined before the measurement of Mdr1/*MDR*1 mRNA is incorporated into laboratory practice.

IMMUNOHISTOCHEMISTRY OF MDR1

The primary advantages of qualitative immunohistochemistry are the ability (1) to discriminate Mdr1 expression in tumor cells from expression in normal epithelial, endothelial, and stromal cells, (2) to detect Mdr1 expression in single cells, allowing for small sample size, and (3) to determine subcellular distributions of Mdr1. Concerns over the sensitivity of immunohistochemistry in detecting low levels of protein are warranted. Insensitivity of immunohistochemistry may be an obstacle to detecting Mdr1 in some cases. It remains to be determined if refinements in immunohistochemical methods developed by several groups will sufficiently lower the threshold of detection of Mdr1 to accommodate all cases in which low levels of Mdr1 mediate clinically significant drug resistance.[45,116] Quantitative immunohistochemistry may emerge as the method of choice for assessment of Mdr1 expression in some clinical applications.[116]

Several anti-Mdr1 monoclonal antibodies (MAbs) have been used to detect Mdr1 in pathology specimens. The first MAb, with a high affinity for Mdr1, that proved useful was MAb C219, developed by Ling's group in Toronto.[45,46,145] MAb C219 was prepared against hamster P-glycoprotein and recognizes a conserved carboxyl-terminal epitope near the ATP-binding domain in both human and rodent Mdr1. Unfortunately, the epitope is shared by several P-glycoprotein isoforms, some of which lack efflux pump activity and are irrelevant in multidrug resistance.[101,258] Thus, immunoreactivity with MAb C219 is not necessarily indicative of the presence of a mediator of multidrug resistance. The specificity of MAb C219 for P-glycoproteins is also controversial, since MAb C219 has been reported to cross-react with muscle myosin.[281,298] In most instances, MAb C219 immunostaining patterns have been found to be identical to the immunostaining patterns of other anti-Mdr1 antibodies that are Mdr1 isoform-specific.[315] Ling's group[101,145] has studied MAb C219 and two other MAbs by high-resolution epitope mapping. MAb C494 binds to a sequence present only in the Class I isoforms of P-glycoproteins, and MAb C32 recognizes a sequence that is conserved in hamster Class I and II isoforms but not the Class III isoforms (Table 2.6). MAb C494 has been used in immunohistochemical studies on surgical pathology specimens.[301]

MAb MRK16 is a human-specific MAb with high affinity for the Mdr1 isoform.[121,281] This MAb recognizes an outer surface epitope. MRK16 must be used on unembedded specimens, whereas MAb C219 can be used on both frozen sections and paraffin sections.

The threshold for the immunohistochemical detection of Mdrs by MAbs C219 and MRK16 have been assessed using a series of KB epidermoid carcinoma cell lines selected for graded levels of Mdr1 expression and drug resistance.[2,264] KB cell lines, originally derived from human cervical carcinoma cells, express Mdr1 but not Mdr2.[241] Gottesman *et al.*[113] found that cell lines with a three- to six-fold increased resistance to colchicine or vinblastine and parallel increases in *MDR* mRNA stained negatively with MAb MRK16 (Table 2.8). This shows that relatively small increases in drug resistance, which are of potential significance in patients, may not be reflected in positive immunostaining. This level of insensitivity may represent an inherent limitation of immunohistochemistry in the assessment of drug resistance in tissue sections or cytology preparations. The threshold for MAb C219 immunostaining is increased (*i.e.*, immunoreactivity is decreased) by paraffin embedding. This favors the use of frozen sections for studies on human tissues with low levels of expression of Mdr1.[55] A requirement for frozen tissue would limit the range of studies that could be performed on archival material.

HYB-612 and HYB-241 are anti-Mdr1 MAbs developed by Hybritech, Inc. (San Diego, CA) in collaboration with Biedler and her associates at Memorial Sloan-Kettering in New York. Mouse MAbs HYB-612 and HYB-241 recognize different external epitopes of Mdrs that are not conserved in the Mdr2 isoform.[56]

Another MAb, JSB-1, developed in the Netherlands, recognizes a highly conserved epitope close to, but not overlapping with, the C219 binding epitope.[256] Comparisons of C219 and JSB-1 immunostaining on adjacent sections confirmed

TABLE 2.8. SENSITIVITY OF VARIOUS METHODS FOR DETECTION OF *MDR*1 GENE EXPRESSION[a]

Method	KB-3-1	KB-8	KB-8-5	KB-8-5-11	KB-C1
Fold resistance	1	2	3–6	20–50	100–300
RNA slot blot	1	10	30	800	3000
Protein Western blot	−	−	±	+	+++
Photoaffinity labeling	−	−	±	NT	+++
Immunohistochemistry	−	−	±	+	+++
In situ hybridization (Grain counts)	2	2	8	24	45

[a] From (with permission) Gottesman, M. M., Goldstein, L. J., Bruggemann, E., Currier, S. J., Galski, H., Cardavelli, C., Thiebaut, F., Willingham, M. C., and Pastan, I. Molecular diagnosis of multidrug resistance. *Cancer Cells* 7: 75–80, 1989.

the presence of identical staining patterns.[298,315] JSB-1 is claimed to be useful for detecting Mdr protein in human tumor cells with low levels of drug resistance.[38,256]

The cross-reactivity of anti-Mdr MAbs has been examined by Schinkel *et al.*,[258] who cloned *MDR2* (aka *MDR3*) cDNA into a mammalian expression vector and co-transfected it with a selectable marker into drug-sensitive human melanoma cells. Using stable Mdr2 isoform expressing cells, they tested the cross-reactivity of MAbs C219, C494, JSB-1, HYB-241 and MRK16 by immunohistochemistry and immunoblotting. Only C219 showed detectable cross-reactivity with human Mdr2. They recommended MRK16 and HYB-241 as most suitable for sensitive and specific cytochemical detection of human Mdr1.

Of the anti-Mdr1 MAbs developed to date, MAb C219 has been the most extensively characterized as a surgical pathology research reagent. Limitations have been placed on its usage by its recent withdrawal from the commercial market in the United States and Canada by its vendor, Centocor Diagnostics (Malvern, PA) because of regulatory issues involving the United States Federal Drug Administration. It remains commercially available in Europe and Japan. We have substituted MAb JSB-1, available from SANBIO (Amsterdam, The Netherlands), for some of our current work on surgical pathology specimens.[318]

False-negative immunohistochemical measurements of expression can result from the relatively high threshold of the detection method. Tissue-specific modifications of proteins can interfere with antibody binding. Some determinants may be masked and require predigestion of deparaffinized sections with proteases to expose the determinants to antibody probes. Cordon-Cardo[55] has reported a loss of Mdr1 expression in formalin-fixed, paraffin-embedded tissues. He finds that the determinants recognized by MAbs HYB-241, HYB-612 and C219 are irreversibly masked or lost through routine processing of paraffin sections, and advocates the use of frozen sections. We found that, although staining intensity can be affected by preembedding in paraffin sections, useful information can be derived from deparaffinized sections stained with MAbs C219 and JSB-1.

MEASUREMENTS OF *MDR*1 mRNA LEVELS

The *MDR* mRNA levels can be measured using nucleic acid probes in Northern blots or slot blots,[95,111,142,143] in *in situ* hybridization,[43,266] or the polymerase chain reaction.[49,201,210] Northern blot and slot blot analyses are relatively sensitive. The presence or absence of *MDR*1 RNA can be confirmed with an RNAse protection analysis.[255] This is an extremely stringent assay and is specific for *MDR*1 transcripts that initiate at either an upstream or downstream promoter site. Advantages of measuring message levels rather than Mdr1 protein include higher sensitivity, as evidenced by the observation that elevated levels of *MDR*1 mRNA are detectable in cell lines that are negative for Mdr1 by immunohistochemistry, and reagent specificity.[113] An important limitation is that for slot blot analysis, at least 10^8 tumor cells are needed.

In situ hybridization with nucleic acid probes on tissue sections provides direct morphological confirmation of the presence of *MDR* mRNA in tumor cells, and permits evaluation of the relationship of *MDR* mRNA expression to specific locations within organs.[43,243] Unless the expression in individual cells is relatively high, the results of *in situ* analyses are difficult to interpret. Also, there may not be an exact correlation between levels of message and protein, since low levels of message can be due to relatively slow rates of transcription or rapid rates of RNA degradation. Use of *in situ* hybridization as a laboratory test is further limited because it is laborious and expensive.

Hybridization of nucleic acid probes to transcripts not derived from the *MDR1* gene, but containing homologous sequences, would give rise to false-positive test results. Cordon-Cardo[55] has reported that tissue culture studies have shown the existence of transcripts homologous to but distinct from *MDR1*. The range of molecular weights reported for Mdr1 has raised the possibility of alternative processing in various cell types.

The polymerase chain reaction provides another approach to the identification and quantitation of *MDR* mRNA. This is the most sensitive test for *MDR1* mRNA detection. Quantitative cDNA-PCR methods have been developed and used to analyze *MDR1* and *MDR2* mRNA expression in various tissues.[201,209] The results are essentially in agreement with the tissue-specific distribution of *MDR1* mRNA and Mdr1 protein described by Fojo *et al.*[95] and others using other approaches. PCR products, in quantitative PCR assays, correlate with the amount of the mRNA template. Initial efforts to develop a cDNA-PCR test for *MDR1* mRNA expression in tumors show promise.[209,210] Due to the remarkable sensitivity of PCR, problems of contamination and artifactual amplification remain an obstacle to the implementation of quantitative PCR technology in the clinical laboratory, although these problems are being addressed by hardware and reagent vendors.

Mdr1 PROTEIN IN NORMAL URINARY BLADDER

The expression of the *MDR1* gene was established in urinary bladder by Southern hybridization of DNA with subfragments of *MDR1* cDNA and by cloning and sequencing of genomic fragments.[49] Although *MDR2* is coexpressed with *MDR1* in liver, kidney, adrenal gland, and spleen, it is not co-expressed in other organs including urinary bladder (Table 2.9).

Variability of expression of Mdr1 from person-to-person has not been examined for large populations of patients using quantitative PCR. Some information obtained by other methods is available on heterogeneity and variability of expression. In an immunohistochemical study of transitional epithelium lining ureters using MAb C219, our group examined paraffin sections of tissue blocks obtained from 50 patients without genitourinary pathology noted at autopsy.[318] In 20 patients, immunostaining was in a paranuclear ("Golgi") distribution; in the remaining 30 patients, immunostaining was either diffuse or negative. Similar results were obtained using segments of fresh-frozen ureters obtained at renal transplantation.[318] Anti-Mdr1 Golgi staining was present in all cell layers, with the heaviest staining in superficial cells (Fig. 2.6). The staining corresponded in extent and distribution to Golgi cytomembranes in transitional epithelium described at the ultrastructural level.[219] The Golgi immunostaining was blocked with a MAb C219 epitope-specific 15-mer, providing additional evidence that the immunostaining represented a P-glycoprotein isoform.[101] An unexpected corre-

TABLE 2.9.   *MDR*1 GENE AND MDR1 PROTEIN IN TRANSITIONAL EPITHELIUM

Tissue[a]	Probe or Method	Expression[b]	Reference
Immunohistochemistry			
Normal			
Ureter	MAb C219	20/50[c]	318
Urinary bladder	MABs HYB-241 & -612	0/NR	55
Tumors			
Urinary bladder[d]	MAbs HYB-241 & -612	2/10	57
Urinary bladder	MAbs HYB-241 & -612	4/10	55
DNA (Gene) Measurements			
Normal			
Urinary bladder	*MDR*1 cDNA	1/1	49
Tumors			
NR			
*MDR*1 mRNA Measurements			
Normal			
Urinary bladder	Quant. PCR[e]	1/1[f]	210
Tumors			
Urinary bladder	Slot blot	1/6	111
Urinary bladder	Slot blot	0/10	114
Urinary bladder	Quant. PCR	1/2	210

[a] Tissues were from surgical specimens and autopsies.

[b] Numerator: number of Mdr1 expressors/total number of cases.

[c] Negative staining and diffuse staining were scored together. Plasma membrane staining was rarely encountered.

[d] Tumor type, not classified.

[e] Quantitative PCR.

[f] Positivity reported as + on a scale of 0+ to 5+.

lation was demonstrated between Golgi MAb C219 immunostaining and expression of blood group antigen A. This was also found using a second MAb, JSB-1.[315,318] The significance of this correlation remains unknown and the possibility that it represents an artifact is a matter of considerable concern. Plasma membrane anti-Mdr1 immunostaining was rarely, if ever, observed in normal transitional epithelium.

Few other studies have been reported on Mdr1 in normal transitional epithelium. In a study using MAbs HYB-241 and HYB-612 as probes, Cordon-Cardo *et al.*[57] reported that urothelium is negative for Mdr1. Very few specimens were examined, and it is not stated whether the bladder specimens were obtained at surgery or autopsy.

Quantitative PCR has been used to measure *MDR*1 message in normal transitional epithelium. Noonan *et al.*[210] found weakly positive expression (+) of *MDR*1 (on a scale of 0+ to 5+). This was based on the analysis of a single specimen. Urothelium was not separated from the muscular bladder wall causing the epithelial *MDR*1 component to be diluted by irrelevant nonepithelial tissue, including muscle.

Interpretation of data on Mdr1 in normal bladder will benefit from information

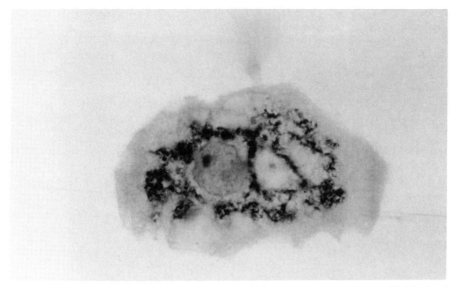

FIG. 2.6. Immunoperoxidase demonstration of MAb C219 reactivity in a human bladder luminal ("umbrella") epithelial cell. The reactivity is in a paranuclear, Golgi-type, pattern of distribution. There is no plasma membrane staining. Cytospin preparation. Hematoxylin counterstain, ×1200.

on the variability and heterogeneity of Mdr1 expression from person to person. Operationally, variability is defined as differences in levels of expression of *MDR* mRNA or Mdr isoforms among people. Heterogeneity is defined as differences in levels of expression within an organ or tumor.

Fojo *et al.*[95] first demonstrated a broad range of *MDR1* mRNA levels in "normal" human colon adjacent to colonic tumor in eight patients. Subsequently, a 14-fold difference in levels of *MDR1* mRNA expression has been found in normal-appearing colonic epithelium.[114] In four of eight cases, levels of expression of *MDR1* mRNA were greater in normal colonic epithelium than in the adjacent tumor. All of the specimens had detectable levels of message. In kidney, normal tissue tended to have higher levels of *MDR1* mRNA than adjacent renal cell carcinomas, and in breast, low levels of *MDR1* mRNA were found in both tumors and adjacent normal tissue. Similar studies on *MDR1* mRNA distributions have not been published for urinary bladder.

We have examined Mdr1 expression in normal organs and tumors from various sites in over 300 patients using immunohistochemistry. For all organs examined, including urinary bladder, both variability and heterogeneity of anti-Mdr staining is the rule rather than the exception. Staining ranged from strongly positive to negative among patients as well as within single tissue sections.

No studies have been published on the prevalence of Mdr1 in normal human tissues in large populations. The relationship of levels of expression of Mdr1 protein in normal and hyperplastic bladder epithelium, in individual patients, to the development of bladder cancer with intrinsic multidrug resistance has not been explored.

Mdr1 PROTEIN IN BLADDER CARCINOMA

Mdr1 has been evaluated in transitional cell carcinomas, in surgical pathology specimens,[111,210] and in tissue cultures derived from transitional cell carcinomas[175] (Table 2.9). As part of a study measuring *MDR1* mRNA levels in over 400 human cancers from various organ sites, Goldstein *et al.*[111] evaluated six bladder tumors and found low-level expression in one tumor. Using MAbs HYB-241 and HYB-612 in an immunohistochemical study, Cordon-Cardo[55] reported anti-Mdr1 reactivity in 40% (4 of 10) bladder cancer cases. In a quantitative PCR study, Noonan *et al.*[210] evaluated *MDR1* expression and found 2+ (on a scale of 0 to 5+) expression in one of two bladder tumors.

While these survey studies point to the fact that some bladder tumors are expressors of Mdr1, these series are small and the descriptions are inadequate to draw conclusions with regard to several crucial parameters, including heterogeneity of expression among tumors and within tumors, and relationships of Mdr1 expression to bladder cancer differentiation and stage.

Mdr1 PROTEIN IN OTHER ORGANS

Although reports of Mdr1 expression in urinary bladder are just beginning to appear, many papers have been published that deal with multidrug resistance and other types of drug resistance in other organs. Some of these studies are relevant to the theme of this chapter on urinary bladder since they describe methodology and study design that may be appropriate for future bladder cancer studies.

In one of the first studies aimed at determining if Mdr1 abnormalities occurred in human cancer patients, Mdr1 overexpression was demonstrated in malignant cells in ascitic fluid from two of five women with clinically-advanced, drug-resistant ovarian cancer.[21] In another early study, human solid tumors were surveyed for evidence of Mdr1 expression using immunoblot assays.[102] Solid tumors from 46 patients, representing 12 tumor types, were included in the study. The only tumors overexpressing Mdr1 protein were 4 of 11 sarcomas. An additional 14 sarcomas were tested and 2 were positive for overexpression of Mdrs. Three of the six Mdr1 protein-positive sarcoma patients had not received chemotherapy so that the Mdr1 expression may have reflected the intrinsic drug resistance of these tumors. The high prevalence of Mdr1 protein expression in sarcomas has been confirmed using quantitative PCR.[210]

In several early studies, the *MDR1* gene in normal tissues and human tumors was quantitated using probes prepared from *MDR1* cDNA.[94,95] Northern and slot blot analyses were used to quantitate *MDR1* mRNA levels. High levels of the message were detected in several human tumors, including some, but not all, tumors of epithelial origin arising in the adrenal gland and colon. In a comparison of primary tumors and recurrent tumors, increased expression of *MDR1* mRNA was found in a few recurrent tumors that appeared following courses of chemotherapy.[95] This provided evidence of the existence of *acquired* multidrug resistance in patient material.

The NIH group headed by Gottesman and Pastan has published the largest study of Mdr1 in human tumors.[111] They analyzed over 400 tumor samples representing a wide spectrum of human malignancies. *MDR*1 mRNA was measured in bulk tumor samples using slot blot hybridization. They found that many tumors from untreated cancer patients had relatively high levels of *MDR*1 mRNA expression. Generally, these tumors arose in organs with Mdr1 as a normal component, including liver, colon, and kidney. Other tumors had intermediate or low levels of *MDR*1 mRNA expression. Recurrent tumors in patients who developed resistance to chemotherapy tended to have higher levels of Mdr1 expression than initial tumors from the same patients. *MDR*1 mRNA was not detected in a large number of tumors, particularly in carcinomas arising in organs that are normally low expressors of Mdr1.

*MDR*1 and *MDR*2 mRNAs have been quantitated by Roninson's group using PCR to detect low levels of message.[210] *MDR*1 and *MDR*2 mRNAs were detected in the majority of sarcomas, compared with Mdr1 detection in 24% of sarcomas in the series of Gerlach *et al.*[102] The highest frequency of *MDR*1 mRNA negativity was demonstrated in Ewing's sarcomas, which are tumors that are relatively sensitive to chemotherapy as compared with other types of sarcomas.

The relationship of Mdr1 levels to tumor histopathology and responses to chemotherapeutic intervention was examined by Kanamaru *et al.*[143] in a series of 42 renal cell carcinomas. *MDR*1 mRNA levels were higher in well-differentiated renal cell carcinomas as compared with poorly differentiated tumors. *In vitro* chemosensitivity assays were performed on 16 of the renal cell carcinoma samples. Using quinidine as a chemosensitizing agent, it was shown that chemosensitivity to doxorubicin was enhanced in the group of tumors that were high expressors of *MDR*1 mRNA, but not in the low expressors. This work and the earlier study of Fojo *et al.*[95] suggested that quantification of *MDR*1 mRNA levels could be useful in developing strategies to overcome clinically significant Mdr1-mediated drug resistance.

Studies on Mdr1 expression in breast carcinomas illustrate the variability in results obtained by different laboratories and suggest a need to standardize methodology before Mdr1 measurements are offered as a laboratory test. Whereas several groups found low incidences of Mdr1 expression in breast cancers by immunohistochemistry,[261,276] Western hybridization,[190] and by RNA detection,[111,190] others have reported higher incidences of *MDR*1 gene expression.[148,250] Verrelle and co-workers found that 85% of breast cancer patients expressed Mdr1 in at least some of their tumor cells, using immunohistochemistry with a different anti-Mdr1 MAb. There are many plausible explanations for these discrepancies, including differences in tumor etiology and carcinogen exposure in different geographic locations.[301] Technical explanations might include a low signal-to-background ratio for the Verrelle's immunohistochemical method that might produce false-positive test results, as suggested by Dalton and Grogan.[64] On the other hand, methods of other investigations may have inappropriately high thresholds of Mdr1 detection.

Many groups have measured Mdr1 proteins and *MDR*1 mRNA levels in hematopoietic dyscrasias. In an early study, Mdr1 was detected in two cases of refractory acute nonlymphoblastic leukemia, using an immunocytochemical assay.[177] The percentage of peripheral blood cells that stained with anti-Mdr1 antibodies increased with subsequent treatment. In another early study using an *MDR1* gene probe, increased *MDR1* mRNA expression was found in 1 of 10 patients with acute lymphoblastic leukemia.[95] The elevated level was obtained from a patient at the time of a second relapse, raising the possibility that this increase was acquired during therapy. Ito *et al.*[137] used immunocytochemistry, Southern hybridization analysis, and Northern hybridization analysis in a study of 19 cases of adult acute leukemia. They found that Mdr1 expression and *MDR1* gene amplification occurred infrequently in leukemic cells at the time of initial presentation as well as at relapse. They concluded that classic multidrug resistance cannot account for the refractoriness to antileukemia drugs in most patients with adult acute leukemia.

Holmes *et al.*[132] screened peripheral blood or bone marrow from 66 patients with myelodysplastic syndromes (MDS) and acute myeloblastic leukemia (AML) for *MDR1* gene amplification, and 40 cases for increased *MDR1* mRNA expression. They found increased *MDR1* mRNA levels in 18 of 40 patients, but not gene amplification. List *et al.*[174] also examined, by immunocytochemistry, Mdr1 protein in MDS and AML following MDS. Mdr1 was detected in 22% of cases of primary MDS, 57% of cases evolving from MDS, and 83% of cases of therapy-related hematological disorders. List *et al.* have reported that multidrug resistance in MDS and karyotypically-related hematological disorders is closely linked to a stem cell phenotype.

Rothenberg *et al.*[244] detected increased *MDR1* gene expression in 4 of 28 patients with acute lymphoblastic leukemia but no evidence of *MDR1* gene amplification. In comprehensive studies using RNA *in situ* hybridization, immunocytochemistry and drug-uptake analyses, they showed that *MDR1* gene expression and Mdr1 protein levels were heterogeneous within the populations of malignant lymphoblasts. Marie *et al.*[179] found similar incidences of increased *MDR1* expression in ALL and AML. They found a significant inverse association of *MDR1* expression and the achievement of complete remissions in adult patients with acute leukemias. In their series, patients with low *MDR1* expression achieved complete remissions in 67% of cases versus 29% of patients *with* higher *MDR1* expression levels. Remissions in the 29% of patients, who were high *MDR1* expressors, may have been related to the treatment of these patients with non-MDR drugs such as araC, prednisone, and cyclophosphamide. Remission durations for patients with Mdr1-positive and Mdr1-negative leukemia cells were not statistically different.

Sato *et al.*[255] measured RNA transcript levels in leukemic cells obtained from 15 adult acute nonlymphocytic leukemia (ANLL) and 15 cases of chronic myelogenous leukemia (CML). Expression of *MDR1* RNA was detected in 12 of 15 cases of ANLL. In patients with CML, *MDR1* RNA was not detected in RNA extracted from chronic phase cells but was found in blastic crisis cells in four patients, usually in trace amounts. They observed that *MDR1* expression was most frequent in leukemic cells of patients who were clinically classified as falling into the "high risk" or "poor prognosis" group on the basis of a history of toxic exposure to chemotherapeutic drugs, leukemia evolving from MDS, or relapsed disease. They showed that, in leukemia, *MDR*1 gene expression is associated with a poor clinical prognosis. In an immunocytochemical study, Kuwazuru *et al.*[162] also found *Mdr*1 gene expression in CML cells from patients in blast crisis.

Studies on multiple myeloma have made important contributions to the development of laboratory methods for quantitating multidrug resistance.[116] In an early study, Dalton *et al.*[66] at the University of Arizona, analyzed the myeloma cells of 13 patients with prior chemotherapy and current drug-refractory disease and found Mdr1-positive cells in 7 of the patients, using MAb JSB-1 for immunostaining. Anti-Mdr1-immunoperoxidase staining was quantitated, using a Cell Analysis System (CAS) image analysis system and methodology developed by Grogan *et al.*[116] An inverse correlation was demonstrated for doxorubicin accumulation and optical density of MAb JSB-1 immunostained cells. This assay can be used to perform a differential count on tumor cells to determine both the percentage of cells that are positive for Mdr1 and the relative staining intensity of individual cells. These studies showed that quantitative microscopy is a useful method for establishing Mdr1 levels.

In a follow-up study by the same group, Grogan *et al.* did a prospective study on consecutive bone marrow samples from 104 myeloma patients, with samples coming both prior to therapy or at the time of relapse. Results showed that myeloma patients with no prior therapy had a 6% incidence of Mdr1 expression, whereas groups of patients exposed to high dosages of either vincristine or doxorubicin had higher incidences of Mdr1 expression (50% and 83% respectively). One hundred percent of patients who received high doses of *both* vincristine and doxorubicin had Mdr1 expression in their malignant plasma cells. The data of Grogan *et al.* also showed that disease duration was not a significant variable between the Mdr1-nonexpressing and Mdr1-expressing groups of patients. The study showed that Mdr1 expression is usually an acquired trait in myeloma, and provided a basis for a predictive mathematical model from which dose-related Mdr1 expression normograms were generated (T. M. Grogan, unpublished observations). The methodology used in these studies on myeloma may be useful for measuring Mdr1 protein levels in tumor cells obtained in bladder washings or, possibly, voided urines.

COMMENTS AND PERSPECTIVE

Major goals of cancer pathobiologists include the identification of markers that will flag patients at high risk for the development of cancers, and the characterization of tumors with respect to their invasive and metastatic potential, in order to provide a rational basis for customizing therapy. The elegant work of Vogelstein and his colleagues provides a framework for the development of a strategy for evaluating putative markers on the basis of their temporal appearance. Although much of the work was performed on colorectal lesions, their model of carcinogenesis serves as guide for research in other organs, including bladder.

Vogelstein's logic is illustrated by several examples. In the evolution of colorectal carcinomas, hypomethylation and deactivation of the APC gene on chromosome 5 are early events. Although potentially important in the pathogenesis of colonic adenomas and precursor lesions for carcinomas, these abnormalities are ubiquitous in colonic polyps and, thus, of little value in identifying polyps with a high risk for progression. Similarly, *ras* gene mutations are not of high prognostic value in colon, since such mutations are found in approximately 50% of intermediate and late stage adenomas, as well as in carcinomas.[304] On the other hand, mutations occurring later in the process of carcinogenesis, such as those involving p53 or DCC, are more likely to affect the metastatic capabilities of tumors. It remains to be shown if these late changes precede invasion or occur concomitantly; this would limit their usefulness as prognosticators.

The applicability of the Vogelstein paradigm to bladder cancer remains to be established. While some groups of bladder cancer patients seem to fit the temporal predictions of the model reasonably well, others seem to diverge from it. Those patients whose clinical courses are most consistent with Vogelstein's model of accumulated genetic abnormalities (Fig. 2.2*B*, curve B) should benefit most from laboratory tests that can predict the aggressive potential of their tumors. Patients who present initially with deeply invasive bladder cancers, a common occurrence, would not benefit from such assays, since their tumors are advanced at the time of diagnosis (Fig. 2.2*B*, curve A).

The search continues for early genetic or epigenetic changes in relatively normal-appearing urothelium that has undergone early events in transformation, which are not apparent cytologically but could be detected in the laboratory with molecular probes. Ideally, these changes in latent lesions would herald the development of the highly aggressive transitional cell carcinomas that would otherwise present with deeply invasive disease. Because of the importance of early detection of lesions with high malignant potential, before they traverse the basement membrane in bladder, clues obtained from Vogelstein's studies on colon and rectum should be pursued with vigor. For example, a reevaluation of screening for *ras* mutations might make sense for certain high-risk patients despite the results of earlier studies showing low *ras* mutation rates in bladder cancers.

In the multidrug resistance field, basic scientists are studying novel mechanisms of action of Mdr1, in addition to its plasma membrane transporter function. For example, there is evidence that suggests that Mdr1 increases fluid-phase endocytosis,[262,263] possibly by destabilizing the membrane in such a way as to increase membrane trafficking.[17] Vesicle transport could provide an alternative pathway for drug excretion. Mdr1 enrichment of membranes could have other effects on cellular physiology and may influence tumor cell interactions.[317] Roles of proteins, other than Mdr1, that are overproduced by many, but not all, multidrug resistant cells merit further study.[191] And, finally, many issues related to binding and transport of drugs, mechanisms of modulation, and questions of functions of Mdr1 in normal tissues, remain to be resolved.

Clinical investigations are aimed at examining relationships between Mdr1 expression in a variety of tumors and responses to therapy. More clinical trials examining the efficacy of using novel Mdr1 pump inhibitors, such as verapamil analogs, for the purpose of converting drug-resistant tumors into drug-sensitive tumors are being planned. It should be mentioned that, in addition to using Mdr1 pump inhibitors as chemosensitizers, there are many other approaches to overcoming drug resistance including increasing drug-dose intensity, exploiting collateral sensitivity, using noncross-resistant drug combinations, and inhibiting cellular growth factors.[63] Recently, an alternative approach, involving the use of therapeutic doses of anti-Mdr1 MAbs, has been proposed that capitalizes on the increased Mdr1 expression on drug-resistant tumor cells. MAbs or MAb-toxin conjugates, directed against Mdr1 extracellular domains on cancer cells, are used to either inhibit Mdr1-mediated drug efflux or to destroy tumor cells via membrane lysis.[93,161,220,291] Although interesting preliminary results have been reported,[220] there are many potential obstacles to implementation of these forms of immunotherapy.[19]

As the field of cancer drug sensitivity testing matures, new opportunities may emerge for pathologists interested in evaluating human tumors.[116,144,314,316] The development of the field of cancer drug sensitivity testing will require comprehensive information on the prevalence and levels of expression of the human *MDR*1 and *MDR*2 genes and their protein products. Data is needed on Mdr1 expression in subpopulations defined by age, sex, race, diet, medical history, drug history, and other parameters.

Several issues came out of the initial tissue-distribution studies on solid tumors. The first relates to the issue of the nonuniformity of Mdr1 protein expression in tumors. Our experience with Mdr1 immunohistochemistry of tumors is that Mdr1 expression is typically heterogeneous. Although we found a few tumors that showed a reasonably uniform level of Mdr1 protein expression throughout the specimen, that was unusual. More typically, Mdr1 expression is patchy. It may even be restricted to a few cancer cells that are isolated deep within the connective tissue stroma near the invasive front of the tumor.[317]

Nonuniform distributions of Mdr1 positive cells in tumors have implications with respect to the use of bulk tumor samples for measuring levels of *MDR*1 mRNA/Mdr1. Heterogeneity also complicates efforts to establish threshold levels of Mdr1 expression that are required to define the multidrug resistance phenotype. Detailed comparative studies on various approaches to Mdr1 diagnostic testing are needed to establish the best methods for Mdr1 measurements in surgical and cytology specimens.

Clinical studies are also needed, in which patients are stratified into chemotherapy protocols, based on levels of *MDR*1 mRNA or Mdr1 protein expression in the primary tumors. Since early studies showed some success in identifying patients with multidrug resistance, those who might be responsive to chemosensitization for a few types of tumors, it can be anticipated that clinical research will be expanded in this area, as parallel studies are initiated for other organ systems. The next set of clinical studies should provide pathologists with opportunities to develop, evaluate, and compare Mdr1 tests and correlate test results with clinical outcomes.

Finally, the multidrug resistance story is probably the tip of the iceberg. Although a large literature on cancer drug resistance is already in existence, we sense that many of the major discoveries that will affect clinical care and circumvent failures of therapy are yet to be made. New features of Mdr1 may be elucidated that could suggest alternative approaches to inhibiting its pump function. Additional genes may emerge, expanding the current menu of drug resistant genes. The challenge to the clinical pathologist will be to devise better tests to establish drug sensitivity profiles for individual tumors. Bringing this form of sensitivity testing into routine practice will pose many challenges, and will require a special partnership in patient care between the pathologist and the oncologist.

ACKNOWLEDGMENTS

I thank Drs. William T. Bellamy, Claire M. Payne, and Thomas M. Grogan for useful discussions and suggestions; Drs. Anna R. Graham and Diane K. Ecklund for critically reading the manuscript; Ms. Sandy Beinar, Ms. Janice Steele, and Ms. Toni Lester for editorial assistance; and Ms. Jeanne Bushell for preparing the figures. This study was supported in part by Grant CA 41183 from the National Cancer Institute.

REFERENCES

1. Ahuja, H., Bar-Eli, M., Advani, S. H., Benchimol, S., and Cline, M. J. Alterations in the p53 gene and the clonal evolution of the blast crisis of chronic myelocytic leukemia. *Proc. Natl. Acad. Sci. USA 86:* 6783–6787, 1989.

2. Akiyama, S.-I., Fojo, A., Hanover, J. A., Pastan, I., and Gottesman, M. M. Isolation and genetic characterization of human KB cell lines resistant to multiple drugs. *Soma Cell Mol. Gen. II:* 117–126, 1985.

3. Albrecht, A. M., Biedler, J. L., and Hutchison, D. J. Two different species of dihydrofolate reductase in mammalian cells differentially resistant to amethopterin and methasquin. *Cancer Res. 32:* 1539–1546, 1972.

4. Althausen, A. F., Prout, G. R., Jr., and Daley, J. J. Non-invasive papillary carcinoma of the bladder associated with carcinoma in situ. *J. Urol. 116:* 575–580, 1976.

5. Ames, G. F-L. The basis of multidrug resistance in mammalian cells: Homology with bacterial transport. *Cell 47:* 323–324, 1986.

6. Ardalan, B., Cooney, D. A., Jayaram, H. N., Carrico, C. K., Glazer, R. I., MacDonald, J., and Schein, P. S. Mechanisms of sensitivity and resistant of murine tumors to 5-fluorouracil. *Cancer Res. 40:* 1431–1437, 1980.

7. Aso, Y., Anderson, L., Soloway, M., Bouffioux, C., Chisholm, G., Debruyne, F., Kawai, T., Kurth, K. H., Maru, A., and Straffon, W. G. E. Prognostic factors in superficial bladder cancer. *Prog. Clin. Biol. Res. 221:* 257–269, 1986.

8. Atkin, N. B., and Fox, M. F. 5q Deletion: The sole chromosome change in a carcinoma of the bladder. *Cancer Genet Cytogenet 46:* 129–131, 1990.

9. Baas, F., and Borst, P. The tissue dependent expression of hamster P-glycoprotein genes. *FEBS Letters 229:* 329–332, 1988.

10. Baas, F., Jongsma, A. P. M., Broxterman, H. J., Arceci, R. J., Housman, D., Scheffer, G. L., Riethorst, A., Van Groenigen, M., Nieuwint, A. W. M., and Joenje, H. Non-P-glycoprotein mediated mechanism for multidrug resistance precedes P-glycoprotein expression during *in vitro* selection for doxorubicin resistance in a human lung cancer line. *Cancer Res. 50:* 5392–5398, 1990.

11. Babu, V. R., Lutz, M. D., Miles, B. J., Farah, R. N., Weiss, L., and Van Dyke, D. L. Tumor behavior in transitional cell carcinoma of the bladder in relation to chromosomal markers and histopathology. *Cancer Res. 47:* 6800–6805, 1987.

12. Babu, V. R., Miles, B. J., Cerney, J. C., Weiss, L., and Van Dyke, D. L. Chromosome 21q22 deletion: A specific chromosome change in a new bladder cancer subgroup. *Cancer Genet. Cytogenet. 38:* 127–129, 1989.

13. Baker, S. J., Fearon, E. R., Nigro, J. M., Hamilton, S. R., Preisinger, A. C., Jessup, J. M., van Tuinen, P., Ledbetter, D. H., Barker, D. F., Nakamura, Y., White, R., and Vogelstein, B.

Chromosome 17 deletions and p53 gene mutations in colorectal carcinomas. *Science 244:* 217–221, 1989.

14. Baker, S. J., Markowitz, S., Fearon, E. R., Willson, J. K., and Vogelstein, B. Suppression of human colorectal carcinoma cell growth by wild-type p53. *Science 249:* 912–915, 1990.

15. Balmain, A., Ramsden, M., Bowen, G. T., and Smith, J. Activation of the mouse cellular Harvey-*ras* gene in chemically induced benign skin papillomas. *Nature (Lond.) 307:* 658–660, 1984.

16. Barbacid, M. Ras genes. *Annu. Rev. Biochem. 56:* 779–827, 1987.

17. Beck, W. T. The cell biology of multiple drug resistance. *Biochem. Pharm. 36:* 2879–2887, 1987.

18. Beck, W. T. Unknotting the complexities of multidrug resistance: The involvement of DNA topoisomerases in drug action and resistance. *J. Natl. Cancer Inst. 81:* 5285–5287, 1989.

19. Beck, W. T. Do anti-P-glycoprotein antibodies have a future in the circumvention of multidrug resistance? *J. Natl. Cancer Inst. 83:* 1364–1366, 1991.

20. Beck, W. T., and Danks, M. K. Characteristics of multidrug resistance in human tumor cells. In *Molecular and Cellular Biology of Multidrug Resistance in Tumor Cells,* edited by I. B. Roninson. New York, Plenum Press, 1991, pp. 3–55.

21. Bell, D. R., Gerlach, J. H., Kartner, N., Buick, R. N., and Ling, V. Detection of P-glycoprotein in ovarian cancer: A molecular marker associated with multidrug resistance. *J. Clin. Oncol. 3:* 311–315, 1985.

22. Berenblum, I. Sequential aspects of chemical carcinogenesis. In *Cancer Etiology,* edited by F. Becker. New York, Plenum Press, 1975, pp. 323–344.

23. Berger, C. S., Sandberg, A. A., Todd, I. A. D., Pennington, R. D., Haddad, F. S., Hecht, B. K., and Hecht, F. Chromosomes in kidney, ureter, and bladder cancer. *Cancer Genet Cytogenet 23:* 1–24, 1986.

24. Berger, M. S., Greenfield, C., Gullick, W. J., Haley, J., Downward, J., Neal, D. E., Harris, A. L., and Waterfield, M. D. Evaluation of epidermal growth factor receptors in bladder tumours. *Br. J. Cancer 56:* 533–537, 1987.

25. Berridge, M. J. Inositol lipids and cell proliferation. *Biochim. Biophys. Acta 907:* 33–45, 1987.

26. Biedler, J. L., Albrecht, A. M., Hutchison, D. J., and Spengler, B. A. Drug response, dihydrofolate reductase, and cytogenetics of amethopterin-resistant Chinese hamster cells *in vitro. Cancer Res. 32:* 153–161, 1972.

27. Bishop, J. M. The molecular genetics of cancer. *Science 235:* 305–311, 1987.

28. Bishop, J. M. Molecular themes in oncogenesis. *Cell 64:* 235–248, 1991.

29. Bodmer, W. F., Bailey, C. J., Bodmer, J., Bussey, H. J. R., Ellis, A., Gorman, P., Lucibello, F. C., Murday, V. A., Rider, S. H., Scambler, P., Sheer, D., Solomon, E., and Spurr, N. K. Localization of the gene for familial adenomatous polyposis on chromosome 5. *Nature (Lond.) 328:* 614–616, 1987.

30. Bos, J. L. The *ras* gene family and human carcinogenesis. *Mutat. Res. 195:* 255–271, 1988.

31. Bos, J. L., Fearon, E. R., Hamilton, S. R., Verlaan-de Vries, M., Van Boom, J. H., Van Der Eb, A. J., and Vogelstein, B. Prevalence of *ras* gene mutations in human colorectal cancers. *Nature (Lond.) 327:* 293–297, 1987.

32. Bos, J. L., Verlaan-de Vries, M., Marshall, C. J., Veeneman, G. H., Van Boom, J. H., and Van Der Eb, A. J. A human gastric carcinoma contains a single mutated and an amplified normal allele of the Ki-*ras* oncogene. *Nucleic Acids Res. 14:* 1209–1217, 1986.

33. Bradley, G., Juranka, P. F., and Ling, V. Mechanism of multidrug resistance. *Biochim. Biophys. Acta 948:* 87–128, 1988.

34. Bradley, G., Naik, M., and Ling, V. P-glycoprotein expression in multidrug-resistant human ovarian carcinoma cell lines. *Cancer Res. 49:* 2790–2796, 1989.

35. Brawn, P. N. The origin of invasive carcinoma of the bladder. *Cancer 50:* 515–519, 1982.

36. Bressac, B., Galvin, K. M., Liang, T. J., Isselbacher, K. J., Wands, J. R., and Ozturk, M. Abnormal structure and expression of p53 gene in human hepatocellular carcinoma. *Proc. Natl. Acad. Sci. USA 87:* 1973–1977, 1990.

37. Broxterman, H. J., Pinedo, H. M., and Kuiper, C. M. Immunohistochemical detection of P-glycoprotein in human tumor cells with low degree of drug resistance. *Int. J. Cancer 43:* 340–343, 1989.

38. Broxterman, H. J., Pinedo, H. M., Kuiper, C. M., van der hoeven, J. J. M., de Lange, P., Quak,

J. J., Scheper, R. J., Keizer, H. G., Schuurhuis, G. J., and Lankelma, J. Immunohistochemical detection of P-glycoprotein in human tumor cells with low degree of drug resistance. *Int. J. Cancer 43:* 340–343, 1989.

39. Cabral, F., Sobel, M. E., and Gottesman, M. M. CHO mutants resistant to colchicine, colcemid or griseofulvin have an altered beta-tubulin. *Cell 20:* 29–36, 1980.
40. Callen, D. F., Baker, E., Simmers, R. N., Seshadri, R., and Roninson, I. B. Localization of the human multiple drug resistance gene, *MDR*1, to 7q21.1. *Hum. Genet. 77:* 142–144, 1987.
41. Carlsen, S. A., Till, J. E., and Ling, V. Modulation of membrane drug permeability in Chinese hamster ovary cells. *Biochem. Biophys. Acta 455:* 900–912, 1976.
42. Carr, F. J., and Fox, B. W. DNA strand breaks and repair synthesis in Yoshida sarcoma: Cells with differential sensitivities to bifunctional alkylating agents and UV light. *Mutat. Res. 83:* 233–249, 1981.
43. Chabner, B. A., and Fojo, A. Multidrug resistance: P-glycoprotein and its allies-the elusive foes. *J. Nat. Cancer Inst. 81:* 910–913, 1989.
44. Chabner, B. A., and Wilson, W. Reversal of multidrug resistance. *J. Clin. Oncol. 9:* 4–6, 1991.
45. Chan, H. S. L., Bradley, G., Thorner, P., Haddad, G., Gallie, B. L., and Ling, V. A sensitive method for immunocytochemical detection of P-glycoprotein in multidrug-resistant human ovarian carcinoma cell lines. *Lab. Invest. 59:* 870–875, 1988.
46. Chan, H. S. L., Thorner, P. S., Haddad, G., and Ling, V. Immunohistochemical detection of P-glycoprotein: Prognostic correlation in soft tissue sarcoma of childhood. *J. Clin. Oncol. 8:* 689–704, 1990.
47. Chen, C-J., Chin, J. E., Ueda, K., Clark, D. P., Pastan, I., Gottesman, M. M., and Roninson, I. B. Internal duplication and homology with bacterial transport proteins in the *mdr*1 (P-glycoprotein) gene from multidrug-resistant human cells. *Cell 47:* 381–389, 1986.
48. Chen, C-J., Clark, D., Ueda, K., Pastan, I., Gottesman, M. M., and Roninson, I. B. Genomic organization of the human multidrug resistance (MDR1) gene and origin of P-glycoproteins. *J. Biol. Chem. 265:* 506–514, 1990.
49. Chin, J. E., Soffir, R., Noonan, K. E., Choi, K., and Roninson, I. B. Structure and expression of the human *MDR* (P-glyoprotein) gene family. *Mol. Cell. Biol. 9:* 3808–3820, 1989.
50. Choi, K., Chen, C-J., Kriegler, M., and Roninson, I. B. An altered pattern of cross-resistance in multidrug-resistant human cells results from spontaneous mutations in the *mdr*1 (P-glyco-protein) gene. *Cell 53:* 519–529, 1988.
51. Cline, M. J. Biology of disease: Molecular diagnosis of human cancer. *Lab. Invest. 61:* 368–380, 1989.
52. Cohen, J. B., and Levinson, A. D. A point mutation in the last intron responsible for increased expression and transforming activity of the c-Ha-*ras* oncogene. *Nature (Lond.) 334:* 119–124, 1988.
53. Coon, J. S., Pauli, B. U., and Weinstein, R. S. Precancer of the urinary bladder. *Cancer Surv 2:* 479–494, 1983.
54. Coon, J. S., Schwartz, D., and Weinstein, R. S. Markers in the analysis of human bladder cancer. *Advances Path 1:* 201–228, 1988.
55. Cordon-Cardo, C. Immunohistochemical analysis of P-glycoprotein expression in normal and tumor tissues in humans. In *Molecular and Cellular Biology of Multidrug Resistance in Tumor Cells,* edited by I. B. Roninson. New York, Plenum Press, 1991, pp. 303–318.
56. Cordon-Cardo, C., O'Brien, J. P., Boccia, J., Casals, D., Bertino, J. R., and Melamed, M. R. Expression of the multidrug resistance gene product (P-glycoprotein) in human normal and tumor tissues. *J. Histochem. Cytochem. 38:* 1277–1287, 1990.
57. Cordon-Cardo, C., O'Brien, J. P., Casals, D., Boccia, J., and Bertino, J. R. Immunoanatomic and immunopathologic expression of the multidrug resistance gene product. *Cancer Cells 7:* 87–93, 1989.
58. Cordon-Cardo, C., O'Brien, J. P., Casals, D., Rittman-Grauer, L., Biedler, J. L., Melamed, M. R., and Bertino, J. R. Multidrug-resistance gene (P-glycoprotein) is expressed by endothelial cells at blood-brain barrier sites. *Proc. Natl. Acad. Sci. USA 86:* 695–698, 1989.
59. Cornwell, M. M., Pastan, I., and Gottesman, M. M. Binding of drugs and ATP by P-glycoprotein

and transport of drugs by vesicles from human multidrug-resistant cells. In *Molecular and Cellular Biology of Multidrug Resistance in Tumor Cells*, edited by I. B. Roninson. New York, Plenum Press, 1991, pp. 229–242.

60. Croop, J. M., Raymond, M., Haber, D., Devault, A., Arceci, R. J., Gros, P., and Housman, D. E. The three mouse multidrug resistance (*mdr*) genes are expressed in tissue-specific manner in normal mouse tissues. *Mol. Cell Biol. 9:* 1346–1350, 1989.

61. Cutler, S. J., Heney, N. M., and Friedell, G. H. Longitudinal study of patients with bladder cancer: Factors associated with disease recurrence and progression. In *Bladder Cancer*, edited by W. W. Bonney. Baltimore, Williams & Wilkins, 1982, pp. 35–46.

62. D'Arpa, P., and Liu, L. F. Topoisomerase-targeting antitumor drugs. *Biochim. Biophys. Acta 989:* 163–177, 1989.

63. Dalton, W. S. Mechanisms of drug resistance in breast cancer. *Sem. Oncol. 17:* 37–39, 1990.

64. Dalton, W. S., and Grogan, T. M. Does P-glycoprotein predict response to chemotherapy, and if so, is there a reliable way to detect it? *J. Natl. Cancer Inst. 83:* 80–81, 1991.

65. Dalton, W. S., Grogan, T. M., Meltzer, P. S., Scheper, R. J., Durie, B. G. M., Taylor, C. W., Miller, T. P., and Salmon, S. E. Drug-resistance in multiple myeloma and non-Hodgkin's lymphoma: Detection of P-glycoprotein and potential circumvention by addition of verapamil to chemotherapy. *J. Clin. Oncol. 7:* 415–424, 1989.

66. Dalton, W. S., Grogan, T. M., Rybski, J. A., Scheper, R. J., Richter, L., Kailey, J. M., Broxterman, H. J., Pinedo, H. M., and Salmon, S. E. Immunohistochemical detection and quantitation of P-glycoprotein in multiple drug-resistant human myeloma cells: Association with level of drug resistance and drug accumulation. *Blood 73:* 747–752, 1989. Abstract.

67. Danks, M. K., Yalowich, J. C., and Beck, W. T. Atypical multiple drug resistance in a human leukemic cell line selected for resistance to teniposide (VM-26). *Cancer Res. 47:* 1297–1301, 1987.

68. Dano, K. Active outward transport of daunomycin in resistant Ehrlich ascites tumor cell. *Biochim. Biophys. Acta 323:* 1466–1483, 1973.

69. Deverson, E. V., Gow, I. R., Coadwell, W. J., Monaco, J. J., Butcher, G. W., and Howard, J. C. MHC class II region encoding proteins related to the multidrug resistance family of transmembrane transporters. *Nature (Lond.) 348:* 738–741, 1990.

70. DeVita, V. T., Jr. Principles of chemotherapy. In *Cancer. Principles & Practice of Oncology*, edited by V. T. DeVita, Jr., S. Hellman, and S. A. Rosenberg. Philadelphia, J. B. Lippincott, Co., 1989, pp. 276–300.

71. Diller, L., Kassel, J., Nelson, C. E., Gryka, M. A., Litwak, G., Gebhardt, M., Bressac, B., Ozturk, M., Baker, S. J., Vogelstein, B., and Friend, S. H. p53 functions as a cell cycle control protein in osteosarcomas. *Mol. Cell. Biol. 10:* 5772–5781, 1990.

72. Droller, M. J. Transitional cell cancer: Upper tracts and bladder. In *Campbell's Urology*, edited by P. C. Walsh, R. F. Gittes, A. D. Perlmutter, and T. A. Stamey. Philadelphia, W. B. Saunders, 1986, pp. 1343–1440.

73. Edelman, G. M. Morphoregulatory molecules. *Biochemistry 27:* 3533–3543, 1988.

74. Egan, S. E., Wright, J. A., Jarolim, L., Yanagihara, K., Bassin, R. H., and Greenberg, A. H. Transformation by oncogenes encoding protein kinases induces the metastatic phenotype. *Science 238:* 202–205, 1987.

75. Eliyahu, D., Goldfinger, N., Pinhasi-Kimhi, O., Shaulski, G., Skurnik, Y., Arai, N., Rotter, V., and Oren, M. Meth a fibrosarcoma cells express two transforming mutant p53 species. *Oncogene 3:* 313–321, 1988.

76. Eliyahu, D., Michalovitz, D., Eliyahu, S., Pinhasi-Kimhi, O., and Oren, M. Wild-type p53 can inhibit oncogene-mediated focus formation. *Proc. Natl. Acad. Sci. USA 86:* 8763–8767, 1989.

77. Eliyahu, D., Raz, A., Gruss, P., Givol, D., and Oven, M. Participation of p53 cellular tumor antigen in transformation of normal embryonic cells. *Nature (Lond.) 312:* 647–649, 1984.

78. Endicott, J. A., and Ling, V. The biochemistry of P-glycoprotein-mediated multidrug resistance. *Annu. Rev. Biochem. 58:* 137–171, 1989.

79. Erickson, L. C., Laurent, G., Sharkey, N. A., and Kohn, K. W. DNA cross-linking and

monoadduct repair in nitrosourea-treated human tumor cells. *Nature (Lond.) 288:* 727–729, 1980.

80. Farber, E. Cellular biochemistry of the stepwise development of cancer with chemicals: G. H. A. Clowes Memorial Lecture. *Cancer Res. 44:* 5463–5474, 1984.

81. Farber, E., and Sarma, D. S. R. Hepatocarcinogenesis: A dynamic cellular prespective. *Lab. Invest. 56:* 4–22, 1987.

82. Farrow, G. M., Utz, D. C., and Rife, C. C. Morphological and clinical observations of patients with early bladder cancer treated with total cystectomy. *Cancer Res. 36:* 2495–2501, 1976.

83. Farrow, G. M., Utz, D. C., Rife, C. C., and Greene, L. F. Clinical observations on sixty-nine cases of in situ carcinoma of the urinary bladder. *Cancer Res. 37:* 2794–2798, 1977.

84. Fearon, E. R., Cho, K. R., Nigro, J. M., Kern, S. E., Simons, J. W., Ruppert, J. M., Hamilton, S. R., Preisinger, A. C., Thomas, G., Kinzler, K. W., and Vogelstein, B. Identification of a chromosome 18q gene that is altered in colorectal cancers. *Science 247:* 49–56, 1990.

85. Fearon, E. R., Feinberg, A. P., Hamilton, S. H., and Vogelstein, B. Loss of genes on the short arm of chromosome 11 in bladder cancer. *Nature (Lond.) 318:* 377–380, 1985.

86. Fearon, E. R., Hamilton, S. R., and Vogelstein, B. Clonal analysis of human colorectal tumors. *Science 238:* 193–197, 1987.

87. Fearon, E. R., and Vogelstein, B. A genetic model for colorectal tumorigenesis. *Cell 61:* 759–767, 1990.

88. Feinberg, A. P., Gehrke, C. W., Kuo, K. C., and Ehrlich, M. Reduced genomic 5-methylcytosine content in human colonic neoplasia. *Cancer Res. 48:* 1159–1161, 1988.

89. Feinberg, A. P., Vogelstein, B., Droller, M. J., Baylin, S. B., and Nelkin, B. D. Mutation affecting the 12th amino acid of c-Ha-*ras* oncogene product occurs infrequently in human cancer. *Science 220:* 1175–1177, 1983.

90. Fenoglio-Preiser, C. M., and Listrom, M. B. Oncogenes: Introduction. In *Molecular Diagnostics in Pathology*, edited by C. M. Fenoglio-Preiser and C. L. Willman. Baltimore, Williams & Wilkins, 1991, pp. 81–110.

91. Fenoglio-Preiser, C. M., Longacre, T. A., and Linstrom, M. G. Oncogenes and tumor suppressor genes in solid tumors: Breast, gynecologic, and urologic tumors. In *Molecular Diagnostics in Pathology*, edited by C. M. Fenoglio-Preiser and C. L. Willman. Baltimore, Williams & Wilkins, 1991, pp. 219–259.

92. Finlay, C. A., Hinds, P. W., and Levine, A. J. The p53 proto-oncogene can act as a suppressor of transformation. *Cell 57:* 1083–1093, 1989.

93. Fitzgerald, D. J., Willingham, M. C., Cardarelli, C. O., Hamada, H., Tsuruo, T., Gottesman, M. M., and Pastan, I. A monoclonal antibody-*pseudomonas* toxin conjugate that specifically kills multidrug-resistant cells. *Proc. Natl. Acad. Sci. USA 84:* 4288–4292, 1987.

94. Fojo, A. T., Shen, D-w., Mickley, L. A., Pastan, I., and Gottesman, M. M. Intrinsic drug resistance in human kidney cancer is associated with expression of a human multidrug-resistance gene. *J. Clin. Oncol. 5:* 1922–1927, 1987.

95. Fojo, A. T., Ueda, K., Slamon, D. J., Poplack, D. G., Gottesman, M. M., and Pastan, I. Expression of a multidrug-resistance gene in human tumors and tissues. *Proc. Natl. Acad. Sci. USA 84:* 265–269, 1987.

96. Foote, S. J., Thompson, J. K., Cowman, A. F., and Kemp, D. J. Amplification of the multidrug resistance gene in some chloroquine-resistant isolates of *P. falciparum. Cell 57:* 921–930, 1989.

97. Foulds, L. The experimental study of tumor progression: A review. *Cancer Res. 14:* 327–339, 1954.

98. Foulds, L. Neoplastic Development 1. New York, Academic Press, 1969, pp. 1–439.

99. Fujita, J., Srivastava, S. K., Kraus, M. H., Rhim, J. S., Tronick, S. R., and Aaronson, S. A. Frequency of molecular alterations affecting *ras* protooncogenes in human urinary tract tumors. *Proc. Natl. Acad. Sci. USA 82:* 3849–3853, 1985.

100. Fujita, J., Yoshida, O., Yuasa, Y., Rhim, J. S., Hatanaka, M., and Aaronson, S. A. Ha-*ras* oncogenes are activated by somatic alterations in human urinary tract tumours. *Nature (Lond.) 309:* 464–466, 1984.

101. Georges, E., Bradley, G., Gariepy, J., and Ling, V. Detection of P-glycoprotein isoforms by gene-specific monoclonal antibodies. *Proc. Natl. Acad. Sci. USA 87:* 152–156, 1990.

102. Gerlach, J. H., Bell, D. R., Karakousis, C., Slocum, H. K., Kartner, N., Rustum, Y. M., Ling, V., and Baker, R. M. P-glycoprotein in human sarcoma: Evidence for multidrug resistance. *J. Clin. Oncol. 5:* 1452–1460, 1987.

103. Gerlach, J. H., Endicott, J. A., Juranka, P. F., Henderson, G., Sarangi, F., Deuchars, K. L., and Ling, V. Homology between P-glycoprotein and a bacterial haemolysin transport protein suggests a model for multidrug resistance. *Nature (Lond.) 324:* 485–489, 1986.

104. Gervasoni, J. E., Jr., Fields, S. Z., Krishna, S., Baker, M. A., Rosado, M., Thuraisamy, K., Hindenberg, A. A., and Taub, R. N. Subcellular distribution of daunorubicin in P-glycoprotein-positive and -negative drug-resistant cell lines using laser-assisted confocal microscopy. *Cancer Res. 51:* 4955–4963, 1991.

105. Gibas, Z., Prout, G. R., Pontes, J. E., Connolly, J. G., and Sandberg, A. A. A possible specific chromosome change in transitional cell carcinoma of the bladder. *Cancer Genet. Cytogenet. 19:* 229–238, 1986.

106. Goelz, S. E., Vogelstein, B., Hamilton, S. R., and Feinberg, A. P. Hypomethylation of DNA from benign and malignant human colon neoplasms. *Science 228:* 187–190, 1985.

107. Goldenberg, G. J., Vanstone, C. L., Israels, L. G., Iise, D., and Bihler, I. Evidence for a transport carrier of nitrogen mustard in nitrogen mustard-sensitive and -resistant L5178Y lymphoblasts. *Cancer Res. 30:* 2285–2291, 1970.

108. Goldie, J. H., and Coldman, A. J. The genetic origin of drug resistance in neoplasms: implications for systemic therapy. *Cancer Res. 44:* 3643–3653, 1984.

109. Goldie, J. H., and Coldman, A. J. Genetic instability in the development of drug resistance. *Sem. Oncol. 12:* 222–230, 1985.

110. Goldie, J. H., Krystal, G., Hartley, D., Gudausks, G., and Dedhar, S. A methotrexate insensitive variant of folate reductase present in two lines of methotrexate-resistant L5178Y cells. *Eur. J. Cancer 16:* 1539–1546, 1980.

111. Goldstein, L. J., Galski, H., Fojo, A., Willingham, M., Lai, S-L., Gazdar, A., Pirker, R., Green, A., Crist, W., Brodeur, G. M., Lieber, M., Cossman, J., Gottesman, M. M., and Pastan, I. Expression of a multidrug resistance gene in human cancers. *J. Natl. Cancer Inst. 81:* 116–124, 1989.

112. Gottesman, M. M. Multidrug resistance during chemical carcinogenesis: A mechanism revealed? *J. Natl. Cancer Inst. 80:* 1352–1353, 1988.

113. Gottesman, M. M., Goldstein, L. J., Bruggemann, E., Currier, S. J., Galski, H., Cardarelli, C., Thiebaut, F., Willingham, M. C., and Pastan, I. Molecular diagnosis of multidrug resistance. *Cancer Cells 7:* 75–80, 1989.

114. Gottesman, M. M., Goldstein, L. J., Fojo, A., Galski, H., and Pastan, I. Expression of the multidrug resistance gene in human cancer. In *Molecular and Cellular Biology of Multidrug Resistance in Tumor Cells,* edited by I. B. Roninson. New York, Plenum Press, 1991, pp. 291–301.

115. Greenberger, L. M., Williams, S. S., and Horwitz, S. B. Biosynthesis of heterogeneous forms of multidrug resistance-associated glycoproteins. *J. Biol. Chem. 262:* 13685–13689, 1987.

116. Grogan, T., Dalton, W., Rybski, J., Spier, C., Meltzer, P., Richter, L., Gleason, M., Pindur, J., Cline, A., Scheper, R., Tsuruo, T., and Salmon, S. Optimization of immunocytochemical P-glycoprotein assessment in multidrug-resistant plasma cell myeloma using three antibodies. *Lab. Invest. 63:* 815–824, 1990.

117. Gros, P., Croop, J., and Housman, D. Mammalian multidrug resistance gene: Complete cDNA sequence indicates strong homology to bacterial transport proteins. *Cell 47:* 371–380, 1986.

118. Gros, P., Raymond, M., and Housman, D. Cloning and characterization of mouse *mdr* genes. In *Molecular and Cellular Biology of Multidrug Resistance in Tumor Cells,* edited by I. B. Roninson. New York, Plenum Press, 1991, pp. 73–89.

119. Haber, D. A., Bevereley, S. M., Kiely, M. L., and Schimke, R. T. Properties of an altered dihydrofolate reductase encoded by amplified genes in cultured mouse fibroblasts. *J. Biol. Chem. 256:* 9501–9510, 1981.

120. Hall, T. C. Prediction of responses to therapy and mechanisms of resistance. *Sem. Oncol. 4:* 193–202, 1977.

121. Hamada, H., and Tsuruo, T. Functional role for the 170- to 180-kDa glycoprotein specific to

drug-resistant tumor cells as revealed by monoclonal antibodies. *Proc. Natl. Acad. Sci. USA* *83:* 7785–7789, 1986.

122. Hamada, H., and Tsuruo, T. Purification of the 170- to 180-kilodalton membrane glycoprotein associated with multidrug resistance. 170- to 180-kilodalton membrane glycoprotein is an ATPase. *J. Biol. Chem. 263:* 1454–1458, 1988.

123. Hansen, M. F., and Cavenee, W. K. Genetics of cancer predisposition. *Cancer Res. 47:* 5518–5527, 1987.

124. Harris, H., Miller, O. J., Klein, G., Worst, P., and Tachibana, T. Suppression of malignancy by cell fusion. *Nature (Lond.) 223:* 363–368, 1969.

125. Hart, I. R., Goode, N. T., and Wilson, R. E. Molecular aspects of the metastatic cascade. *Biochim. Biophys. Acta 989:* 65–84, 1989.

126. Herrera, L., Kakati, S., Gibas, L., Pietrzak, E., and Sandberg, A. A. Brief Clinical Report: Gardner syndrome in a man with an interstitial deletion of 5q. *Am. J. Med. Genet. 25:* 473–476, 1986.

127. Hill, B. T., Deuchars, K., Hosking, L. K., Ling, V., and Whelan, R. D. H. Overexpression of P-glycoprotein in mammalian tumor cell lines after fractionated X irradiation in vitro. *J. Natl. Cancer Inst. 82:* 607–612, 1990.

128. Hindenburg, A. A., Baker, M. A., Gleyzer, E., Stewart, V. J., Case, N., and Taub, R. N. Effect of verapamil and other agents on the distribution of anthracyclines and on reversal of drug resistance. *Cancer Res. 47:* 1421–1425, 1987.

129. Hindenburg, A. A., Gervasoni, J. E., Jr., Krishna, S., Stewart, V. J., Rosado, M., Lutzky, J., Bhalla, K., Baker, M. A., and Taub, R. N. Intracellular distribution and pharmacokinetics of daunorubicin in anthracycline-sensitive and -resistant HL-60 cells. *Cancer Res. 49:* 4607–4614, 1989.

130. Hinds, P., Finlay, C., and Levine, A. J. Mutation is required to activate the p53 gene for cooperation with the *ras* oncogene and transformation. *J. Virol. 63:* 739–746, 1989.

131. Hollstein, M., Sidransky, D., Vogelstein, B., and Harris, C. C. p53 mutations in human cancer. *Science 253:* 49–53, 1991.

132. Holmes, J., Jacobs, A., Carter, G., Janowska-Wieczorek, A., and Padua, R. A. Multidrug resistance in haemopoietic cell lines, myelodysplastic syndromes and acute myeloblastic leukaemia. *Br. J. Haemotol. 72:* 40–44, 1989.

133. Hopman, A. H. N., van Hooren, E., van de Kaa, C. A., Vooijs, P. G. P., and Ramaekers, F. C. S. Detection of numerical chromosome aberrations using *in situ* hybridization in paraffin sections of routinely processed bladder cancers. *Modern Pathol. 4:* 503–513, 1991.

134. Hsu, S. I-H., Lothstein, L., and Horwitz, S. B. Differential overexpression of three *mdr* gene family members in multidrug-resistant J774.2 mouse cells. Evidence that distinct P-glycoprotein precursors are encoded by unique *mdr* genes. *J. Biol. Chem. 264:* 12053–12062, 1989.

135. Hyde, S. C., Emsley, P., Hartshorn, M. J., Mimmack, M. M., Gileadi, U., Pearce, S. R., Gallagher, M. P., Gill, D. R., Hubbard, R. E., and Higgins, C. F. Structural model of ATP-binding proteins associated with cystic fibrosis, multidrug resistance and bacterial transport. *Nature (Lond.) 346:* 362–365, 1990.

136. Ishikawa, J., Maeda, S., Takahashi, R., Kamidono, S., and Sugiyama, T. Lack of correlation between rare ha-*ras* alleles and urothelial cancer in Japan. *Int. J. Cancer 40:* 474–478, 1987.

137. Ito, Y., Tanimoto, M., Kumazawa, T., Okumura, M., Morishima, Y., Ohno, R., and Saito, H. Increased P-glycoprotein expression and multidrug-resistant gene (mdr1) amplification are infrequently found in fresh acute leukemia cells. Sequential analysis of 15 cases of initial presentation and relapsed stage. *Cancer 63:* 1534–1538, 1989.

138. Jordan, A. M., Weingarten, J., and Murphy, W. M. Transitional cell neoplasms of the urinary bladder. Can biologic potential be predicted from histologic grading. *Cancer 60:* 2766–2774, 1987.

139. Joyce, A. D., D'Emilia, J. C., Steele, G., Jr., Libertino, J. A., Silverman, M. L., and Summerhayes, I. C. Detection of altered H-*ras* proteins in human tumors using Western blot analysis. *Lab. Invest. 61:* 212–218, 1989.

140. Juliano, R. L., and Ling, V. A surface glycoprotein modulating drug permeability in Chinese hamster ovary cell mutants. *Biochim. Biophys. Acta 455:* 152–162, 1976.

141. Juranka, P. F., Zastawny, R. L., and Ling, V. P-glycoprotein: Multidrug-resistance and a superfamily of membrane-associated transport proteins. *FASEB J. 3:* 2583–2592, 1989.

142. Kakehi, Y., Kanamaru, H., Yoshida, O., Ohkubo, H., Nakanishi, S., Gottesman, M. M., and Pastan, I. Measurement of multidrug-resistance messenger RNA in urogenital cancers: Elevated expression in renal cell carcinoma is associated with intrinsic drug resistance. *J. Urol. 139:* 862–865, 1988.

143. Kanamaru, H., Kakehi, Y., Yoshida, O., Nakanishi, S., Pastan, I., and Gottesman, M. M. MDR1 RNA levels in human renal cell carcinomas: Correlation with grade and prediction of reversal of doxorubicin resistance by quinidine in tumor explants. *J. Nat. Cancer Inst.* 81: 844–849, 1989.

144. Kane, S. E., and Gottesman, M. M. Multidrug resistance in the laboratory and clinic. *Cancer Cells 1:* 33–36, 1989.

145. Kartner, N., Evernden-Porelle, D., Bradley, G., and Ling, V. Detection of P-glycoprotein in multidrug-resistant cell lines by monoclonal antibodies. *Nature (Lond.) 316:* 820–823, 1985.

146. Kaye, K. W., and Lange, P. H. Mode of presentation of invasive bladder cancer: Reassessment of the problem. *J. Urol. 128:* 31–33, 1982.

147. Keates, R. A. B., Sarangi, F., and Ling, V. Structural and functional alterations in microtubule protein from Chinese hamster ovary cell mutants. *Proc. Natl. Acad. Sci. USA 78:* 5638–5642, 1981.

148. Keith, W. N., Stallard, S., and Brown, R. Expression of *mdr1* and *gst-π* in human breast tumours: Comparison to *in vitro* chemosensitivity. *Br. J. Cancer 61:* 712–716, 1990.

149. Kern, S. E., Fearon, E. R., Tersmette, K. W. F., Enterline, J. P., Leppert, M., Nadamura, Y., White, R., Vogelstein, B., and Hamilton, S. R. Allelic loss in colorectal carcinoma. *JAMA 261:* 3099–3103, 1989.

150. Kern, S. E., Hamilton, S. R., and Vogelstein, B. Clinical implication of colorectal tumor mutations. In *Molecular Foundations of Oncology*, edited by S. Broder. Baltimore, Williams & Wilkins, 1991, pp. 381–390.

151. Kessel, D. Resistance to Antineoplastic Drugs. Boca Raton, Fla., CRC Press, Inc., 1989, pp. 1–448.

152. Kessel, D., Beck, W. T., Kukuruga, D., and Schulz, V. Characterization of multidrug resistance by fluorescent dyes. *Cancer Res. 51:* 4665–4670, 1991.

153. Kessel, D., Hall, T. C., Roberts, D., and Wodinsky, I. Uptake as a determinant of methotrexate response in mouse leukemias. *Science 150:* 752–753, 1965.

154. Kimura, N. and Shimada, N. Membrane-associated nucleoside diphosphate kinase from rat liver. *J. Biol. Chem. 263:* 4647–4653, 1988.

155. Kinzler, K. W., Nilbert, M. C., Su, L-K., Vogelstein, B., Bryan, T. M., Levy, D. B., Smith, K. J., Preisinger, A. C., Hedge, P., McKechnie, D., Finniear, R., Marham, A., Groffen, J., Boguski, M. S., Altschul, S. F., Horii, A., Ando, H., Miyoshi, Y., Miki, Y., Nichisho, I., and Nakamura, Y. Identification of FAP locus genes from chromosome 5q21. *Science 253:* 661–665, 1991.

156. Kinzler, K. W., Nilbert, M. C., Vogelstein, B., Bryan, T. M., Levy, D. B., Smith, K. J., Preisinger, A. C., Hamilton, S. R., Hedge, P., Markham, A., Carlson, M., Joslyn, G., Groden, J., White, R., Miki, Y., Miyoshi, Y., Nishisho, I., and Nakamura, Y. Identification of a gene located at chromosome 5q21 that is mutated in colorectal cancers. *Science 251:* 1366–1370, 1991.

157. Klein, G., and Klein, E. Evolution of tumours and the impact of molecular oncology. *Nature (Lond.) 315:* 190–195, 1985.

158. Knudson, A. G., Jr. Hereditary cancer, oncogenes, and antioncogenes. *Cancer Res. 45:* 1437–1443, 1985.

159. Konen, P. L., Currier, S. J., Rutherford, A. V., Gottesman, M. M., Pastan, I., and Willingham, M. C. The multidrug transporter: rapid modulation of efflux activity monitored in single cells by the morphologic effects of vinblastine and daunomycin. *J. Histochem. Cytochem. 37:* 1141–1145, 1989.

160. Kovnat, A., Buick, R. N., Choo, B., De Harven, E., Kopelyan, I., Trent, J. M., and Tannock, I. F. Malignant properties of sublines selected from a human bladder cancer cell line that contains an activated c-Ha-*ras* oncogene. *Cancer Res. 48:* 4993–5000, 1988.

161. Kulkarni, S. S., Wang, Z., Spitzer, G., Taha, M., Hamada, H., Tsuruo, T., and Dicke, K. A.

Elimination of drug-resistant myeloma tumor cell lines by monoclonal anti-P-glycoprotein antibody and rabbit complement. *Blood 74:* 2244–2251, 1989.

162. Kuwazuru, Y., Yoshimura, A., Hanada, S., Ichikawa, M., Saito, T., Uozumi, K., Utsunomiya, A., Arima, T., and Akiyama, S. Expression of the multidrug transporter, P-glycoprotein, in chronic myelogenous leukaemia cells in blast crisis. *Br. J. Haematol. 74:* 24–29, 1990.

163. Lane, D. P., and Benchimol, S. p53: Oncogene or anti-oncogene? *Genes Dev. 4:* 1–8, 1990.

164. Lange, P. H., and Limas, C. Molecular markers in the diagnosis and prognosis of bladder cancer. *Urology 23 (4 Suppl.):* 46–54, 1984.

165. Layton, M. G., and Franks, L. M. Selective suppression of metastasis but not tumorigenicity of a mouse lung carcinoma by cell hybridization. *Int. J. Cancer 37:* 723–730, 1986.

166. Leppert, M., Burt, R., Hughes, J. P., Samowitz, W., Nakamura, Y., Woodward, S., Gardner, E., Lalouel, J-M., and White, R. Genetic analysis of an inherited predisposition to colon cancer in a family with a variable number of adenomatous polyps. *N. Engl. J. Med. 322:* 904–908, 1990.

167. Leppert, M., Dobbs, M., Scambler, P., O'Connell, P., Nakamura, Y., Stauffer, D., Woodward, S., Burt, R., Hughes, J., Gardner, E., Lathrop, M., Wasmuth, J., Lalouel, J-M., and White, R. The gene for familial polyposis coli maps to the long arm of chromosome 5. *Science 238:* 1411–1413, 1987.

168. Lerman, R. I., Hutter, V. P., and Whitmore, W. F. Papilloma of the urinary bladder. *Cancer 25:* 333–342, 1970.

169. Levinson, B. B., Ullman, B., and Martin, D. W., Jr. Pyrimidine pathway variants of cultured mouse lymphoma cells with altered levels of both orotate phosphoribosyltransferase and orotidylate decarboxylase. *J. Biol. Chem. 254:* 4396–4401, 1979.

170. Limas, C., and Lange, P. A, B, H antigen detectability in normal and neoplastic urothelium. Influence of methodologic factors. *Cancer 49:* 2476–2484, 1982.

171. Ling, V., and Thompson, L. H. Reduced permeability in CHO cells as a mechanism of resistance to colchicine. *J. Cell Physiol. 83:* 103–116, 1973.

172. Linzer, D. I. H. The marriage of oncogenes and anti-oncogenes. *Trends Genet. 4:* 245–247, 1988.

173. Liotta, L. A., Kohn, E., Steeg, P. S., and Stegler-Stevenson, W. Molecular biology of metastasis. In *Molecular Foundations of Oncology*, edited by S. Broder. Baltimore, Williams & Wilkins, 1991, pp. 57–81.

174. List, A. F., Spier, C. M., Cline, A., Doll, D. C., Garewal, H., Morgan, R., and Sandberg, A. A. Expression of the multidrug resistance gene product (P-glycoprotein) in myelodysplasia is associated with a stem cell phenotype. *Br. J. Haematol. 78:* 28–34, 1991.

175. Long, J. P., Jr., Prout, G. R., Jr., Wong, Y. K., and Lin, C-W. The effect of verapamil on a multi-drug resistant bladder carcinoma cell line and its potential as an intravesical chemotherapeutic agent. *J. Urol. 143:* 1053–1056, 1990.

176. Ludescher, C., Gattringer, C., Drach, J., Hofmann, J., and Grunicke, H. Rapid functional assay for the detection of multidrug-resistant cells using the fluorescent dye rhodamine 123. *Blood 78:* 1385–1387, 1991.

177. Ma, D. D. F., Davey, R. A., Harman, D. H., Isbister, J. P., Scurr, R. D., Mackertich, S. M., Dowden, G., and Bell, D. R. Detection of a multidrug resistant phenotype in acute non-lymphoblastic leukaemia. *Lancet 1:* 135–137, 1987.

178. Malone, P. R., Visvanathan, K. V., Ponder, B. A. J., Shearer, R. J., and Summerhayes, I. C. Oncogenes and bladder cancer. *Br. J. Urol. 57:* 664–667, 1985.

179. Marie, J.-P., Zittoun, R., and Sikic, B. I. Multidrug resistance (*mdr*1) gene expression in adult acute leukemias: Correlations with treatment outcome and in vitro drug sensitivity. *Blood 78:* 586–592, 1991.

180. Marshall, C. J. In *RNA Tumor Viruses*. New York, Cold Springs Harbor Press, 1985.

181. Marshall, C. J. Tumor suppressor genes. *Cell 64:* 313–326, 1991.

182. Martin, W. J. Polymerase chain reactions: A tool for the modern pathologist. In *Molecular Diagnostics in Pathology*, edited by C. M. Fenoglio-Preiser and C. L. Willman. Baltimore, Williams & Wilkens, 1991, pp. 21–46.

183. Marx, J. Gene identified for inherited cancer susceptibility. *Science 253:* 616, 1991.

184. Mattern, J., Efferth, T., and Volm, M. Overexpression of P-glycoprotein in human lung carcinoma xenografts after fractionated irradiation *in vivo*. *Radiat. Res. 127:* 335–338, 1991.

185. McGrath, J. P., Capon, D. J., Goeddel, D. V., and Levinson, A. D. Comparative biochemical properties of normal and activated human *ras* p21 protein. *Nature (Lond.) 310:* 644–649, 1984.

186. McGrath, J. P., and Varshavsky, A. The yeast STE6 gene encodes a homologue of the mammalian multidrug resistance P-glycoprotein. *Nature (Lond.) 340:* 400–404, 1989.

187. McNutt, N. S., Hershberg, R. A., and Weinstein, R. S. Further observations on the occurrence of nexuses in benign and malignant human cervical epithelium. *J Cell Biol 51:* 805–825, 1971.

188. McNutt, N. S., and Weinstein, R. S. Carcinoma of the cervix: Deficiency of nexus intercellular junctions. *Science 165:* 597–599, 1969.

189. Mercer, W. E., Shields, M. T., Amin, M., Sauve, G. J., Appella, E., Romano, J. W., and Ullrich, S. J. Negative growth regulation in a glioblastoma tumor cell line that conditionally expresses human wild-type p53. *Proc. Natl. Acad. Sci. USA 87:* 6166–6170, 1990.

190. Merkel, D. E., Fuqua, S. A. W., Tandon, A. K., Hill, S. M., Buzdar, A. U., and McGuire, W. L. Electrophoretic analysis of 248 clinical breast cancer specimens for P-glycoprotein overexpression or gene amplification. *J. Clin. Oncol. 7:* 1129–1136, 1989.

191. Meyers, M. B., and Biedler, J. L. Protein changes in multidrug resistant cells. In *Molecular and Cellular Biology of Multidrug Resistant Tumor Cells*, edited by I. B. Roninson. New York, Plenum Press, 1991, pp. 243–261.

192. Miller, C. W., Aslo, A., Tsay, C., Slamon, D., Ishizaki, K., Toguchida, J., Yamamuro, T., Lampkin, B., and Koeffler, H. P. Frequency and structure of *p53* rearrangements in human osteosarcoma. *Cancer Res. 50:* 7950–7954, 1990.

193. Miller, R. L., Burowski, R. M., Budd, G. T., Purvis, J., Weick, J. K., Shepard, K., Midha, K. K., and Ganapathi, R. Clinical modulation of doxorubicin resistance by the calmodulin-inhibitor, trifluoperazine: A phase I/II trial. *J. Clin. Oncol. 6:* 880–888, 1988.

194. Miller, T. P., Grogan, T. M., Dalton, W. S., Spier, C. M., Scheper, R. J., and Salmon, S. E. P-glycoprotein expression in malignant lymphoma and reversal of clinical drug resistance with chemotherapy plus high-dose verapamil. *J. Clin. Oncol. 9:* 17–24, 1991.

195. Mirski, S. E. L., Gerlach, J. H., and Cole, S. P. C. Multidrug resistance in a human small cell lung cancer cell line selected in adriamycin. *Cancer Res. 47:* 2594–2598, 1987.

196. Monpezat, J.-Ph., Delattre, O., Bernard, A., Grunwald, D., Remvikos, Y., Muleris, M., Salmon, R. J., Frelat, G., Dutrillaux, B., and Thomas, G. Loss of alleles on chromosome 18 and on the short arm of chromosome 17 in polypoid colorectal carcinomas. *Int. J. Cancer 41:* 404–408, 1988.

197. Morgan, S. A., Watson, J. V., Twentyman, P. R., and Smith, P. J. Flow cytometric analysis of Hoechst 33342 uptake as an indicator of multi-drug resistance in human lung cancer. *Br. J. Cancer 60:* 282–287, 1989.

198. Moscow, J. A., and Cowan, K. H. Multidrug resistance. *J. Nat. Cancer Inst. 80:* 14–20, 1988.

199. Muleris, M., Salmon, R. J., Zafrani, B., Girodet, J., and Dutrillaux, B. Consistent deficiencies of chromosome 18 and of the short arm of chromosome 17 in eleven cases of human large bowel cancer: A possible recessive determinism. *Ann. Genet.(Paris) 28:* 206–213, 1985.

200. Murphree, A. L., and Benedict, W. F. Retinoblastoma: Clues to human oncogenesis. *Science 223:* 1028–1033, 1984.

201. Murphy, L. D., Herzog, C. E., Rudick, J. B., Fojo, A. T., and Bates, S. E. Use of the polymerase chain reaction in the quantitation of *mdr*-1 gene expression. *Biochemistry 29:* 10351–10356, 1990.

202. Murphy, W. M. Diseases of the urinary bladder, urethra, ureters, and renal pelves. In *Urological Pathology*, edited by W. M. Murphy. Philadelphia, W. B. Saunders Company, 1989, pp. 34–146.

203. Neal, D. E., Marsh, C., Bennett, M. K., Abel, P. D., Hall, R. R., Sainsbury, J. R. C., and Harris, A. L. Epidermal-growth-factor receptors in human bladder cancer: Comparison of invasive and superficial tumours. *Lancet 1:* 366–368, 1985.

204. Ng, W. F., Sarangi, F., Zastawny, R. L., Veinot-Drebot, L., and Ling, V. Identification of members of the P-glycoprotein multigene family. *Mol. Cell Biol. 9:* 1224–1232, 1989.

205. Nickerson, J. A., and Wells, W. W. The microtubule-associated nucleoside diphosphate kinase. *J. Biol. Chem. 259:* 11297–11304, 1984.
206. Nicolson, G. L. Tumor cell instability, diversification and progression to the metastatic phenotype: From oncogene to oncofetal expression. *Cancer Res. 47:* 1473–1487, 1987.
207. Nigro, J. M., Baker, S. J., Preisinger, A. C., Jessup, J. M., Hostetter, R., Cleary, K., Bigner, S. H., Davidson, N., Baylin, S., Devilee, P., et al. Mutations in the p53 gene occur in diverse human tumour types. *Nature (Lond.) 342:* 705–708, 1989.
208. Nishisho, I., Nakamura, Y., Miyoshi, Y., Miki, Y., Ando, H., Horii, A., Koyama, K., Utsunomiya, J., Baba, S., Hedge, P., Markham, A., Krush, A. J., Petersen, G., Hamilton, S. R., Nilbert, M. C., Levy, D. B., Bryan, T. M., Preisinger, A. C., Smith, K. J., Su, L.-K., Kinzler, K. W., and Vogelstein, B. Mutations of chromosome 5q21 genes in FAP and colorectal cancer patients. *Science 253:* 665–669, 1991.
209. Noonan, K. E., and Roninson, I. B. Quantitative estimation of MDRL1 of mRNA level by polymerase chain reaction. In *Molecular and Cellular Biology of Multidrug Resistance in Tumor Cells,* edited by I. B. Roninson. New York, Plenum Press, 1991, pp. 319–333.
210. Noonan, K. E., Beck, C., Holzmayer, T. A., Chin, J. E., Wunder, J. S., Andrulis, I. L., Gazdar, A. F., Willman, C. L., Griffith, B., Von Hoff, D. D., and Roninson, I. B. Quantitative analysis of *MDR1* (multidrug resistance) gene expression in human tumors by polymerase chain reaction. *Proc. Natl. Acad. Sci. USA 87:* 7160–7164, 1990.
211. Norming, U., Nyman, C. R., and Tribukait, B. Comparative flow cytometric deoxyribonucleic acid studies on exophytic tumor and random mucosal biopsies in untreated carcinoma of the bladder. *J. Urol. 142:* 1442–1447, 1989.
212. Nowell, P. C. The clonal evolution of tumor cell populations. *Science 194:* 23–28, 1976.
213. Nowell, P. C. Mechanisms of tumor progression. *Cancer Res. 46:* 2203–2207, 1986.
214. Ouellette, M., Hettema, E., Wüst, D., Fase-Fowler, F., and Borst, P. Direct and inverted DNA repeats associated with P-glycoprotein gene amplification in drug resistant *Leishmania. EMBO J. 10:* 1009–1016, 1991.
215. Park, M., and Vande Woude, G. F. Oncogenes: Genes associated with neoplastic diseases. In *The Metabolic Basis of Inherited Disease,* edited by C. R. Scriver, A. L. Beaudet, W. S. Syl, and D. Valle. New York, McGraw-Hill, 1989, pp. 251–277.
216. Pastan, I., and Gottesman, M. Multiple-drug resistance in human cancer. *N. Engl. J. Med. 316:* 1388–1393, 1987.
217. Pastan, I., and Gottesman, M. M. Multidrug resistance. *Annu. Rev. Med. 42:* 277–286, 1991.
218. Pastan, I., and Gottesman, M. M. Drug resistance: Biological warfare at the cellular level. In *Molecular Foundations of Oncology,* edited by S. Broder. Baltimore, Williams & Wilkins, 1991, pp. 83–93.
219. Pauli, B. U., Alroy, J., and Weinstein, R. S. The ultrastructure and pathobiology of urinary bladder cancer. In *The Pathology of Bladder Cancer,* edited by G. T. Bryan and S. M. Cohen. Boca Raton, Fla., CRC Press, 1983, pp. 41–140.
220. Pearson, J. W., Fogler, W. E., Volker, K., Usui, N., Goldenberg, S. K., Gruys, E., Riggs, C. W., Komschlies, K., Wiltrout, R. H., Tsuruo, T., Pastan, I., Gottesman, M., and Longo, D. L. Reversal of drug resistance in a human colon cancer xenograft expressing MDR1 complementary DNA by in vivo administration of MDK-16 monoclonal antibody. *J. Natl. Cancer Inst. 83:* 1386–1391, 1991.
221. Peehl, D. M., and Stamey, T. A. Oncogenes: A review with relevance to cancers of the urogenital tract. *J. Urol. 135:* 897–904, 1986.
222. Per, S. R., Mattern, M. M., Mirabelli, C. K., Drake, F. H., Johnson, R. K., and Crooke, S. T. Characterization of a subline of P388 leukemia resistant to amscarine: Evidence of altered topoisomerase II function. *Mol. Pharmacol. 32:* 17–25, 1987.
223. Peto, R. Epidemiology, multistage models, and short term mutagenesis tests. Origins of human cancer. *Cold Spring Harbor Conf. Cell Proliferation 4:* 1403–1428, 1977.
224. Pitot, H. C. Chemicals and cancer: Initiation and promotion. *Hosp. Practice 18:* 101–113, 1983.
225. Pohl, J., Goldfinger, N., Radler-Pohl, A., Rotter, V., and Schirrmacher, V. p53 increases experimental metastatic capacity of murine carcinoma cells. *Mol Cell Biol 8:* 2978–2081, 1988.

226. Pozzatti, R., Muschel, R., Williams, J., Padmanabhan, R., Howard, B., Liotta, L., and Khoury, G. Primary rat embryo cells transformed by one or two oncogenes show different metastatic potentials. *Science 232:* 223–227, 1986.

227. Presant, C. A., Kennedy, P. S., Wiseman, C., Gala, K., Bouzaglou, A., Wyres, M., and Naessig, V. Verapamil reversal of clinical doxorubicin resistance in human cancer. *Am. J. Clin. Oncol. 9:* 355–357, 1986.

228. Prout, G. R., Jr., Griffin, P. P., Daly, J. J., and Heney, N. M. *Carcinoma* in situ *of the urinary bladder with and without associated vesical neoplasms. Cancer 52:* 524–532, 1983.

229. Rasman, M., Lee, M., Creasey, W., and et al., Mechanisms of resistance to 6-thiopurines in human leukemia. *Cancer Res. 34:* 1952–1956, 1974.

230. Reddy, E. P., Reynolds, R. K., Santos, E., and Barbacid, M. A point mutation is responsible for the acquisition of transforming properties by the T24 human bladder carcinoma oncogene. *Nature (Lond.) 300:* 149–152, 1982.

231. Reichard, P., Skold, O., Klein, G., Revesz, L., and Magnusson, P-H. Studies on resistance against 5-fluorouracil: I. Enzymes of the uracil pathway during development of resistance. *Cancer Res. 22:* 235–243, 1962.

232. Richards, B., Aso, Y., Bollack, C., Fossa, S., Koontz, W., Matsuda, M., Matsumoto, K., Prout, G., Van der Werf-Messing, B., and Wolf, H. Prognostic factors in infiltrating bladder cancer. *Prog Clin Biol Res 221:* 271–286, 1986.

233. Riehm, H., and Biedler, J. L. Potentiation of drug effect by Tween 80 in Chinese hamster cells resistant to actinomycin D and daunomycin. *Cancer Res. 32:* 1195–1200, 1972.

234. Riordan, J. R., and Ling, V. Genetic and biochemical characterization of multidrug resistance. *Pharmacol. Ther. 28:* 51–75, 1985.

235. Riordan, J. R., Rommens, J. M., Kerem, B-s., Alon, N., Rozmahel, R., Grzelczak, Z., Zielenski, J., Lok, S., Plavsic, N., Chou, J-L., Drumm, M. L., Iannuzzi, M. C., Collins, F. S., and Tsui, L-C. Identification of the cystic fibrosis gene: Cloning and characterization of complementary DNA. *Science 245:* 1066–1073, 1989.

236. Rogon, A. M., Hamilton, T. C., and Young, R. G. Reversal of adriamycin resistance by verapamil in human ovarian cancer. *Science 224:* 994–996, 1984.

237. Ronchi, E., Sanfillippo, O., Di Fonzo, G., Bani, M. R., Torre, G. D., Catania, S., and Silvestrini, R. Detection of the 170 kDa P-glycoprotein in neoplastic and normal tissues. *Tumori 75:* 542–546, 1989.

238. Roninson, I. B. Structure and evolution of P-glycoproteins. In *Molecular and Cellular Biology of Multidrug Resistance in Tumor Cells*, edited by I. B. Roninson. New York, Plenum Press, 1991, pp. 189–211.

239. Roninson, I. B. P-glycoprotein-mediated drug resistance: Puzzles and perspectives. In *Molecular and Cellular Biology of Multidrug Resistance in Tumor Cells*, edited by I. B. Ronison. New York, Plenum Press, 1991, pp. 395–402.

240. Roninson, I. B. *Molecular and Cellular Biology of Multidrug Resistance in Tumor Cells.* New York, Plenum Press, 1991.

241. Roninson, I. B., Chin, J. E., Choi, K., Gros, P., Housman, D. E., Fojo, A., Shen, D-w., Gottesman, M. M., and Pastan, I. Isolation of human *mdr* DNA sequences amplified in multidrug-resistant KB carcinoma cells. *Proc. Natl. Acad. Sci. USA 83:* 4538–4542, 1986.

242. Roninson, I. B., Pastan, I., and Gottesman, M. M. Isolation and characterization of the human *MDR* (P-glycoprotein) genes. In *Molecular and Cellular Biology of Multidrug Resistance in Tumor Cells*, edited by I. B. Roninson. New York, Plenum Press, 1991, pp. 91–106.

243. Roninson, I. B., Patel, M. G., Lee, I., Noonan, K. E., Chen, C-J., Choi, K., Chin, J. E., Kaplan, R., and Tsuruo, T. Molecular mechanisms and diagnostics of multidrug resistance in human tumor cells. *Cancer Cells 7:* 81–86, 1989.

244. Rothenberg, M. L., Mickley, L. A., Cole, D. E., Balis, F. M., Tsuruo, T., Poplack, D. G., and Fojo, A. T. Expression of the *mdr*-1/P-170 gene in patients with acute lymphoblastic leukemia. *Blood 74:* 1388–1395, 1989.

245. Rowley, J. D. Chromosome pattern in animal and human tumors. In *Chromosomes and Cancer: From Molecules to Man*, edited by J. D. Rowley and J. E. Ultmann. New York, Academic Press, 1983, pp. 56–60.

246. Rowley, J. D. Cytogenetics: Past, present and future. In *Molecular Foundations of Oncology*, edited by S. Broder. Baltimore, Williams & Wilkins, 1991, pp. 3–26.
247. Ruoslahti, E. Fibronectin and its receptors. *Annu. Rev. Biochem. 57:* 375–413, 1988.
248. Russell, P. J., Brown, J. L., Grimmond, S. M., and Raghavan, D. Molecular biology of urological tumours. *Br. J. Urol. 65:* 121–130, 1990.
249. Salmon, S. E., Dalton, W. S., Grogan, T. M., Plezia, P., Lehnert, M., Roe, D. J., and Miller, T. P. Multidrug-resistant myeloma: Laboratory and clinical effects of verapamil as a chemosensitizer. *Blood 78:* 44–50, 1991.
250. Salmon, S. E., Grogan, T. M., Miller, T., Scheper, W. S., and Dalton, W. S. Prediction of doxorubicin resistance in vitro in myeloma, lymphoma, and breast cancer by P-glycoprotein staining. *J. Natl. Cancer Inst. 81:* 696–701, 1989.
251. Samowitz, W., Paull, G., and Hamilton, S. R. Reported binding of monoclonal antibody RAP-5 to formalin-fixed tissue sections is not indicative of ras p21 expression. *Human Pathol 19:* 127–132, 1988.
252. Sandberg, A. A. Chromosome changes in bladder cancer: Clinical and other correlations. *Cancer Genet. Cytogenet. 19:* 163–175, 1986.
253. Sandberg, A. A. Chromosomes in solid tumors: Benign and malignant. In *The Chromosomes in Human Cancer and Leukemia*. New York, Elsevier, 1990, pp. 789–966.
254. Santos, E., Reddy, E. P., Pulciani, S., Feldmann, R. J., and Barbacid, M. Spontaneous activation of a human proto-oncogenes. *Proc. Natl. Acad. Sci. USA 80:* 4679–4683, 1983.
255. Sato, H., Gottesman, M. M., Goldstein, L. J., Pastan, I., Block, A. M., Sandberg, A. A., and Preisler, H. D. Expression of the multidrug resistance gene in myeloid leukemias. *Leuk. Res. 14:* 11–22, 1990.
256. Scheper, R. J., Bulte, J. W. M., Brakkee, J. G. P., Quak, J. J., van der Schoot, E., Balm, A. J. M., Meijer, C. J. L. M., Broxertman, H. J., Kuiper, C. M., Lankelma, J., and Pinedo, H. M. Monoclonal antibody JSB-1 detects a highly conserved epitope on the P-glycoprotein associated with multi-drug-resistance. *Int. J. Cancer 42:* 389–394, 1988.
257. Schimke, R. T., Kaufman, R. J., Alt, F. W., and Kellems, R. F. Gene amplification and drug resistance in cultured murine cells. *Science 202:* 1051–1055, 1978.
258. Schinkel, A. H., Roelofs, M. E. M., and Borst, P. Characterization of the human *MDR*3 P-glycoprotein and its recognition by P-glycoprotein-specific monoclonal antibodies. *Cancer Res. 51:* 2628–2635, 1991.
259. Schlaifer, D., Laurent, G., Chittal, S., Tsuruo, T., Soues, S., Muller, C., Charcosset, J. Y., Alard, C., Brousset, P., Mazerrolles, C., and Delsol, G. Immunohistochemical detection of multidrug resistance associated P-glycoprotein in tumour and stromal cells of human cancers. *Br. J. Cancer 62:* 177–182, 1990.
260. Schmid, M., Haaf, T., and Grunert, D. 5-Azacytidine-induced undercondensations in human chromosomes. *Hum. Genet. 67:* 257–263, 1984.
261. Schneider, J., Bak, M., Efferth, T., Kaufmann, M., Mattern, J., and Volm, M. P-glycoprotein expression in treated and untreated human breast cancer. *Br. J. Cancer 60:* 815–818, 1989.
262. Sehested, M., Skovsgaard, T., van Deurs, B., and Winter-Nielsen, H. Increased plasma membrane traffic in daunorubicin resistant P388 leukaemic cells. Effect of daunorubicin and verapamil. *Br. J. Cancer 56:* 747–751, 1987.
263. Sehested, M., Skovsgaard, T., van Deurs, B., and Winther-Nielson, H. Increase in nonspecific absorptive endocytosis in anthracycline- and vinca-alkaloid-resistant Ehrlich ascites tumor cell lines. *J. Natl. Cancer Inst. 78:* 171–179, 1987.
264. Shen, D-W., Cardarelli, C., Hwang, J., Cornwell, M., Richert, N., Ishii, S., Pastan, I., and Gottesman, M. M. Multiple drug-resistant human KB carcinoma cells independently selected for high-level resistance to colchicine, adriamycin, or vinblastine show changes in expression of specific proteins. *J. Biol. Chem. 261:* 7762–7770, 1986.
265. Shen, D.-W., Fojo, A., Chin, J. E., Roninson, I. B., Richert, N., Pastan, I., and Gottesman, M. M. Human multidrug-resistant cell lines: Increased *mdr*1 expression can precede gene amplification. *Science 232:* 643–645, 1986.
266. Shen, D.-W., Pastan, I., and Gottesman, M. M. In situ hybridization analysis of acquisition and loss of the human multidrug-resistance gene. *Cancer Res. 48:* 4334–4339, 1988.

267. Shih, C., Padhy, L. C., Murray, M., and Weinberg, R. A. Transforming genes of carcinomas and neuroblastomas introduced into mouse fibroblasts. *Nature (Lond.) 290:* 261–264, 1981.
268. Sistonen, L., and Alitalo, K. Activation of *c-ras* oncogenes by mutations and amplification. *Ann. Clin. Res. 18:* 297–303, 1986.
269. Skalka, A. M., Reddy, E. P., and Curran, T. *The Oncogene Handbook.* Amsterdam, Elsevier, 1988.
270. Smeets, W., Pauwels, R., Laarakkers, L., Debruyne, F., and Geraedts, J. Chromosomal analysis of bladder cancer. III. Nonrandom alterations. *Cancer Genet. Cytogenet. 29:* 29–41, 1987.
271. Smyth, J. F., Robins, A. B., and Leese, C. L. The metabolism of cytosine arabinoside as a predictive test for clinical response to the drug in acute myeloid leukemia. *Eur. J. Cancer 12:* 567–573, 1976.
272. Stanbridge, E. J. Suppression of malignancy in human cells. *Nature (Lond.) 260:* 17–20, 1976.
273. Stanbridge, E. J. Identifying tumor suppressor genes in human colorectal cancer. *Science 247:* 12–13, 1990.
274. Steeg, P. S., Bevilacqua, G., Kopper, L., Thorgeirsson, U. P., Talmadge, J. E., Liotta, L. A., and Sobel, M. E. Evidence for a novel gene associated with low tumor metastatic potential. *J. Natl. Cancer Inst. 80:* 200–204, 1988.
275. Stock, L. M., Brosman, S. A., Fahey, J. L., and Liu, B. C-S. Ras related oncogene protein as a tumor marker in transitional cell carcinoma of the bladder. *J. Urol. 137:* 789–791, 1987.
276. Sugawara, I., Nakahama, M., and Hamada, H. Tissue distribution of P-glycoprotein encoded by a multidrug-resistant gene as revealed by a monoclonal antibody, MRK16. *Cancer Res. 48:* 1926–1929, 1988.
277. Tabin, C. J., Bradley, S. M., Bargmann, C. I., Weinberg, R. A., Papageorge, A. G., Scolnick, E. M., Dhar, R., Lowy, D. R., and Chand, E. H. Mechanism of activation of a human oncogene. *Nature (Lond.) 300:* 143–149, 1982.
278. Takasahi, T., Nau, M., Chiba, I., Birrer, M. J., Rosenberg, R. K., Vinocour, M., Levitt, M., Pass, H., Gazdar, A. F., and Minna, J. D. p53: A frequent target for genetic abnormalities in lung cancer. *Science 246:* 491–494, 1989.
279. Taparowsky, E., Suard, Y., Fasano, O., Shimizu, K., Goldfarb, M., and Wigler, M. Activation of the T24 bladder carcinoma transforming gene is linked to a single amino acid change. *Nature (Lond.) 300:* 762–765, 1982.
280. Taylor, C. W., Dalton, W. S., Parrish, P. P., Gleason, M. C., Bellamy, W. T., Thompson, F. H., Roe, D. J., and Trent, J. M. Different mechanisms of decreased drug accumulation in doxorubicin and mitoxantrone resistant variants of the MCF-7 human breast cancer cell line. *Br. J. Cancer 63:* 923–929, 1991.
281. Thiebaut, F., Tsuruo, T., Hamada, H., Gottesman, M. M., Pastan, I., and Willingham, M. C. Immunohistochemical localization in normal tissues of different epitopes in a multidrug transport protein P170: Evidence for localization in brain capillaries and crossreactivity of one antibody with a muscle protein. *J. Histochem. Cytochem. 37:* 159–164, 1989.
282. Thorgeirsson, U. P., Turpeenniemi-Hujanen, T., Williams, J. E., Westin, E. H., Heilman, C. A., Talmadge, J. E., and Liotta, L. A. NIH/3T3 cells transfected with human tumor DNA containing activated *ras* oncogenes express the metastatic phenotype in nude mice. *Mol Cell Biol 5:* 259–262, 1985.
283. Tong, L., deVos, A. M., Milburn, M. V., Jancarik, J., Noguchi, S., Nishimura, S., Miura, K., Ohtsuka, E., and Kim, S. Structural differences between a ras oncogene protein and the normal protein. *Nature (Lond.) 337:* 90–93, 1989.
284. Traut, T. W. Do exons code for structural or functional units in proteins. *Proc. Natl. Acad. Sci. USA 85:* 2944–2948, 1988.
285. Tribukait, B. Flow cytometry in surgical pathology and cytology of tumors of the genito-urinary tract. In *Advances In Clinical Cytology Vol. II*, edited by L. G. Koss and D. V. Coleman. New York, Masson, 1984, pp. 163–189.
286. Tribukait, B. Flow cytometry in assessing the clinical aggressiveness of genito-urinary neoplasms. *World J. Urol. 5:* 108–122, 1987.
287. Trowsdale, J., Hanson, I., Mockridge, I., Beck, S., Townsend, A., and Kelly, A. Sequences

encoded in the class II region of the MHC related to the 'ABC' superfamily of transporters. *Nature (Lond.) 348:* 741–744, 1990.

288. Tsai, Y., Nichols, P. W., Hiti, A. L., Williams, Z., Skinner, D. G., and Jones, P. A. Allelic losses of chromosomes 9, 11, and 17 in human bladder cancer. *Cancer Res. 50:* 44–47, 1990.

289. Tsuruo, T. Mechanisms of multidrug resistance and implications for therapy. *Jpn J Cancer Res 79:* 285–296, 1988.

290. Tsuruo, T. Reversal of multidrug resistance by calcium channel blockers and other agents. In *Molecular and Cellular Biology of Multidrug Resistance in Tumor Cells*, edited by I. B. Roninson. New York, Plenum Press, 1991, pp. 349–372.

291. Tsuruo, T., Hamada, H., Sato, S., and Heike, Y. Inhibition of multidrug resistant human tumor growth in athymic nude mice by anti-P-glycoprotein moncloncal antibodies. *Jpn J Cancer Res 80:* 627–631, 1989.

292. Tsuruo, T., Iida, H., Tsukagoshi, S., and Sakurai, Y. Overcoming of vincristine resistance in P388 leukemia in vivo and in vitro through enhanced cytotoxicity of vincristine and vinblastine by verapamil. *Cancer Res. 41:* 1967–1972, 1981.

293. Ueda, K., Cornwell, M. M., Gottesman, M. M., Pastan, I., Roninson, I. B., Ling, V., and Riordan, J. R. The mdr1 gene, responsible for multidrug-resistance, codes for P-glycoprotein. *Biochem. Biophy. Res. Comm. 141:* 956–962, 1986.

294. Valenzuela, D. M., and Croffen, J. Four human carcinoma cell lines with novel mutations in position 12 of c-K-ras oncogenes. *Nucleic Acids Res. 14:* 843–852, 1986.

295. Van der Bliek, A., Baas, F., and Ten Houte de Lange, T. The human *mdr3* gene encodes a novel P-glycoprotein homologue and gives rise to alternatively spliced mRNAs in liver. *Eur. Mol Biol 6:* 3325–3331, 1987.

296. Van der Bliek, A. M., and Borst, P. Multidrug resistance. *Adv. Cancer Res. 52:* 165–201, 1989.

297. Van der Bliek, A. M., Kooiman, P. M., Schneider, C., and Borst, P. Sequence of *mdr3* cDNA encoding a human P-glycoprotein. *Genetics 71:* 401–411, 1988.

298. Van der Valk, F., and Van Kalken. C. K. Distribution of multi-drug resistance-associated P-glycoprotein in normal and neoplastic human tissues. *Ann Oncol 1:* 56–64, 1990.

299. Vanni, R. Nonrandom chromosomal changes in transitional cell carcinoma of the bladder. (Letter to the Editor.) *Cancer Res. 46:* 4873, 1986.

300. Vanni, R., Scarpa, R. M., Nieddu, M., and Usai, E. Identification of marker chromosomes in bladder tumor. *Urol Int 41:* 403–406, 1986.

301. Verrelle, P., Meissonnier, F., Fonck, Y., Feillel, V., Dionet, C., Kwiatkowski, F., Plagne, R., and Chassagne, J. Clinical relevance of immunohistochemical detection of multidrug resistance P-glycoprotein in breast carcinoma. *J. Natl. Cancer Inst. 83:* 111–116, 1991.

302. Viola, M. V., Fromowitz, F., Oravez, S., Deb, S., and Schlom, J. *ras* oncogene p21 expression is increased in premalignant lesions and high grade bladder carcinoma. *J. Exp. Med. 161:* 1213–1218, 1985.

303. Vogelstein, B. A deadly inheritance. *Nature (Lond.) 348:* 681–682, 1990.

304. Vogelstein, B., Fearon, E. R., Hamilton, S. R., Kern, S. E., Preisinger, A. C., Leppert, M., Nakamura, Y., White, R., Smits, A. M. M., and Bos, J. L. Genetic alterations during colorectal-tumor development. *N. Engl. J. Med. 319:* 525–532, 1988.

305. Vogelstein, B., Fearon, E. R., Kern, S. E., Hamilton, S. R., Preisinger, A. C., Nakamura, Y., and White, R. Allelotype of colorectal carcinomas. *Science 244:* 207–211, 1989.

306. Ward, J. M., Hagiwara, A., Tsuda, H., Tatematsu, M., and Ito, N. H-*ras* p21 and peanut lectin immunoreactivity of hyperplastic, preneoplastic and neoplastic urinary bladder lesions in rats. *Jpn J Cancer Res 79:* 152–155, 1988.

307. Ward, J. M., Pardue, R. L., Junker, J. L., Takahashi, K., Shih, T. Y., and Weislow, O. S. Immunocytochemical localization of rasHa p21 in normal and neoplastic cells in fixed tissue sections from harvey sarcoma virus-infected mice. *Carcinogen 7:* 645–665, 1986.

308. Warr, J. R., and Atkinson, G. F. Genetic aspects of resistance to anticancer drugs. *Physiol. Rev. 68:* 1–26, 1988.

309. Weil, M. M., Kavanagh, J. J., and Deisseroth, A. Molecular genetics of genitourinary cancers. In *Molecular Foundations of Oncology*, edited by S. Broder. Baltimore, Williams & Wilkins, 1991, pp. 367–380.

310. Weinberg, R. A. The action of oncogenes in the cytoplasm and nucleus. *Science 230:* 770–776, 1985.
311. Weinberg, R. A. Oncogenes, antioncogenes, and the molecular bases of multistep carcinogenesis. *Cancer Res. 49:* 3713–3721, 1989.
312. Weinberg, R. A. The retinoblastoma gene and cell growth control. *TIBS 15:* 199–202, 1990.
313. Weinberg, R. A. Molecular biology of carcinogenesis: A multistep process. In *Molecular Foundations of Oncology*, edited by S. Broder. Baltimore, Williams & Wilkins, 1991, pp. 27–39.
314. Weinstein, R. S., and Coon, J. S. Laboratory assessment of P-glycoprotein in cancer chemosensitivity testing. *Hum. Pathol. 21:* 785–786, 1990.
315. Weinstein, R. S., Coon, J. S., Dominguez, J. M., Jakate, S. M., Lebovitz, M. D., Chang, M. A., and Kluskens, L. F. Correlation between ABO blood type and Golgi P-glycoprotein expression in epithelia. *Lancet 336:* 54–55, 1990.
316. Weinstein, R. S., Grogan, T. M., Kuszak, J. R., Jakate, S. M., Kluskens, L. F., and Coon, J. S. Multidrug resistance gene product (P-glycoprotein) in normal tissue and tumors. *Adv. Pathol. 4:* 207–234, 1991.
317. Weinstein, R. S., Jakate, S. M., Dominguez, J. M., Lebovitz, M. D., Koukoulis, G. K., Kuszak, J. R., Klusens, L. F., Grogan, T. M., Saclarides, T. J., Roninson, I. B., and Coon, J. S. Relationship of the expression of the multidrug resistance gene product (P-glycoprotein) in human colon carcinoma to local tumor aggressiveness and lymph node metastasis. *Cancer Res. 51:* 2720–2726, 1991.
318. Weinstein, R. S., Kuszak, J. R., Jakate, S. M., Lebovitz, M. D., Kluskens, L. F., and Coon, J. S. ABO blood type predicts the cytolocalization of anti-P-glycoprotein monoclonal antibody reactivity in human colon and ureter. *Hum. Pathol. 21:* 949–958, 1990.
319. Weinstein, R. S., Kuszak, J. R., Kluskens, L. F., and Coon, J. S. P-glycoproteins in pathology: The multidrug resistance gene family in humans. *Hum. Pathol. 21:* 34–48, 1990.
320. Weinstein, R. S., Miller, A. W. III, and Pauli, B. U. Carcinoma in situ: Pathobiology of a paradox. *Urol Clin N Am 7:* 523–531, 1980.
321. Weinstein, R. S., and Pauli, B. U. Cell junctions and the biological behavior of cancer. In *Junctional Complexes in Epithelial Cells*, edited by M. Stoker, G. Bock, and S. Clark. New York, John Wiley & Sons, 1987, pp. 240–260.
322. Weiss, L. Metastatic inefficiency. *Adv. Cancer Res. 54:* 159–211, 1990.
323. Wick, M. R. Immunohistologic detection of ras oncogene products. *Arch Pathol Lab Med 113:* 13–15, 1989.
324. Willingham, M. C., Cornwell, M. M., Cardarelli, C. O., Gottesman, M. M., and Pastan, I. Single cell analysis of daunomycin uptake and efflux in multidrug-resistant and -sensitive KB cells: Effects of verapamil and other drugs. *Cancer Res. 46:* 5941–5946, 1986.
325. Willingham, M. C., Richert, N. D., Cornwell, M. M., Tsuruo, T., Hamada, H., Gottesman, M. M., and Pastan, I. Immunocytochemical localization of P170 at the plasma membrane of multidrug-resistant human cells. *J. Histochem. Cytochem. 35:* 1451–1456, 1987.
326. Yuasa, Y., Srivastava, S. K., Dunn, C. Y., Rhim, J. S., Reddy, E. P., and Aaronson, S. A. Acquisition of transforming properties by alternative point mutations within c-bas/has human proto-oncogene. *Nature (Lond.) 303:* 775–779, 1983.
327. Yusa, K., and Tsuruo, T. Reversal mechanism of multidrug resistance by verapamil: Direct binding of verapamil to P-glycoprotein on specific sites and transport of verapamil outward across the plasma membrane of K562/ADM cells. *Cancer Res. 49:* 5002–5006, 1989.

Chapter 3

Significant Nonmalignant Proliferative and Neoplastic Lesions of the Urinary Bladder

GEORGE M. FARROW

INTRODUCTION

The urinary bladder, composed as it is of a homogeneous epithelial lining of urothelial or transitional cells and a wall of smooth muscle, is an organ that might be expected to exhibit a rather limited number of proliferative and neoplastic possibilities. It is true that the vast majority of the tumors are of transitional cell type, and yet the potential for diverse differentiation of both the epithelial and mesenchymal components of the urinary bladder offers an interesting minority of proliferative and neoplastic lesions, many of which have escaped a solid concept of histogenesis. Among these, many represent metaplastic phenomenon, but others appear to be clearly neoplastic.

SQUAMOUS METAPLASIA

Squamous epithelium histologically similar to that of the vaginal mucosa has been found in the trigone and bladder neck region in up to 85% of women without urological disorders.[2,3,6,11-13] Although this is reported more commonly in the reproductive age group, some have found a similar incidence in pre- and post-menopausal women at autopsy examination of the urinary bladder.[6] This finding is much less common in men.[3]) Patches of squamous epithelium have been observed cytoscopically and the term "pseudomembranous trigonitis" has been applied[2] with the implication of a pathological process. Cytoscopically, squamous metaplasia appears as a white patch on the mucosal surface, usually but not always, well demarcated, and often irregular in shape.[13] The lesions may be finely granular in appearance and extend upward toward the ureteral orifices. There may be a rim of increased vascularity. In bladders obtained at autopsy, the application of Lugol's solution facilitates identification of the metaplastic zones.[6]

Although it has been widely stated that squamous epithelium in this location represents a persistence of squamous epithelium related to a common embryological development of this portion of the bladder and vagina, at least three possibilities for the origin of this epithelium have been offered.[12] It may result from metaplasia from preexisting transitional epithelium or develop from primitive cells capable of forming either transitional epithelium or squamous epithelium. The potentialities for differentiation in bladder epithelium are known to be considerable.[8] It may represent embryologically displaced squamous epithelium or it could be that squamous epithelium from the urethra extends into the bladder and displaces the transitional epithelium.

The squamous epithelium may present a single contiguous sheet, or there may be a mosaic of microscopic islands separated by transitional epithelium of normal appearance.[6] Microscopically, the urothelium is replaced by well-differentiated mature squamous epithelium (Fig. 3.1). Hyperkeratinization of the surface is not a feature of pure squamous metaplasia. Depending on the age and hormonal status of the subject, the stage in the menstrual cycle, and the pre- or postmenopausal status, the squamous epithelium may be more or less glycogenated, which is represented by cytoplasmic clearing in H & E sections, more advanced in the superficial layers of the epithelium. This glycogenation must be distinguished from the koilocytotic change of condylomatous lesions, which differs in that the cytologic clearing is perinuclear and characteristically well demarcated in the cytoplasm (Fig. 3.2). The nuclear changes of condyloma are not a feature of simple metaplasia. Cyclical hormonal-induced changes in squamous cellular glycogenation and maturation are similar to those of vaginal mucosa[12] and can be evaluated using urine cytology preparations.[4,7,9]

The term "pseudomembranous trigonitis" suggests a pathological process. Associated chronic inflammation has been found in about a third of the cases.[6] It is not clear in these cells whether the inflammation is related to the evolution of the metaplasia or whether the inflammation is the result of a decreased efficiency of the squamous epithelium in presenting a barrier to irritative substances in the urine.

Atypical squamous metaplasia, often termed "leukoplakia," is an important pathological condition that must be distinguished from simple squamous metaplasia. In addition to replacement of the normal urothelium by squamous epithelium, leukoplakia is characterized by abnormal maturation with the formation of a prominent surface layer of hyperkeratinization. There is epithelial thickening, some degree of acanthosis, and nuclear and cytoplasmic abnormalities classified as varying degrees of dysplasia (Fig. 3.3).

Leukoplakia is as common in men as in women and distribution of the lesions is not limited to the trigone or bladder neck regions. The abnormality is often widespread, involving a large portion of the bladder mucosal surface. The patients are typically older, give a long history of lower urinary tract symptoms usually related to decreased ability to empty the urinary bladder associated with chronic bladder infections, and often bladder calculi. Neurogenic bladder is a risk factor for leukoplakia. Cystoscopically and grossly, leukoplakia is grayish-white and the lesions are described as parchment- or coral-like.[10]

Leukoplakia is now accepted as an important precursor of squamous cell carcinoma of the urinary collecting system, particularly the bladder.[1,5,10] A simultaneous association with carcinoma, usually squamous but occasionally transitional type, is reported in 10–21% of cases, and another 21% have been documented as progressing from leukoplakia to carcinoma.[1]

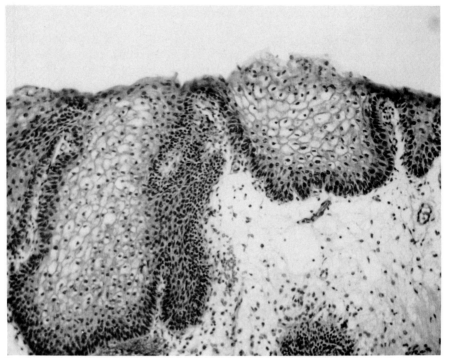

FIG. 3.1. Squamous metaplasia of the type found normally in the trigone of women. Cytoplasmic clearing is due to glycogenation under estrogen stimulation. H & E, × 250.

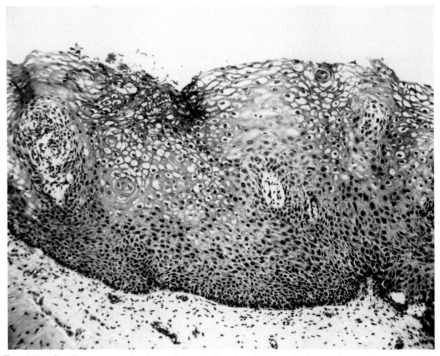

FIG. 3.2. Condyloma acuminatum. There is basal cell hyperplasia, nuclear enlargement, hyperchromasia, and binucleation. Koilocytotic cytoplasmic clearing is prominent in the more superficial cells. H & E, × 250.

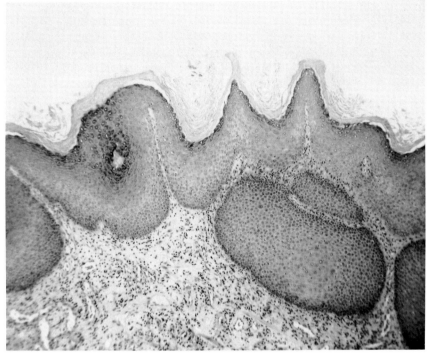

FIG. 3.3.   Leukoplakia. There is hyperkeratosis, papillomatosis, acanthosis, and inflammation in the lamina propria. H & E, × 125.

INTESTINAL/COLONIC METAPLASIA

This terminology describes the appearance of colonic type or mucin-producing goblet cells in the bladder epithelium. When these mucinous or goblet cells are admixed with proliferations of Brunn's nests in the lamina propria, the condition is more properly described as cystitis glandularis; however, a confusion of terminology exists. Colonic metaplasia is usually a focal phenomenon, but diffuse forms may be associated with a diversion of urine away from the urothelial lining of the bladder as seen in exstrophy of the bladder[17,21] and other diverting conditions.[23] Colonic metaplasia may also be associated with other underlying pathological states such as a chronic cystitis, bladder calculi, parasitic infections, and fistulous connections.[15,22] In some instances, the condition exists without any known precipitating factors and may be extensive or diffuse.[14,32]

The epithelium of the urinary tract is derived from two germ layers. The epithelium of the renal pelvis, ureter, and possibly the trigone of the bladder are of mesodermal derivation, but the remainder of the bladder is of endodermal origin.[22] The urothelium, under normal conditions, contains cells with cytoplasmic mucin,[16,19] which may increase in inflammatory states. Although the surface urothelium is normally devoid of glandular tissue structures, mucus-producing subepithelial glands in the region of the trigone have been known for many years as the so-called glands of Albarran.

persist.[31] In spite of the name, any significant degree of inflammation is unusual (Fig. 3.5).

Cystitis glandularis, as already noted, describes the appearance of glandular structures in the lamina propria, often admixed with cystitis cystica (Fig. 3.5). These glandular structures are lined by mucus-producing goblet cells.[34] Cystitis glandularis should be distinguished from intestinal metaplasia, a surface phenomenon, by the subepithelial localization beneath an intact transitional epithelium, although overlapping features occur. If one limits the term cystitis glandularis to those structures in a subepithelial localization, then the relationship to adenocarcinoma is not clear cut, but it is not likely that cystitis glandularis is a significant risk factor for adenocarcinoma, since most cancer cases actually arise in intestinal metaplasia.[30] Cystitis glandularis may occasionally reach a degree of focal prominence in the bladder so as to simulate a neoplasm.[25,26,28,29] Conversely, true carcinomas with extension into lamina propria may exhibit a deceptively benign appearance and be mistaken for Brunn's nests, cystitis cystica, or cystitis glandularis.[33] The process of cystitis glandularis and intestinal metaplasia is apparently reversible in some cases with restitution of normal transitional epithelium after ablation of the glandular epithelium by such modalities as laser coagulation.[32]

NEPHROGENIC METAPLASIA/ADENOMA

An unusual urinary bladder epithelial proliferative lesion forming structures resembling renal tubules was first described by Davis in 1949.[37] Almost simultaneously, in 1950, Friedman and Kuhlenbeck[41] reported eight similar cases that they analyzed in greater detail. They characterized the lesions as "adenomatoid" tumors of the urinary bladder and coined the term "nephrogenic adenoma." These lesions all had the common feature of the formation in the lamina propria of the lining of the urinary bladder epithelial tubules lined by a single layer of cuboidal or columnar epithelium. They noted that the lesions also contain papillary structures and the biological behavior was that of a benign process. A recent review article[47] found 272 case reports detailed in 52 publications in the English literature. About 80% of the reported cases have been located in the urinary bladder,[35,39,43,48] but other sites include the urethra, both male[44,46] and female,[36] and rarely the ureter and renal pelvis.[45] Although the term adenoma was used initially to describe the condition, the process is generally regarded as metaplastic rather than neoplastic.[40,42,45,46,51]

The condition has been reported about twice as frequently in men than women in a wide range of ages, including children. In the majority of cases, the development of the lesion has followed an episode of trauma of some type to the urinary bladder, including surgical trauma, blunt trauma, calculi, and usually attended by long-term catheter drainage. Overdistension of the urinary bladder in the treatment of chronic interstitial cystitis has been associated with the development of the lesion.[49]

Symptoms are nonspecific and include hematuria (40%), dysuria (35%), frequency and urgency (35%), and suprapubic (15%) and flank pain (5%). The cystoscopic appearance is that of a papillary and polypoid tumor, which can

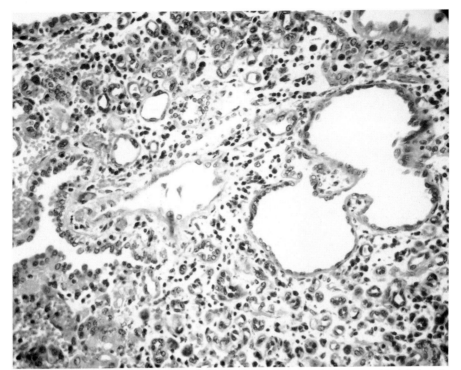

FIG. 3.6. Nephrogenic adenoma/metaplasia. In the lamina propria, innumerable tubular structures of variable diameter are lined by a single layer of low cuboidal epithelial cells. H & E, × 400.

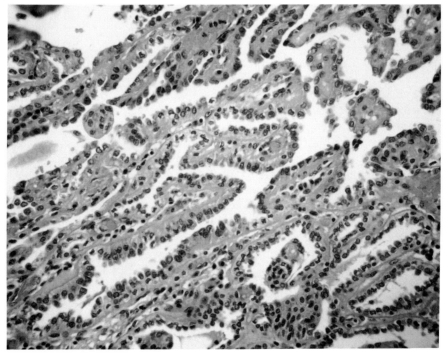

FIG. 3.7. Nephrogenic adenoma/metaplasia. On the lining surface of the bladder, exophytic papillary structures are covered by a single layer of low cuboidal epithelial cells. H & E, × 400.

resemble transitional cell carcinoma. The lesions may be solitary and discrete or multifocal, typically on the trigone and bladder base, but lesions may be extensive and involve large areas of the bladder surface.

Histopathologically, the lesion features a combination of papillary fronds and tubules. The tubules are situated in the lamina propria by the bladder mucosa and are never observed deeper in the muscular layers of the bladder. The tubules are extremely variable in size, ranging from a few dozen micrometers in diameter to large cystically dilated structures up to a millimeter. The lining cells form a single layer and are typically cuboidal with scant cytoplasm. There is characteristically a hobnail appearance to the cuboidal cells lining the tubules (Fig. 3.6). Goblet cells and mucin are not found within these tubules, but zones of urothelial colonic metaplasia are commonly associated with nephrogenic metaplasia. Similar hobnail cells line the delicate frond-like papillary structures in single layer extending outward from the mucosal surface (Fig. 3.7). Mitoses are absent or rare.

The initial observation by Friedman and Kuhlenbeck of the resemblance of the tubular structures to renal tubules led to a theory of histogenesis related to adenomatous proliferation of vestigial mesonephric tubular remnants in the urinary bladder. Beyond the rather superficial resemblance of these structures to renal tubules, examination of surface lectins of normal urothelium, embryonic kidney, cystitis cystica and glandularis, and squamous metaplasia has demonstrated similarities between the structures of nephrogenic adenoma and embryonic renal tubules.[38] In spite of this, the condition is now more commonly regarded as a form of urothelial metaplasia. The occasional finding of replacement of the surface urothelium adjacent to gross lesions by the single-layered hobnail epithelium may support this concept (Fig. 3.8).

Treatment has been most often surgical resection and fulguration. In many instances the lesions regressed after time and after removal of the precipitating stimuli. In rare cases the lesions may persist and progress and require extensive surgical ablation. Twenty-seven cases of nephrogenic adenoma have been associated with bladder carcinoma, usually transitional type.[47]

In 1968 the apparent first case report of mesonephric adenocarcinoma of the bladder appeared.[39] This neoplasm metastasized widely. The histopathological features of this neoplasm exhibited a resemblance to nephrogenic adenoma and suggested a malignant counterpart to this lesion. A recent review article of clear cell adenocarcinoma of the urinary bladder,[52] a term now preferred to mesonephric adenocarcinoma, found 19 reported cases in the literature. These tumors must be distinguished from nephrogenic adenoma, which they may resemble.[53] Clear cell carcinomas generally occur in an older age group, have a strong predilection for women, and are usually solitary, large, and invasive.[50] There is significant nuclear enlargement and atypia, the cytoplasm is abundant, mitoses may be plentiful, but tubular and papillary structures resembling nephrogenic adenoma may be prominent (Fig. 3.9).

PAPILLOMA

The term papilloma implies a true epithelial neoplasm, and in the urinary bladder several varieties occur. Most are transitional cell type and are exophytic.[59]

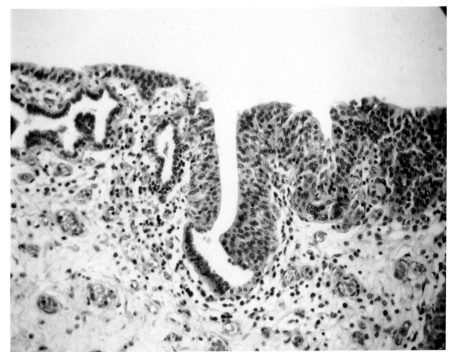

FIG. 3.8. Nephrogenic metaplasia. Normal urothelium interfaces with a surface component of low cuboidal epithelial cells. H & E, × 250.

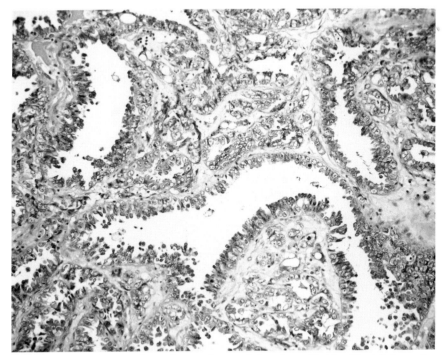

FIG. 3.9. Clear cell/mesonephric adenocarcinoma of the urinary bladder. The tubular and papillary structures exhibit a resemblance to nephrogenic adenoma. The papillae and tubules are lined by more than one layer of cells, and there are nuclear characteristics of malignancy. H & E, × 250.

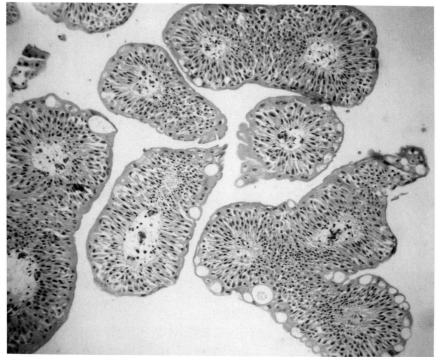

FIG. 3.10. Transitional papilloma. Each of the papillae is covered by an entirely normal urothelium. Surface umbrella cells are evident on the luminal aspect. H & E, × 125.

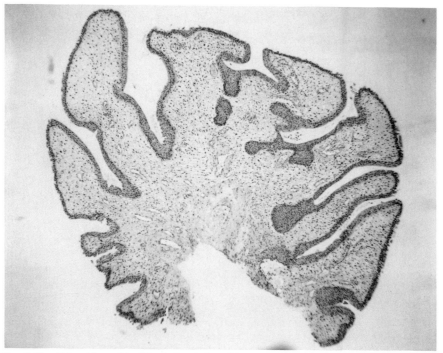

FIG. 3.11. Polypoid cystitis. The lesion is broad based. The papillary structures are thick and consist of edematous lamina propria instead of a fibrovascular core. H & E, × 25.

The distinction from well-differentiated papillary transitional cell carcinoma is an area in which confusion and disagreement exists.[60,61] This is dealt with in detail in another chapter of this volume and the subject has recently been reviewed in detail.[58] There is a small number of exophytic papillary lesions, however, that can be clearly separated morphologically from other papillary lesions and that are clearly benign. These tumors occur in a much younger age group than transitional cell carcinoma, usually in the second to fourth decades. They are usually small, localized, and are composed of exophytic epithelial papillary structures covered by perfectly normal urothelial cells of four to seven layers. Each papilla is covered by an outer luminal layer of normal large surface cells, the umbrella cells (Fig. 3.10). Rare reoccurrence of the neoplasms can occur. The risk factors for the development of a true transitional carcinoma later has not been observed.

POLYPOID AND PAPILLARY CYSTITIS

A proliferative lesion, which is not a true neoplasm but which may simulate a papillary tumor, is polypoid or papillary cystitis.[54,57] In these cases, inflammation and edema of the lamina propria associated with proliferation of surface urothelium leads to polypoid- or even papillary-appearing lesions. The underlying causes of the inflammation and edema are variable, but these lesions are frequently seen in association with indwelling catheters.[55,56] Other cases have been associated with vesicle fistulas.

Microscopically, the lesions are broad-based (Fig. 3.11). The bulk of the lesion is accounted for by the edema and inflammation in the lamina propria. The broad papillary structures are covered by normal urothelium (Fig. 3.12). Cystitis cystica is often an associated lesion. The lesions are usually spontaneously reversible when the inciting stimulus is removed.

INVERTED PAPILLOMA

In 1963, Potts and Hirst[73] reported a case of an epithelial lesion of the urinary bladder that exhibited a unique histological feature of an inverted growth pattern, and they were the first to use the term "inverted papilloma." Adult males, average age around 60, are the predominant population, although the lesion has also been reported in women. The lesions appear to be acquired rather than congenital. The lesions are much less common than the exophytic types of transitional cell neoplasms or invasive carcinomas, accounting for about 2.2% of lesions originating in the urothelium.[67] Most tumors are located in the urinary bladder, usually in the inferior aspect near the trigone or vesicle neck,[63,65–77] but inverted papilloma has also been reported in the urethra, ureters, and renal pelvis.[67,68,70,75] In the bladder, the lesions appear cystoscopically as solitary pedunculated and polypoid tumors with a smooth rounded surface on a broad base. The average size is 2 cm, but lesions up to 8 cm have been described.

The histological features are those of an invaginating proliferation of transitional cells extending and appearing to arise from an attenuated, nonpapillary surface epithelium (Fig. 3.13). In contrast to exophytic papillary transitional cell neoplasm, the fibrovascular supportive stroma surrounds the epithelial elements

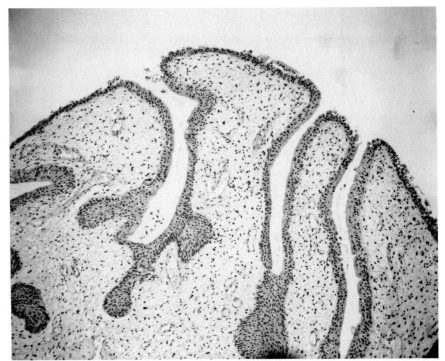

FIG. 3.12. Polypoid cystitis. The broad papillary structures contain an edematous stroma with chronic inflammatory cells and each papillae is covered by normal urothelial cells. H & E, × 80.

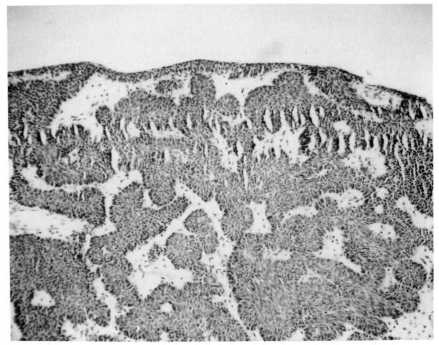

FIG. 3.13. Inverted urothelial papilloma. There is an endophytic proliferation of cells in the lamina propria arranged in a trabecular architecture. H & E, × 40.

rather than forming a central core. The epithelial cells are arrayed in a characteristic fashion that is virtually diagnostic of the lesion. The outer cells are arranged with their long axes perpendicular to the enveloping basement membrane, and this orientation changes to a parallel orientation in the center of the tissue core (Fig. 3.14). The central cells may exhibit cytological features of differentiation into squamous cells. Microcysts are often present within the epithelial cores and these contain an eosinophilic, PAS-positive substance. The connective tissue stroma may appear loose textured, almost myxomatous (Fig. 3.15). No significant degree of nuclear hyperchromasia or enlargement is noted among the epithelial cells. Mitotic figures are very rarely observed. The neoplasm is located in the lamina propria and does not extend into the bladder wall muscle.

The precise histogenesis of this lesion is not known. The resemblance of the epithelium in the region of microcysts to the epithelium of cystitis cystica suggests a possible histogenetic relationship. Ultrastructurally, the cells comprising the solid parts of the lesion exhibit cytoplasmic processes and frequently desmosomes with a cytoplasm rich in microfilaments with free ribosomes, glycogen, and mitochondria. The cells that form the microcysts differ in the feature of microvilli on the luminal surface.[62]

Case reports have appeared from time to time associating inverted papillomas with carcinoma of the urothelium.[64,69–72,74–76] In many instances, it would appear that the association is fortuitous with the carcinoma developing independently from the inverted papilloma; however, there are several reports of carcinoma purportedly developing in an inverted papilloma. It is known that some transitional carcinomas may exhibit an inverted growth pattern from their very inception. If strict criteria are maintained for the histopathological diagnosis of inverted papilloma, then simple excision is almost always curative.

CONDYLOMA ACUMINATUM

Case reports of involvement of the urinary bladder with lesions of condyloma acuminatum continue to appear,[78,80,82–84] comprising at the time of this writing about 16 cases.[78] Most cases have been associated with lesions in other sites such as the urethra, vulva, vagina, anus, and perineum. Women outnumber men about two to one in the bladder cases, and most patients have been immunosuppressed. The bladder lesions may be solitary or diffuse and multifocal. Cystoscopically, the lesions have the typical papillary or verrucous configuration.

Microscopically, the lesions must be distinguished from squamous metaplasia on the one hand and leukoplakia or verrucous squamous cell carcinoma on the other. Verrucous squamous cell carcinomas have been reported in the urinary bladder.[79] In a recent case, it is believed that verrucous squamous cell carcinoma developed from condyloma acuminatum.[85] The histopathological features are those of epithelial thickening, squamous metaplasia, hyperkeratinization, and prominent koilocytotic cytoplasmic change, associated with nuclear enlargement, hyperchromasia, irregularities of nuclear shape, and binucleation (Fig. 3.2).

Human papilloma virus Types 6 and 11 are the causative agents in the urinary bladder lesions. In a recent report in which a search was made for HPV in 22 cases of bladder cancer, in one case of invasive squamous carcinoma, HPV Type

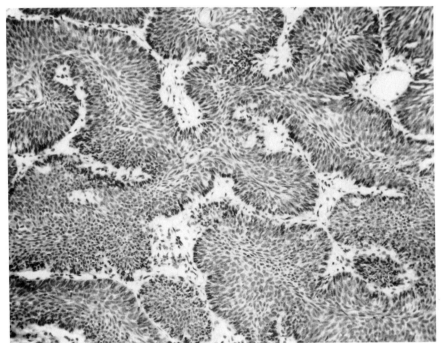

FIG. 3.14. Inverted urothelial papilloma. The fibrovascular stroma surrounds the epithelial structures. The elongated epithelial cells are arranged peripherally with the long axis perpendicular to the stroma and centrally in a parallel fashion. H & E, × 160.

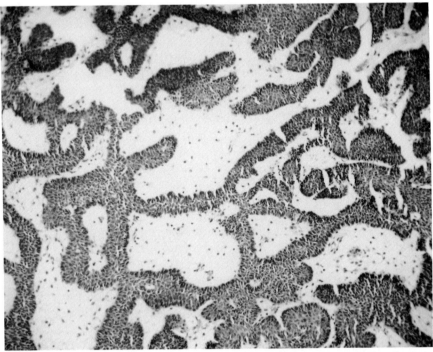

FIG. 3.15. Inverted urothelial papilloma. The connective tissue stroma has a loosely textured, almost myxoid, appearance. H & E, × 100.

11 was found by the *in situ* hybridization technique within the neoplastic cells.[81] The bladder lesions of condyloma acuminatum typically recur at least once and are difficult to treat.

FIBROBLASTIC PSEUDOTUMOR

A number of reports have appeared in the literature since 1980 of spindled cell lesions in the urinary bladder with microscopic features similar to a sarcoma, but in which the subsequent clinical course indicated a benign process.[87,88,91-94,96,100] Although the majority of the cases have occurred among adults, at least 10 cases have been reported in children.[86] The cases fall into two general categories: those with a previous history of some surgical insult to the urinary bladder and those with no apparent precipitating cause. The former lesions have also been termed "postoperative spindled cell nodules" and have typically occurred in adult patients, both men and women, at various intervals, usually in weeks or months following a surgical procedure such as a transurethral resection of the prostate gland or of a bladder tumor.

Cystoscopically, the lesions have been described as circumscribed, solid, polypoid masses, "heaped-up tumors," or as a protruding friable vegetant mass. A size of about 4 cm is average. In those cases that have been resected, there is an intramural bladder wall component that may extend deeply into the muscular wall of the bladder.

Microscopically, the urothelial surface overlying the lesion is usually ulcerated with an inflammatory exudate. The lesion itself is composed of plump, fibroblastic cells, often arranged in interlacing fascicles with a delicate stroma of small blood vessels (Fig. 3.16). Inflammatory cells are scattered throughout the lesion, but inflammation is not a prominent feature except on the ulcerated surface. Necrosis is not a feature, although foci of intralesional hemorrhage may be prominent. Stromal edema may be present creating a loosely textured pattern of elongated spindled cells (Fig. 3.17). Mitotic figures may be abundant. Studies have demonstrated the constituent cells to be fibroblasts[93] or myofibroblasts.[87] The postoperative lesions and the apparently spontaneous lesions exhibit such a degree of resemblance and overlapping features as to suggest a common pathogenesis.

The degree of cellularity is such as to suggest sarcoma (Fig. 3.18). In adults, the common sarcoma of the urinary bladder is leiomyosarcoma[90,95,97] and in children rhabdomyosarcoma. Myxoid variants of leiomyosarcoma of the urinary bladder might be expected to pose a significant problem in the differential because of some overlapping histopathological features.[99] Since many of these patients have recently been treated for urinary bladder carcinoma, the differential diagnosis must include a pseudosarcomatous stromal reaction associated with an invasive carcinoma.[89,101] Rarely, benign fibroepithelial polyps of the urinary bladder may exhibit stromal cells with atypical features.[98] The recognition of the proliferative nature of the pseudotumor is based on the resemblance to other fibroblastic proliferative lesions such as nodular fasciitis. This is the major clue to the correct interpretation. One does not find the cigar-shaped nuclei of the leiomyosarcoma nor the degree of nuclear anaplasia in these lesions, and, in the

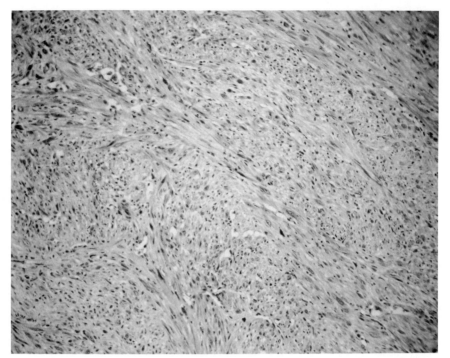

FIG. 3.16. Fibroblastic pseudotumor. Plump fibroblastic cells are arranged in interlacing fascicles. H & E, × 125.

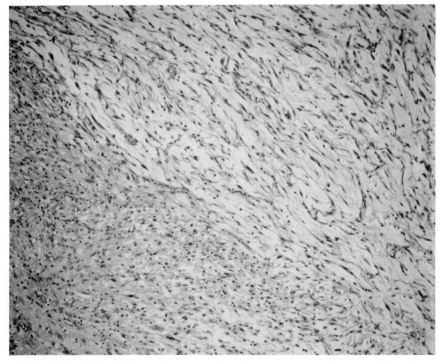

FIG. 3.17. Postoperative fibroblastic pseudotumor. Elongated spindled cells are loosely arranged in an edematous stroma. H & E, × 125.

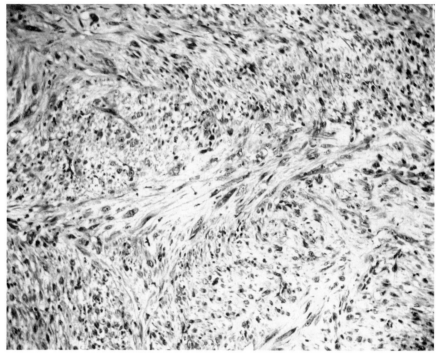

FIG. 3.18.   Fibroblastic pseudotumor. Bizarre spindled cells exhibit a degree of cellularity that suggests sarcoma. H & E, × 250.

childhood cases, the lack of eosinophilic myogenic cytoplasm or cross-striated cells is a major point.

In most cases, the fibroblastic pseudotumor has been resected, either by open segmental cystectomy or more often by transurethral resection. When the diagnosis is correct, the course has been that of a benign process, and recurrence of the lesion after the first episode is distinctly uncommon. It must be remembered that many of these patients have previously harbored urinary bladder carcinoma and are still at significant risk for recurrence of this tumor.

REFERENCES

Squamous Metaplasia

1. Benson, R. C., Swanson, S. K., and Farrow, G. M. Relationship of leukoplakia to urothelial malignancy. *J. Urol. 131:* 507–511, 1984.
2. Henry, L., and Fox, M. Histological findings in pseudomembranous trigonitis. *J. Clin. Pathol. 24:* 605–608, 1971.
3. Ito, N., Hirose, M., Shirai, T., Tsuda, H., Nokanishi , K., and Fukushima, S. Lesions of the urinary bladder epithelium in 125 autopsy cases. *Acta. Pathol. Japan 31:* 545–557, 1981.
4. Lancioni, L. J., Martinez Amézaga, L. A., and Lo Biano, V. S. Urocytogram and pregnancy. I. Methods and normal values. *Acta. Cytol. 13:* 279–287, 1969.
5. Locke, J. R., Hill, D. E., and Walzer, Y. Incidence of squamous cell carcinoma in patients with long-term catheter drainage. *J. Urol. 133:* 1034–1035, 1985.

6. Long, E. D., and Shepherd, R. T. The incidence and significance of vaginal metaplasia of the bladder trigone in adult women. *Br. J. Urol. 55:* 189–194, 1983.
7. McRae, D. J. Correlation between vaginal cytology and urinary hormone assays in pregnancy. *Acta. Cytol. 11:* 45–50, 1967.
8. Mostofi, F. K. Potentialities of bladder epithelium. *J. Urol. 71:* 705–714, 1954.
9. O'Morchoe, P. J., and O'Morchoe, C. C. C. Method for urinary cytology in endocrine assessment. *Acta. Cytol. 11:* 145–149, 1967.
10. Reece, R. W., and Koontz, W. W. Leukoplakia of the urinary tract: A review. *J. Urol. 114:* 165–171, 1975.
11. Streitz, J. M. Squamous epithelium in the female trigone. *J. Urol. 90:* 62–66, 1963.
12. Tyler, D. E. Stratified squamous epithelium in the vesical trigone and urethra: Findings correlated with the menstrual cycle and age. *Am. J. Anat. 111:* 319–335, 1962.
13. Widran, J., Sanchez, R., and Gruhn, J. Squamous metaplasia of the bladder: A study of 450 patients. *J. Urol. 112:* 479–482, 1974.

Intestinal/Colonic Metaplasia

14. Bullock, P. S., Thoni, D. E., and Murphy, W. M. The significance of colonic mucosa (intestinal metaplasia) involving the urinary tract. *Cancer 59:* 2086–2090, 1987.
15. Davis, E. L., Goldstein, A. M. B., and Morrow, J. W. Unusual bladder mucosal metaplasia in a case of chronic prostatitis and cystitis. *J. Urol. 111:* 767–769, 1974.
16. Gordon, A. Intestinal metaplasia of the urinary tract epithelium. *J. Pathol. Bact. 85:* 441–444, 1963.
17. Goyanna, R., Emmett, J. L., and McDonald, J. R. Exstrophy of the bladder complicated by adenocarcinoma. *J. Urol. 65:* 391–399, 1951.
18. Jacob, N. H., and Mau, W. Metaplasia of ureteral epithelium resulting in intestinal mucosa and adenocarcinomatous transformation: Report of two cases. *J. Urol. 65:* 20–24, 1951.
19. Mende, T. J., and Chambers, E. L. Distribution of mucopolysaccharide and alkaline phosphatase in transitional epithelia. *J. Histochem. Cytochem. 5:* 99–104, 1957.
20. Miller, D. C., Gang, D. L., Gavris, V., Alroy, J., Ucci, A. A., and Parkhurst, E. C. Villous adenoma of the urinary bladder: A morphologic or biologic entity? *Am. J. Clin. Pathol. 79:* 728–731, 1983.
21. O'Kane, H. O., and Megaw, J. M. Carcinoma in the exstrophic bladder. *Br. J. Surg. 55:* 631–635, 1968.
22. Ward, A. M. Glandular neoplasia within the urinary tract. The aetiology of adenocarcinoma of the urothelium with a review of the literature. I. Introduction: The origin of glandular epithelium in the renal pelvis, ureter, and bladder. *Virchows Arch. Abt. A Path. Anat. 352:* 296–311, 1971.
23. Young, R. H., and Parkhurst, E. C. Mucinous adenocarcinoma of the bladder. Case associated with extensive intestinal metaplasia of urothelium in patient with nonfunctioning bladder for twelve years. *Urology 24:* 192–195, 1984.

Brunn's Nests, Cystitis Cystica, and Cystitis Glandularis

24. Andersen, J. A., and Hansen, B. F. The incidence of cell nests, cystitis cystica and cystitis glandularis in the lower urinary tract revealed by autopsies. *J. Urol. 108:* 421–424, 1972.
25. Dann, R. H., Arger, P. H., and Enterline, H. T. Benign proliferation processes presenting as mass lesions in the urinary bladder. *AJR 116:* 822–829, 1972.
26. Emmett, J. L., and McDonald, J. R. Proliferation of glands of the urinary bladder simulating malignant neoplasm. *J. Urol. 48:* 257–265, 1942.
27. Goldstein, A. M. B., Fauer, R. B., and Chinn, M., et al. New concepts on formation of Brunn's nests and cysts in urinary tract mucosa. *Urology 11:* 513–517, 1978.
28. Lane, T. J. D. An uncommon bladder condition simulating carcinoma. Glandular proliferation

in the epithelium of the urinary tract, with special reference to cystitis cystica and cystitis glandularis. *Br. J. Urol. 20:* 175–179, 1948.

29. Lowry, E. C., Hamm, F. C., and Beard, D. E. Extensive glandular proliferation of the urinary bladder resembling malignant neoplasm. *J. Urol. 52:* 133–138, 1944.

30. Lin, J. I., Tseng, C. H., Choy, C., Yong, H. S., Marsidi, P. S., and Pilloff, B. Diffuse cystitis glandularis: Associated with adenocarcinomatous change. *Urology 15:* 411–415, 1980.

31. Parker, C. Cystitis cystica and glandularis: A study of 40 cases. *Proc. R. Soc. Med. 63:* 239–242, 1970.

32. Stillwell, T. J., Patterson, D. E., Rife, C. C., and Farrow, G. M. Neodymium: yag laser treatment of cystitis glandularis. *J. Urol. 139:* 1298–1299, 1988.

33. Talbert, M. L., and Young, R. H. Carcinomas of the urinary bladder with deceptively benign-appearing foci: A report of three cases. *Am. J. Surg. Pathol. 13:* 374–381, 1989.

34. Wells, M., and Anderson, K. Mucin histochemistry of cystitis glandularis and primary adenocarcinoma of the urinary bladder. *Arch. Pathol. Lab. Med. 109:* 59–61, 1985.

Nephrogenic Metaplasia/Adenoma

35. Berger, B. W., Bhagavan, B. S., Reiner, W., Engel, R., and Lepor, H. Nephrogenic adenoma: Clinical features and therapeutic considerations. *J. Urol. 126:* 824–826, 1981.

36. Bhagavan, B. S., Tiamson, E. M., Wenk, R. E., Berger, B. W., Hamamoto, G., and Eggleston, J. C. Nephrogenic adenoma of the urinary bladder and urethra. *Hum. Pathol. 12:* 907–916, 1981.

37. Davis, T. A. Hamartoma of the urinary bladder. *Northwest Medicine 48:* 182–185, 1949.

38. Devine, P., Ucci, A. A., Krain, H., Gavris, V. E., Bhagavan, B. S., Heaney, J. A., and Alroy, J. Nephrogenic adenoma and embryonic kidney tubules share PNA receptor sites. *Am. J. Clin. Pathol. 81:* 728–732, 1984.

39. Dow, J. A., and Young, J. D. Mesonephric adenocarcinoma of the bladder. *J. Urol. 100:* 466–469, 1968.

40. Ford, T. F., Watson, G. M., and Cameron, K. M. Adenomatous metaplasia (nephrogenic adenoma) of urothelium. An analysis of 70 cases. *Br. J. Urol. 57:* 427–433, 1985.

41. Friedman, N., and Kuhlenbeck, H. Adenomatoid tumors of the bladder reproducing renal structures (nephrogenic adenomas). *J. Urol. 64:* 657–670, 1950.

42. Goldman, R. L. Nephrogenic metaplasia (nephrogenic adenoma, adenomatoid tumor) of the bladder. *J. Urol. 108:* 565–567, 1972.

43. Hasen, H. B. Nephrogenic adenoma of the bladder. *J. Urol. 88:* 629–630, 1962.

44. Ingram, E. A., and DePauw, P. Adenocarcinoma of the male urethra with associated nephrogenic metaplasia. Case report and review of the literature. *Cancer 55:* 160–164, 1985.

45. Lugo, M., Petersen, R. O., Elfenbein, I. B., Stein, B. S., and Duker, N. J. Nephrogenic metaplasia of the ureter. *Am. J. Clin. Pathol. 80:* 92–97, 1983.

46. Martin, S. A., and Santa Cruz, D. J. Adenomatoid metaplasia of prostatic urethra. *Am. J. Clin. Pathol. 75:* 185–189, 1981.

47. McIntire, T. L., Soloway, M. S., and Murphy, W. M. Nephrogenic adenoma. *Urology 29:* 237–241, 1987.

48. Navarre, R. J., Loening, S. A., Platz, C., Narayana, A., and Culp, D. A. Nephrogenic adenoma: A report of nine cases and review of the literature. *J. Urol. 127:* 775–779, 1982.

49. Plimpton, H. W., Crawford, E. D., and Goldhaln, R. T. Nephrogenic adenoma associated with interstitial cystitis. *Urology 26:* 498–500, 1985.

50. Schultz, R. E., Block, M. J., Tomaszewski, J. E., Brooks, J. S. J., and Hanno, P. M. Mesonephric adenocarcinoma of the bladder. *J. Urol. 132:* 263–265, 1984.

51. Sussman, E. B., Brice, M., and Gray, G. F. Nephrogenic metaplasia of the bladder. *J. Urol. 111:* 34–35, 1974.

52. Young, R. H., and Scully, R. E. Clear cell adenocarcinoma of the bladder and urethra. A report of three cases and review of the literature. *Am. J. Surg. Pathol. 9:* 816–826, 1985.

53. Young, R. H., and Scully, R. E. Nephrogenic adenoma. A report of 15 cases, review of the

literature and comparison with clear cell adenocarcinoma of the urinary tract. *Am. J. Surg. Pathol. 10:* 268–275, 1986.

Polypoid Cystitis

54. Buck, E. G. Polypoid cystitis mimicking transitional cell carcinoma. *J. Urol. 131:* 963–965, 1984.
55. Ekelund, P., Anderstrom, C., Johansson, S. L., and Larsson, P. The reversibility of catheter-associated polypoid cystitis. *J. Urol. 130:* 456–459, 1983.
56. Ekelund, P., and Johansson, S. Polypoid cystitis. A catheter associated lesion of the human bladder. *Acta. Pathol. Microbiol. Scand. Sect. A, 87:* 179–184, 1979.
57. Young, R. H. Papillary and polypoid cystitis. A report of eight cases. *Am. J. Surg. Pathol. 12:* 542–546, 1988.

Transitional Cell Papilloma

58. Eble, J. N., and Young, R. H. Benign and low grade papillary lesions of the urinary bladder: A review of the papilloma-papillary carcinoma controversy, and a report of five typical papillomas. *Sem. Diag. Pathol. 6:* 351–371, 1989.
59. Farrow, G. M. Histopathology and cytopathology of bladder cancer. In *Surgical Pathology of Urologic Disease,* edited by N. Javadpour and S. H. Barsky. Baltimore, Williams & Wilkins, 1987, pp. 156–182.
60. Greene, L. F., Hanash, K. A., and Farrow, G. M. Benign papilloma or papillary carcinoma of the bladder. *J. Urol. 110:* 205–207, 1973.
61. Jordan, A. M., Weingarten, J., and Murphy, W. M. Transitional cell neoplasms of the urinary bladder: Can biologic potential be predicted from histologic grading? *Cancer 60:* 2766–2774, 1987.

Inverted Papilloma

62. Alroy, J., Miller, A. W., III, Coon, J. S., James, K. K., and Gould, V. E. Inverted papilloma of the urinary bladder: Ultrastructural and immunologic studies. *Cancer 46:* 64–70, 1980.
63. Anderstrom, C., Johansson, S., and Pettersson, S. Inverted papilloma of the urinary tract. *J. Urol. 127:* 1132–1134, 1982.
64. Altaffer, L. F., III, Wilkerson, S. Y., Jordan, G. H., and Lynch, D. F. Malignant inverted papilloma and carcinoma in situ of the bladder. *J. Urol. 128:* 816–818, 1982.
65. Camerson, K. M., and Lupton, C. H. Inverted papilloma of the lower urinary tract. *Br. J. Urol. 48:* 567–577, 1976.
66. DeMeester, L. J., Farrow, G. M., and Utz, D. C. Inverted papillomas of the urinary bladder. *Cancer 36:* 505–513, 1975.
67. Kunze, E., Schauer, A., and Schmitt, M. Histology and histogenesis of two different types of inverted urothelial papillomas. *Cancer 51:* 348–358, 1983.
68. Kyriakos, M., and Royce, R. K. Multiple simultaneous inverted papillomas of the upper urinary tract. A case report with a review of ureteral and renal pelvic inverted papillomas. *Cancer 63:* 368–380, 1989.
69. Lazarevic, B., and Garret, R. Inverted papilloma and papillary transitional cell carcinoma of urinary bladder. *Cancer 42:* 1904–1911, 1978.
70. Palvio, D. H. B. Inverted papillomas of the urinary tract, a case of multiple, recurring inverted papillomas of the renal pelvis, ureter, and bladder associated with malignant change. *Scand. J. Urol. Nephrol. 19:* 299–302, 1985.
71. Paulson, J., Metwalli, N., Wu, B., and Nachomovitz, L. Transitional cell carcinoma of bladder with features of inverted papilloma. *Lab. Invest. 58:* 71A, 1988.
72. Phillips, D. E. H., and Blenkinsopp, W. K. Inverted papilloma and papillary transitional cell carcinoma of bladder. *Br. J. Urol. 61:* 162–163, 1988.
73. Potts, I. F., and Hirst, E. Inverted papilloma of the bladder. *J. Urol. 90:* 175–179, 1963.
74. Renfer, L. G., Kelley, J., Belville, W. D. Inverted papilloma of the urinary tract: Histogenesis, recurrence and associated malignancy. *J. Urol. 140:* 832–834, 1988.

75. Schultz, R. E., and Boyle, D. E. Inverted papilloma of renal pelvis associated with contralateral ureteral malignancy and bladder recurrence. *J. Urol. 139:* 111–113, 1988.

76. Stein, D. S., Rosen, S., and Kendall, A. R. The association of inverted papilloma and transitional cell carcinoma of the urothelium. *J. Urol. 131:* 751–752, 1984.

77. Uyama, T., Nakamura, S., and Moriwaki, S. Inverted papilloma of bladder. *Urology 16:* 152–154, 1980.

Condyloma Acuminatum

78. Del Mistro, A., Koss, L. G., Braunstein, J., Bennett, B., Saccomano, G., and Simons, K. M. Condyloma acuminata of the urinary bladder. Natural history, viral typing, and DNA content. *Am. J. Surg. Pathol. 12:* 205–215, 1988.

79. Holck, S., and Jorgensen, L. Verrucous carcinoma of urinary bladder. *Urology 22:* 435–437, 1983.

80. Keating, M. A., Young, R. H., Carr, C. P., Nikrui, N., Heney, N. M. Condyma acuminatum of the bladder and ureter. Case report and review of the literature. *J. Urol. 133:* 465–467, 1985.

81. Kerley, S. W., Person, D. L., Fishback, J. L. Human papillomavirus and carcinoma of the urinary bladder. *Mod. Pathol.*, in press 1991.

82. Massé, S., Tosi-Kruse, A., Carmel, M., and Elhilali, M. Condyloma acuminatum of bladder. *Urology 17:* 381–382, 1981.

83. McClure, J., and Young, R. H. Infectious disease of the urinary bladder, including malacoplakia. In *Pathology of the Urinary Bladder*, edited by R. H. Young. New York, Churchill Livingstone, 1989, pp. 350–373.

84. van Poppel, H., Stessens, R., de Vos, R., and von Damme, B. Isolated condyloma acuminatum of the bladder in a patient with multiple sclerosis: Etiological and pathological considerations. *J. Urol. 136:* 1071–1073, 1986.

85. Walther, M., O'Brien, D. P., and Birch, H. W. Condylomata acuminata and verrucous carcinoma of the bladder: Case report and literature review. *J. Urol. 135:* 362–365, 1986.

Fibroblastic Pseudotumor

86. Albores-Saavedra, J., Manivel, C., Essenfeld, H., Dehner, L. P., Drut, R., Gould, E., and Rosai, J. Pseudosarcomatous myofibroblastic proliferation of the urinary bladder of children. *Cancer 66:* 1234–1241, 1990.

87. Forrest, J. B., King, G. S., and Pittman, G. B. An atypical myofibroblastic tumor of the bladder resembling a sarcoma. *J. Okla. State Med. Assoc. 81:* 222–224, 1988.

88. Goussot, J. F., Coindre, J. M., Merlio, J. P., and de Mascarel, A. An adult atypical fibromyxoid tumor of the urinary bladder. *Tumori 75:* 79–81, 1989.

89. Mahadevia, P. S., Alexander, T. F., Rojas-Corona, R., and Koss, I. C. Pseudosaromatous stromal reaction in primary and metastatic urothelial carcinoma. A source of diagnostic difficulty. *Am. J. Surg. Pathol. 13:* 782–790, 1989.

90. Mills, S. E., Bova, S. G., Wick, M. R., and Young, R. H. Leiomyosarcoma of the urinary bladder. A clinicopathologic study of 15 cases. *Am. J. Surg. Pathol. 13:* 480–489, 1989.

91. Nochomovitz, L. E., and Orenstein, J. M. Inflammatory pseudotumor of the urinary bladder— possible relationship to nodular fasciitis. *Am. J. Surg. Pathol. 9:* 366–373, 1985.

92. Proppe, K. H., Scully, R. E., and Rosai, J. Postoperative spindle cell nodules of the genitourinary tract resembling sarcoma. *Am. J. Surg. Pathol. 8:* 101–108, 1984.

93. Ro, J. Y., Ayala, A. G., Ordonez, N. G., Swanson, D. A., and Babaian, R. I. Pseudosarcomatous fibromyxoid tumor of the urinary bladder. *Am. J. Clin. Pathol. 86:* 583–590, 1986.

94. Roth, J. A. Reactive pseudosarcomatous response in urinary bladder. *Urology 16:* 635–637, 1980.

95. Sen, S., Malek, R. S., Farrow, G. M., and Lieber, M. M. Sarcoma and carcinosarcoma of the urinary bladder in adults. *J. Urol. 133:* 29–30, 1985.

96. Stark, G. I., Fedderson, R., Lower, B. A., Benson, C. T., Black, W., and Borden, T. A. Inflammatory pseudotumor (pseudosarcoma) of the bladder. *J. Urol. 141:* 610–612, 1989.

97. Tsukamoto, T., and Lieber, M. M. Sarcomas of the kidney, urinary bladder, prostate, spermatic cord, paratestis, and testis in adults. In *Management of Soft Tissue Sarcomas*, edited by J. H. Raff. Chicago, Year Book Medical Publishers, 1984.

98. Young, R. H. Fibroepithelial polyp of the bladder with atypical stroma cells. *Arch. Pathol. Lab. Med. 110:* 241–242, 1986.

99. Young, R. H., Proppe, K. H., Dickersin, G. R., and Skully, R. E. Myxoid leiomyosarcoma of the urinary bladder: Report of a case. *Arch. Pathol. Lab. Med. 111:* 359–362, 1987.

100. Young, R. H., and Scully, R. E. Pseudosarcomatous lesions of the urinary bladder, prostate gland, and urethra. A report of three cases and the review of the literature. *Arch. Pathol. Lab. Med. 111:* 354–358, 1987.

101. Young, R. H., and Wick, M. R. Transitional cell carcinoma of the urinary bladder with pseudosarcomatous stroma. *Am. J. Clin. Pathol. 89:* 216–219, 1988.

Chapter 4

Urothelial Neoplasia

WILLIAM M. MURPHY

Urothelial neoplasia is an extremely complex subject that is difficult to study. The optimal experiment, in which a cohort of human beings could be completely examined at multiple intervals throughout their lives and neoplastic lesions documented but observed without treatment, can never be done, even if we knew what to look for and had the technical means to perform the correct studies. Lacking the ability to observe the process directly, our knowledge of urothelial carcinogenesis stems largely from four sources: (1) observations of the tissues of experimental animals exposed to such large doses of chemicals that host factors are negated and only the effects of the drugs themselves can be studied; (2) clinical observations of humans who select themselves according to their perception of the severity of their symptoms and who are promptly treated once a neoplastic lesion is discovered; (3) studies of human neoplasms isolated from their normal environment and grown either in tissue culture or in immunologically deficient animals; and (4) comparisons of the growth patterns, phenotypic features, antigenic compositions, DNA contents, and genetic constitutions of tissues and cells that we have previously determined to be either normal or neoplastic. Information from these sources is incomplete and sometimes confusing, so we must attempt to make sense of the subject by creating conceptual schemes and theories that must be constantly revised as new information challenges some of their tenets.

If all this were not problem enough, our knowledge about any individual patient's reaction to neoplastic events is so rudimentary that we are tempted to leave host-related processes out of our theories. Given the circumstances, it is little wonder that we struggle to understand neoplasia. We seek the guidance of those who have written on the subject of cancer and carcinogenesis, but should not be surprised if these "experts" interpret the available data differently, each trying to make sense of the subject through his or her personal perspective composed from his own clinical and experimental observations combined with selections from the published experience of others glued together with intuition.

This Chapter will describe and discuss urothelial neoplasms in a conceptual framework of carcinogenesis. Those readers interested primarily in the diagnostic features of bladder neoplasms will find ample descriptions and illustrations as well as references to recently published textbooks and monographs. Those who

77

find themselves frustrated by the constant redefinition and reclassification of these tumors might find comfort in explanations of the sources of controversy. Those who question the biology, as opposed to the morphology, of various urothelial neoplasms may benefit from a personal frame of reference that represents a synthesis of many ideas and continues to evolve.

Our concepts of the nature of cancer and carcinogenesis have changed greatly over the years. No single theory has been able to explain all observations and none has been universally accepted. Not too long ago, many of us were taught that cancer is a foreign event superimposed upon a normal person who just happened to find himself in a dangerous environment. For bladders, such an environment might include breathing air rich in cigarette smoke or fumes from petrochemicals. On a more general scale, the unlucky individual might have been struck by a haphazard x-ray that caused a mutation in a gene. Cells harboring mutated genes are abnormal and, if they survive and proliferate, can create malignant clones. Perhaps mimicking the maturation of the human, these clones could evolve through various immature forms that could be recognized by astute pathologists using light microscopy if only they could see representative specimens early enough. This thinking implied that carcinogenesis produced cells foreign to the host. They had their own peculiar antigens, elicited an immune response similar to that produced by infectious organisms, and were usually ugly-looking under the light microscope. All of the functions necessary for growth, differentiation, and dissemination resided in these cancer cells. The host might try, but had no effective defenses. Once established, death from cancer was inevitable, although the time course was determined by the tumor cells and might be so prolonged that many patients died of old age or other diseases first. Since the host was defenseless, only early medical intervention offered any hope of cure.

It is currently recognized that human carcinogenesis is not a foreign event superimposed upon a normal person. At the very least, multiple events are required to initiate the process, initiated cells must be promoted, and further events must occur before these initiated and promoted cells can progress.[21] We now understand that clonal heterogeneity is the rule among carcinomas and that the process occurs very early as a function of proliferation.[28,75] We know that carcinogenesis is a highly regulated event and suspect that it utilizes normal cell mechanisms and structures to achieve growth and dissemination.[19,49,63,74] We are not so sure that we can recognize the earliest carcinogenic events or that all ugly cells are aggressive.[82] Most of us still believe that the process is totally engineered by the tumor itself; that the host may be effective only in preventing the initial events; and that dissemination depends on the appearance of a superclone of cancer cells with the ability to invade nonepithelial tissues, travel in the systemic circulation, adhere to tissues at distant sites, and proliferate in foreign environments.[44]

Still, there are nagging questions. If epithelial neoplasia results totally from the genetic ingenuity of the tumor cells and the host plays no effective role, then why are cancers not more prevalent in areas with high concentrations of suspected carcinogenic chemicals? After all, the vast majority of smokers and individuals in the petrochemical industry never develop bladder cancer. Why does the entire human urothelium not develop neoplastic changes, as occurs in rodents exposed to chemical carcinogens? Why do most human urothelial neoplasms differentiate toward transitional cell epithelium? If the host is unimportant, how do the tumor cells know where they are? Why do the majority of cells in any single tumor look alike? Why not have an array of glandular, squamous, neuroendocrine, or other phenotypes in every tumor? If all of the functions necessary for invasion and metastasis can reside in one cell, why do metastases rarely become detectable before the primary tumor is at least 1 cm^3 in size? These types of questions could go on and on.

Neoplasms are much easier to study than the hosts in whom they arise and it is not surprising that most of our current knowledge of carcinogenesis comes from examining the characteristics of tumor cells. Yet it seems that the above questions cannot be adequately answered without devoting more of our collective energy to examining the host. After all, the greatest genetic diversity resides in the host's cells and our current studies seem to point toward alterations in normal host functions as the basis for many types of cancer. In fact, evidence that normal host systems are essential for the growth and dissemination of cancer cells is gradually accumulating. It appears that every oncogene function has a suppressor gene antithesis.[49,74] Under certain conditions, fibroblasts can be made to secrete proteases that break down normal stromal matrix, perhaps facilitating tumor cell motility in these areas.[6,61,68] Cancer cells often have increased numbers of receptors for growth factors that are normally produced by the host.[48] Alterations in the environment of tumor cells can alter their phenotype and may even cause them to return to normal function.[29,36]

If the tumor cells can simulate or subvert all of these normal host functions, the host must certainly be able to affect the process at every level simply by reacting appropriately or not cooperating. Could it be that the absence of disseminated cancers represents effective host resistance rather than the absence of carcinogenic stimuli or the presence of cancers with defective growth? One might speculate that the histological type and degree of cellular anaplasia of any particular neoplasm represents the relative success of host defenses at the time of examination so that high-grade, invasive cancers reveal multiple host system failures and low-grade, noninvasive lesions indicate considerable host system success. At the extremes, complete host success results in no clinical disease, whereas complete host failure is manifested by death from disease. It is unlikely that all factors necessary for growth, differentiation, invasion, and metastasis can be expressed by any single cancer cell so that progressive disease requires clonal heterogeneity of neoplastic cells, probable cooperation among clones of tumor cells, and even the utilization of normal host systems.[6,28,68,75] It is equally unlikely that the host has only one method (*e.g.,* the systemic immune system) for combating neoplastic clones. Most likely, the host-tumor relationship is a never-ending dynamic that can be influenced by environmental factors and ameliorated by medical intervention.

ETIOLOGY AND PATHOGENESIS

Neither the etiology nor the pathogenesis of urothelial neoplasms is exactly known.[53] The only environmental chemicals that have been proven to cause human bladder cancer are arylamines, and almost no one is currently exposed to them.[10] Nevertheless, the relatively high incidence of bladder neoplasms among cigarette smokers and in areas where people might be exposed to industrial petrochemicals suggests more than a casual relationship.[34,45] World-wide, most bladder cancers can be attributed to infestation with the calcified eggs of *Schistosoma haematobium*, a situation that predisposes to bladder dysfunction, infection, and chronic physical irritation.[20] Other suspected etiological factors for urothelial neoplasia include: cyclophosphamide, phenacetin, chronic irritation, benzidine, auramine, bladder outlet obstruction, cyclamates, coffee, dietary fats and oils, vitamin A deficiency, nitrate and its metabolites, tryptophan, azathioprine, opium, viruses, motor exhaust fumes, and bracken fern.[10,53]

Urine itself has often been shown to contain substances that enhance and might even be essential for the development of urothelial neoplasms.[87] Once neoplasia has arisen, certain substances in urine might be important for tumor growth or progression. Urine is rich in epidermal growth factor (EGF), but urothelial cells normally manifest only a few receptor sites for EGF.[48] The number of receptors increases in association with increasing degrees of cellular anaplasia so that high-grade transitional cell neoplasms have more receptors than normal urothelium or low-grade tumors. Autocrine motility factor (AMF) is a 50 kd cytokine found in the urine of patients with transitional cell carcinoma.[32] This substance can stimulate motility *in vitro* using cultured tumor cells and may be important in facilitating invasion *in vivo*.

Recent studies of the chromosomal structure of transitional cell tumors have uncovered certain abnormalities that occur so frequently as to be considered at least nonrandom if not specific aberrations. Among these are an isochromosome of the short arm of chromosome 5, monosomy of chromosome 9, and deletion of the short arm of chromosome 11.[30,71] Other chromosomal abnormalities often found in bladder tumors include: deletions in 6q, 8p, 10q, 13, and 17p; duplications in 1 and 3; trisomy in 1, 7, and 20.[1,30,71,79]

Abnormalities of oncogene expression have been identified in certain bladder tumors. These include hypomethylation of c-*myc* and expression of the p21 gene product of c-Ha-*ras*.[15,81] It has long been known that transitional cell carcinomas are relatively antigenically deficient with regard to their blood group antigen expression.[43]

The relationship of any of these phenomena to the development or enhancement of neoplastic growth is difficult to assess. Many of our observations probably represent epiphenomena and only further studies will determine which factors are important. In attempting to determine factors essential for the initiation and growth of tumor cells, we usually find ourselves very much in the situation of a person who wants to determine the composition of the soil but is only able to examine the flowers.

CLINICAL FEATURES

Most urothelial neoplasms arise in the urinary bladder and occur with the following frequency: transitional cell (76–90%); squamous cell (2–15%); mixed (4–6%); undifferentiated (<2%); adenocarcinoma (<1%).[26,53] They may occur at almost any age, but the majority of patients are men between 50 and 70 years old (mean and median = 64–68 years). Tumors arising in patients under 40 years of age are usually of low grade and stage and are therefore associated with a very good prognosis.[41] Age itself is apparently not an important prognostic factor compared to grade and stage, however. The incidence among whites is twice that of blacks but race does not affect the behavior of the tumors once they are present. Bladder neoplasms account for less than 10% of all carcinomas in the United States and cause approximately 5% of cancer-related deaths.[8] Although the incidence in the Surveillance, Epidemiology, and End Results (SEER) statistics has steadily risen from 30,000 to approximately 50,000 new cases per year over the past 2 decades, the death rate has remained constant at approximately 10,000 per year. The implications of these figures are not easy to understand. They suggest either more efficient detection, an increase in the detection of biologically benign lesions, more effective treatment, a more cancer-resistant patient population, or other factors.[46]

The signs and symptoms of urothelial neoplasms vary somewhat with the histological type of lesion.[17] Papillary and invasive transitional cell tumors and many adenocarcinomas are usually associated with hematuria, either gross or microscopic, but this finding must be regarded as nonspecific since bladder lesions of almost every type result in an increase in urinary red blood cells. Pure squamous cell carcinomas are almost always associated with chronic irritation and/or infection and any individual with long-standing obstructive disease, urinary stones, diverticula, or neurogenic bladder is at increased risk.[53] Excretion of keratinous debris may also occur. Occasionally, patients with adenocarcinomas may complain of slimy urine, but mucus excretion is generally found by the physician, the patient being aware of either hematuria or the full feeling associated with a mass lesion. Urothelial carcinoma *in situ* is characteristically associated with painful urination, urgency, frequency, nocturia, and suprapubic pain symptoms identical to those of interstitial cystitis.[80] Any significant structural or functional abnormality of the urinary bladder may raise the risk for neoplasia but in most instances the risk is probably low.

Urothelial tumors (except urachal carcinomas) are localized to the bladder at diagnosis in 72% of cases.[13] The most common site for urothelial neoplasia is the bladder base, an area more closely related to elements of Müllerian, mesonephric, and hindgut embryologic anlage than any other part of the urinary system. Our experience indicates that, contrary to most publications, the majority of neoplasms are of high cytologic grade and potentially aggressive. This discrepancy arises from the tendency of pathologists to lump 50% of transitional cell lesions into an intermediate grade that is then further included among low-grade tumors. A large percentage of intermediate grade transitional cell tumors are composed of at least some anaplastic cells and behave like high-grade cancers.[78] Prognosis varies with the distribution of lesions at the initial diagnosis, the histologic type, and the cytologic grade.[53,69]

The adverse outcome associated with metastatic and locally disseminated disease needs no explanation except to comment that these circumstances might be considered to identify patients with multiple deficiencies in host defense mechanisms rather than particularly virulent cancer cell clones. Invasion into the muscular wall is a particularly poor prognostic sign, with 10 year actuarial survivals in the range of only 30% for transitional cell carcinomas and less for squamous and adenocarcinomas.[38,53] Multifocal or large tumors tend to be high grade and associated with worse outcomes, perhaps because of the existence of clever tumors or possibly because ordinary neoplastic processes have occurred in individuals that have deficiencies in their ability to control local growth. Among transitional cell neoplasms, cytologic grade is a very important indicator of biological behavior.[33,38,76] Almost all deeply invasive transitional cell carcinomas have at least some foci of high cytologic grade and prognosis is relatively poor even among those high-grade cancers that are papillary, noninvasive, or only superficially invasive lesions at initial diagnosis.[38,76] In contrast, papillary transitional cell neoplasms of very low cytologic grade have rarely if ever been observed to invade muscle or metastasize and are probably biologically benign.[33,38,42]

The prognosis for patients who develop squamous, glandular, and undifferentiated carcinomas is poor even if differentiation among the tumor cells themselves is good. This makes sense if one accepts the concept that differentiation is a host-controlled event that occurs at the local level. Only neoplasms differentiating toward normal transitional cell epithelium can be considered under good host control. Put another way, the more the tumor looks like skin or colon (given that metaplasias are not neoplasms), the more undifferentiated it is.

When considering prognosis, urologists often speak of "superficial carcinoma." Empirical observations over many years have given urologists the impression that any bladder tumor that has not yet invaded the muscular wall can be controlled by local therapy and will be associated with a good prognosis. Since so-called "superficial" bladder neoplasms are not a pure entity, this clinical conclusion should be called into question by pathologists. The majority of superficial bladder tumors are papillary lesions of low cytologic grade. These lesions are not aggressive and respond well to any form of treatment. Carcinoma *in situ* is a high-grade lesion that has a relatively good prognosis, especially over the short term. In contrast, papillary and focally invasive nodular cancers are sometimes of high cytologic grade. These carcinomas are not necessarily associated with a good long-term prognosis and this fact should be brought to the attention of urologists.[76]

DETECTION AND MONITORING

There is no single technique that will reliably reveal the presence of a urothelial neoplasm at every examination. The most useful methods are cystoscopy, histology, and cytology. Cystoscopy allows the examiner to detect and localize papillary and nodular lesions in most but not all areas of the urothelium. Tiny tumors and flat areas of cancer are difficult or even impossible to identify with this method. Nor can the cystoscopist accurately predict the cytologic grade of bladder neoplasms. Histology is particularly valuable in determining the nature of cystoscopic abnormalities and, if they are neoplastic, in evaluating their cytologic grade. This technique is dependent upon the skill of the cystoscopist since the pathologist can only evaluate those portions of urothelium selected by the urologist.

Cytology can be used to detect true carcinomas, *i.e.*, neoplasms with anaplastic cells. The sampling method, exfoliated cells in urine or avulsed cells in bladder washings, provides specimens more representative of the entire urothelium than either cystoscopy or cytology, and cytology can detect tiny lesions or flat carcinomas better than cystoscopy. Cytology is the best single method for monitoring carcinomas *in situ* and lesions treated with topical therapy.[57] It suffers from an inability to localize the neoplasms and inaccuracy in both grading and determination of invasion. The poor performance of cytology in the detection of low-grade papillary and flat urothelial lesions reflects the near normal phenotypic appearance of the cells comprising these tumors rather than deficiencies in the technique itself and can actually be used to advantage in follow-up. As long as the cytology remains normal or equivocal, it is unlikely that the patient has developed a life-threatening tumor and few attempts at localization with cystoscopy and selected site biopsies are necessary.[50] Many urologists currently accept this thinking and are willing to increase the intervals between cystoscopic examinations as long as urinary cytology specimens remain free of high-grade malignant cells.[72] Paradoxically, the main drawback to the widespread implementation of cytology in an organized follow-up program of bladder cancer patients has resided in the lack of confidence among pathologists in their ability to use the method accurately. Cystoscopy, histology, and cytology are all valuable tests for the detection and monitoring of bladder neoplasms. Each complements the other and there is no reason not to use all three whenever possible.

Other methods for detection and monitoring are less established but might also be valuable. Chief among these is flow cytometry. The value of this method rests with the fact that aggressive neoplasms usually contain relatively large populations of cells with abnormal amounts of DNA and that the presence of these abnormal cell populations correlates strongly with the potential for an adverse outcome.[47,78] The notion that flow cytometry provides a more objective measure of urothelial neoplasia than histology or cytology is widespread among clinicians but is not completely true. If only distinct populations of cells with abnormal DNA are accepted as neoplastic and only carefully prepared histograms are used, then objectivity in the interpretation of the results can be high. However, a relatively large percentage of bladder neoplasms has either no aneuploid cells or populations of cells with near diploid (hyperdiploid) DNA and these cases require considerable medical skill for accurate interpretation.[11,56] Further, the creation of the histograms usually seen in publications may border on a technical art form and could hardly be considered to be the result of the technical prowess of the unaided instrument. Lastly, aneuploidy is not always a measure of malignancy and many neoplastic cells have normal amounts of DNA.[56,78] Nevertheless, skillful flow cytometry can be valuable in the detection and monitoring of bladder carcinomas and its incorporation into a battery of tests used for the purpose is justified.[2]

Methods such as digitizing image analysis can provide DNA ploidy analysis as well as morphometric data and are rapidly finding a niche in the diagnostic armamentarium of the pathologist.[67] New generation expert systems are on the horizon.[84] Monoclonal antibodies directed against antigens found in various grades of transitional cell tumors may be helpful.[25] Methods to evaluate tumor cell kinetics and determine the chromosomal structure and gene expression of urothelial neoplasms are too new for routine diagnostic use.[1,30,62,64,71,79]

CLASSIFICATION

Urothelial neoplasms are classified according to their histological differentiation into transitional cell, squamous, mixed (usually transitional cell and squamous), undifferentiated, and adenocarcinoma. As previously stated, transitional cell tumors comprise 76–90% of all urothelial neoplasms and most of the rest are pure squamous cell tumors. All other types are uncommon. Variants of each histological type have been recognized.[86] Only transitional cell neoplasms can be considered truly differentiated and it is not surprising that grouping urothelial tumors according to their degree of cytologic anaplasia and the extent to which the arrangement of their cells resembles that of normal urothelium (*i.e.,* grading) has only been clearly important for transitional cell tumors.

Over the years, several grading schemes have been popular and many are still in use. (Table 4.1)[5,9,18,27,38,39,51] All have certain common features: (1) urothelial neoplasms are grouped according to histological differentiation; (2) only transitional cell neoplasms are graded; (3) transitional cell lesions are divided into three to five categories depending on the degree to which the tumor recapitulates normal transitional cell epithelium; and (4) grading is heavily influenced by cytologic features so that tumors composed of almost normal-appearing cells are classified in the lowest grade and tumors composed of anaplastic cells comprise the highest grade.

Considering the variation of histological types and the subtleties of evaluating cytologic anaplasia, there is very good agreement among pathologists required to classify urothelial neoplasms. The oft-quoted 30% intra- and interobserver variation occurs when we are asked to grade transitional cell neoplasms, not when

TABLE 4.1. COMMON GRADING SYSTEMS FOR TRANSITIONAL CELL NEOPLASMS

	WHO[51]	Bergkvist[5]	Broders[9]	Murphy[38]
Papilloma	X			X
Carcinoma				
0		X		
1	X	X	X	
				(Low grade) X
2	X	X	X	
				(High grade) X
3	X	X	X	
4		X	X	

we are determining whether or not a given lesion is a neoplasm.[65] In fact, the classification of any individual tumor provides only a rough estimate of the future behavior of that lesion in that patient and this pathological function should not be overemphasized.

Ideally, one would like to classify urinary cytology specimens using the same nomenclature as that preferred for histological samples. In our experience, the information available from examination of the disaggregated cells in a urinary specimen is such that accurate correlations between cytologic and histologic specimens are not always possible.[54] The cytologic sample contains cells from all parts of the bladder urothelium, whereas the histological specimen represents only a small focus. In the absence of the stalk, the cells of transitional cell papillomas often lack significant abnormalities and are difficult to recognize as neoplastic.[52]

It is not usually possible to determine the presence of invasion by examination of urinary cells alone so that the distinction between invasive and *in situ* high-grade lesions is usually not possible. Adenocarcinomas are difficult to distinguish from high-grade transitional cell cancers in urinary specimens. Maturation normally occurs in a transitional cell tumor so that the cells at the surface may be better differentiated than those in the base. Under these circumstances, the urinary specimen may contain only low-grade neoplastic cells, whereas the histological preparation reveals a high-grade lesion. For all of these reasons, we have adopted the following nomenclature in reporting cytologic specimens[54]:

Negative cytology, (including reactive states)
Dysplastic cells
Abnormal cells suspicious for neoplasia
Neoplastic cells
    Low-grade neoplasm
    High-grade neoplasm
    Squamous cell carcinoma
    Adenocarcinoma
    Nonepithelial neoplasm.

The most popular current classification scheme for urothelial neoplasms is that of the World Health Organization.[51] In this formulation, almost all lesions are considered malignant, benign papillomas being relatively rare. More recent empirical observations have provided data in support of what many urologists and pathologists have long suspected, namely that benign transitional cell neoplasms are rather common and may comprise as much as 25% of transitional cell tumors.[38]

The discrepancy can be explained by a brief review of the evolution of knowledge concerning carcinogenesis. Until relatively recently, most investigators and practitioners believed that aggressive epithelial cancers arose through an orderly and time-sequenced series of graded cytologic changes that could be detected with diligent application of relatively simple techniques involving screening and light microscopy. Tumors arising subsequent to resection of the primary lesion were termed "recurrences" and considered to be a sign of uncontrolled growth potential. Lesions of low cytologic grade and good differentiation were regarded as young or early lesions to be contrasted to the old, late cancers of high grade and poor differentiation. Using this concept, all transitional cell neoplasms were cancers since all had the potential to recur and the achievement of high cytologic grade and poor differentiation was only a matter of time.

Experimental and empirical observations over the last 2 decades have provided new insight into carcinogenesis and required major revisions in our concepts. We have begun to appreciate the complexities of the process and to understand that the evolution of an epithelial malignancy probably does not proceed in a time-sequenced manner and does not necessarily manifest a series of morphological changes that can be easily recognized through the light microscope.[21] In the bladder, truly recurrent tumors are uncommon, most being new tumors arising in locations different from that of the primary lesion. More importantly, an orderly series of progressive cytologic anaplasia cannot be readily detected during clinical observation, suggesting that whatever events have produced the particular grade of transitional cell tumor seen at the initial diagnosis have occurred before diagnosis and are now relatively stable. Patients presenting with very low-grade papillary tumors may indeed develop new lesions, but the new tumors are usually of the same grade and stage. Recurrences of high-grade lesions usually represent persistence of the primary cancer through previous dissemination of tumor cells or multifocal carcinoma *in situ*.[23,40] Lastly, there is mounting evidence that the host has multiple ways of resisting the development of cancer.[74,83] Using these new concepts of carcinogenesis, the notion of a benign transitional cell neoplasm becomes more palatable.

The following paragraphs will describe the essential diagnostic features of the major types of urothelial neoplasms. Transitional cell lesions will be graded according to our modification of the WHO scheme.[38,53] Variants of the major histological types will not be detailed. Anyone reading a description of an epithelial neoplasm must be aware that the information is at best a distillation of features that have been important to the author. Neoplasms are composed of millions of cells representing heterogeneous differentiation and every cell will not conform to the general description. It is the ability to appropriately weigh the myriad features present in almost every neoplasm that identifies the superior diagnostician, and it is the presence of so much visual information in these cases that inhibits reproducibility among different observers. The following descriptions are offered as guidelines for evaluation of histological and cytologic specimens from patients with urothelial neoplasms.

Transitional cell neoplasms can be separated into three grades based on light microscopic features alone (Table 4.2). The lowest grade lesions cannot be recognized as neoplastic unless the cells are arranged on a delicate fibrovascular stalk. These lesions are probably benign in the sense that their component cells retain many features of normal urothelium, invasion of the lamina propria may not be possible, and invasion of the muscular wall, metastases, and death from this lesion have not been observed. We recommend the term "papilloma" but would not quarrel with equivalent terminology such as "low-grade papillary tumor." The majority of transitional cell neoplasms are carcinomas in the sense

TABLE 4.2. GUIDELINES FOR EVALUATING TRANSITIONAL CELL NEOPLASMS[a]

	Configuration		Cell Distribution		Nuclear Features			
	Papillary	Nodular	Even	Clustered	Pleomorphism	Chromatin		Large Nucleoli
						Fine	Coarse	
Papilloma	+++	0	+++	0	±	+++	0	±
Carcinoma								
Low grade	++	+	+++	0	+	++	±	+
High grade	+	+++	0	+++	+++	+	+++	++

[a] Key to features: 0 = absent; ± may occur sporadically; + = occurs in some tumors but not constant; ++ = occurs in most tumors; +++ = characteristic feature that occurs in all or almost all cases.

that their cells lack most of the features of normal urothelium and deep invasion, metastases, and death from these lesions have been observed. Even so, a small proportion of carcinomas are of low cytologic grade and identify a patient population that is at considerably lower risk for death from disease than patients having lesions of high cytologic grade.

TRANSITIONAL CELL PAPILLOMA

Transitional cell papillomas are exophytic tumors composed of well-differentiated transitional cells arranged on a delicate fibrovascular stalk (Fig. 4.1). Most bladder lesions with this histology have been called "carcinoma" in the WHO scheme, although exact extrapolations cannot be made and it would be inaccurate to say that all neoplasms classified as TCC-I in WHO terminology are actually papillomas. The exact frequency of these tumors is unknown but they may comprise as much as 25% of transitional cell neoplasms.[38] Only 24–60% of transitional cell papillomas have been detected using urinary cytology.[53] Over 80% retain their normal blood group antigens. DNA ploidy and chromosomal structure are normal in almost all, as is the expression of epidermal growth factor receptors and c-HA-ras oncogene.[48,81] Proliferative activity is similar to that of normal urothelium.[64] In fact, these lesions would probably not be considered neoplastic at all except for the clinical observations that papillary bladder tumors tend to recur and patients harboring such tumors are at increased risk for the development of invasive and metastatic carcinomas. Applying our present concepts, one might theorize that the appearance of transitional cell papillomas represents failure of the host to prevent abnormal cell proliferation but success in controlling growth rate, differentiation, and the development of significant clonal heterogeneity of the tumor cell population.

Papillomas usually appear cystoscopically as single lesions at the bladder base. Histologically, multiple layers of well-differentiated transitional cells are arranged on a delicate fibrovascular stalk. The number of layers is only important in defining a neoplasm in the rare instance where the cells themselves appear completely normal through the light microscope. At low magnification, the cells of papillomas appear evenly distributed with little nuclear crowding and variable preservation of cytoplasmic clearing. Nuclei may be ovoid, rounded, or elliptical

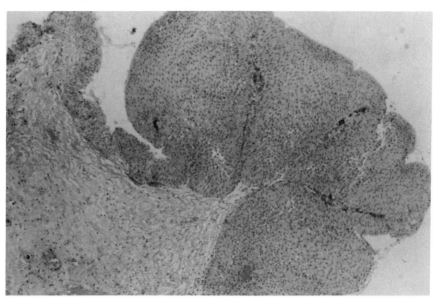

FIG. 4.1.   Transitional cell papilloma. Note the uniform distribution of nuclei in cells arranged on delicate fibrovascular stalks. H & E, × 60.

but many retain a semblance of normal orientation toward the surface. The superficial cell layer is retained. Unlike colon polyps, the neoplastic cells commonly cover the stalk and adjacent flat epithelium. At higher magnification, the nuclei have slight irregularities in their borders, usually manifested by shallow depressions or sharp indentations (abnormal nuclear shape index to the morphometrist) (Fig. 4.2). Chromatin is finely granular and evenly distributed. Nucleoli are small or absent. Mitoses are usually sparse and normal in configuration. Fine structural details are best appreciated after fixation in picric acid-based solutions such as Hollande's, but may be seen after formalin fixation provided that care is taken to properly preserve the pH. In our experience, the most important histological features of transitional cell papillomas are the even cellular distribution (probably a reflection of low nuclear:cytoplasmic ratios), the nuclear shape, and the chromatin characteristics. Neither the number nor distribution of mitoses has been particularly helpful in grading these tumors.

When disaggregated into cytologic samples, the cells of transitional cell papillomas often lack significant abnormalities and it may not be possible to recognize them using light microscopy alone. Monoclonal antibodies targeted to these elements are being developed and tested but their importance in diagnostic work remains to be determined.[35] In many instances, the best clue to the presence of a transitional cell papilloma will be an increased number of urothelial cells in a randomly voided urine sample.[12] Despite the difficulties of rendering an unequivocal diagnosis, the cells comprising transitional cell papillomas are rarely entirely normal (Fig. 4.3). They may aggregate in loose clusters or cohesive papillary configurations. More importantly, the cells of papillomas are larger than the normal basal and intermediate cells almost always found in the same sample.

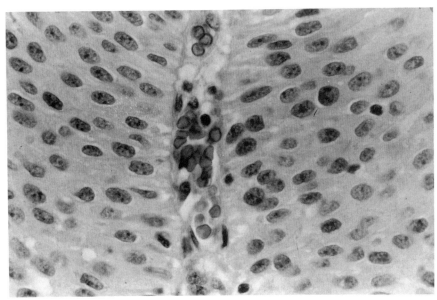

FIG. 4.2. Higher magnification of the neoplasm in Figure 4.1. The nuclei tend to retain their polarization and tend to be evenly distributed throughout the tumor. Many have irregularities of their borders. H & E, × 600.

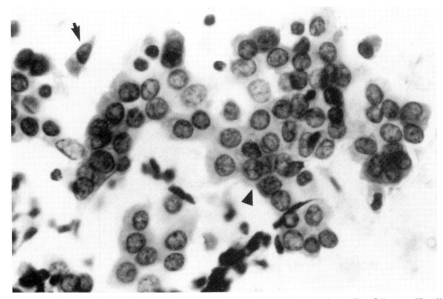

FIG. 4.3. Cytology from the tumor in Figures 4.1 and 4.2. One of the isolated "normal" cells is indicated by the *arrow*. Clusters of atypical (dysplastic) cells comprise most of the photograph. One of these clusters is indicated by the *arrowhead*. Note that the atypical nuclei are slightly larger and more rounded than the normal nuclei. They have a more granular chromatin and many have irregularities of their nuclear borders. EA, × 600.

Their nuclei tend to be eccentric and their nuclear:cytoplasmic ratios are increased compared to normal. Irregularities of nuclear borders are often apparent and the chromatin is more granular than normal. Neither cytoplasmic vacuolization nor large nucleoli are features of transitional cell papillomas and their presence indicates a reactive/reparative/regenerative process. The most common pitfall in assessing a urinary sample for low-grade neoplastic cells is overreliance on papillary aggregation.[53] Not all papillary aggregates are neoplastic and one must examine the features of the component cells to determine the true nature of the process. The main purpose of urinary cytology in a case of clinically suspected transitional cell papilloma is to exclude a more aggressive neoplasm, *i.e.*, one composed of easily recognized high-grade malignant cells.

The determination of DNA ploidy by flow cytometry on transitional cell papillomas themselves is of limited value.[55] At least 95% of lesions have normal DNA content and the prognosis of those few cases with DNA aneuploidy has been unpredictable. In contrast, DNA ploidy determinations using flow cytometry have been more useful when performed on urinary specimens from patients with transitional cell papillomas.[2,56] Since urinary samples are more representative of the urothelium than are selected tissue biopsies, there is a greater chance of detecting abnormal cells, perhaps in a co-existing carcinoma *in situ*. DNA ploidy determinations are especially valuable when used in conjunction with light microscopy on the same urinary sample.

The differential diagnosis of transitional cell papillomas includes inflammatory lesions, inverted papilloma, and true carcinomas. Inflammatory lesions may have multiple cell layers but are distinguished from papillomas by a stalk broadened by connective tissue with or without inflammatory cells. The papillary projections of these lesions are rarely long and almost never branched. Inverted papilloma is a closely defined neoplasm with a distinctive growth pattern.[16] In addition to a smooth outer surface to the tumor, the neoplastic cells are arranged opposite to that of an exophytic lesion. Differentiation proceeds *toward* rather than away from the center of the papilla and the connective tissue is on the outside rather than the inside. On the other hand, an inverting pattern may comprise a portion of a transitional cell papilloma. Carcinomas can be distinguished from papillomas primarily by their cytologic features. Low-grade carcinomas lack cytoplasmic clearing, have higher nuclear:cytoplasmic ratios, and more crowded nuclei. When seen in cytologic preparations, the cells of almost all low-grade carcinomas have recognizable features of neoplasia, manifesting in chromatin granularity, high nuclear:cytoplasmic ratio, and nuclear eccentricity. High-grade transitional cell cancers differ from papillomas by the tendency of their nuclei to cluster and overlap in addition to their coarsely granular chromatin and prominent nucleoli. Problems in differentiating papillomas from carcinomas occur primarily when a papillary tumor consists mostly of papilloma cells with only a few areas of carcinoma (Fig. 4.4). In such cases, one should examine the stromal interface and be aware of the cytologic findings before rendering a diagnosis. Clusters of high-grade cells tend to occur at the invasive margin. High-grade bladder cancers almost always exfoliate cells with malignant features.

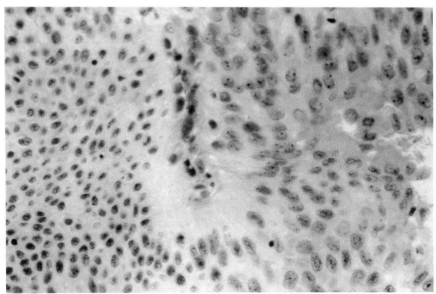

FIG. 4.4. A predominantly low-grade transitional cell tumor (left) that contains foci composed of high-grade cells (right). Tumors with this morphology should not be considered papillomas. In fact, the cytology from this case contained high-grade cancer cells. H & E, × 300.

TRANSITIONAL CELL CARCINOMA

If transitional cell papillomas are excluded, the majority of transitional cell neoplasms of the urinary bladder are carcinomas, *i.e.*, they are composed of cells with significant anaplasia and have demonstrated the ability, at least in some individuals, to invade and metastasize. If defined according to our previous guidelines, these lesions can be divided into low- and high-grade tumors with the low-grade carcinomas comprising only a small proportion.[38] Most low-grade carcinomas would be recognized as TCC-II using WHO terminology, but a few might be called TCC-1, perhaps accounting for the rare case of metastasis from a TCC-1 (WHO) and the justification for including all papillomas among the malignancies.

Transitional cell carcinomas, low grade, are almost always papillary, but neoplasms of similar cytology may compose nodular invasive and flat, noninvasive lesions. The nodular invasive tumors retain the designation transitional cell carcinoma, low grade, but the flat noninvasive lesions are included among the range of histological change recognized as carcinoma *in situ*. In most reports, transitional cell carcinomas of intermediate grade comprise almost half the cases, a classification tendency of pathologists that can be avoided and probably should be discouraged since it is not particularly helpful to the patient. If low-grade transitional cell carcinomas are an entity rendered distinctive by both histological features and biological behavior, they may comprise as few as 13% of cases but the proportion recognized in daily practice is probably closer to 20–25%.[38] Accurate information is very difficult to obtain since low-grade (or G2) tumors have not been closely defined in most of the literature and the number of cases assigned to this category is most likely unnecessarily large. One might theorize, however, that it is possible for the host to fail at preventing abnormal cellular proliferation and to partially fail at controlling differentiation while succeeding for prolonged periods at inhibiting the development of the clonal components necessary for invasion and dissemination.

We have attempted to define and describe the features of low-grade transitional cell carcinomas as a distinct histologic entity (Fig. 4.5). At low magnification, the cells are close together but uniformly distributed. Their nuclei retain some orientation to the surface but the superficial cell layer is usually absent, attenuated, or only focally retained. At higher magnification, the nuclei are similar to those of transitional cell papilloma in their even distribution of finely granular chromatin, small nucleoli, and border irregularities, but all features seem slightly more accentuated and more cells do not conform to the norm (Fig. 4.6). Most importantly, the cells of low-grade transitional cell carcinoma do not cluster and their nuclei do not overlap in the pattern of a high-grade tumor. Mitoses are usually numerous.

Cytologically, cells from a low-grade carcinoma may be isolated or appear in loose clusters (Fig. 4.7). They have high nuclear:cytoplasmic ratios and nuclei so eccentric that the cytoplasm often appears at only one rim of the cell. Irregularities of nuclear borders are usually prominent. They are focal, however, and only one notch or crease or shallow indentation occurs in any particular nucleus. The nuclei have distinctly granular but evenly distributed chromatin that can most easily be identified by focusing the microscope through the various planes of the

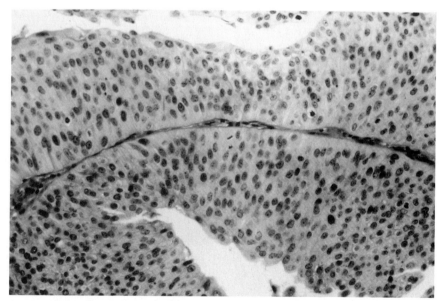

FIG. 4.5. Transitional cell carcinoma, low grade. At low magnification, the nuclei are evenly distributed but more crowded than in a papilloma. H & E, × 192.

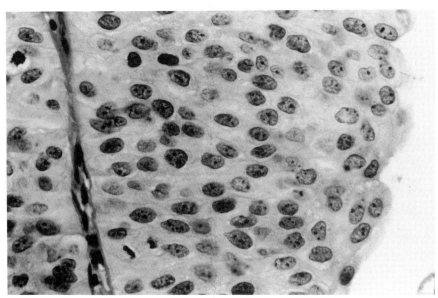

FIG. 4.6. Higher magnification of the tumor in Figure 4.5. Most of the nuclei have become rounded. Their nuclear chromatin seems slightly more granular than in Figure 4.2, but it is still evenly distributed. Note the absence of large nucleoli. H & E, × 480.

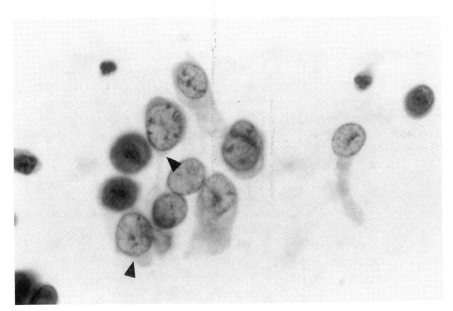

FIG. 4.7. Cytologic sample from the tumor in Figures 4.5 and 4.6. *Arrowheads* mark the whispy cytoplasm that tends to trail out from the neoplastic nuclei. These nuclei have considerable volume and are difficult to focus completely in one plane. Therefore, they seem to have areas of nuclear clearing when in fact the chromatin is evenly distributed. EA, × 756.

nuclei. In any particular plane, the chromatin may appear washed out. Nucleoli are not a prominent feature of low-grade carcinoma cells.

Determination of DNA ploidy using flow cytometry has been particularly useful in those situations where most of the transitional cell neoplasms have been classified in the intermediate grade.[78] Approximately 50% of so-called G2 carcinomas have DNA aneuploidy and these lesions, though not identical to G3 tumors, tend to act like them. If a more restrictive histological definition of low-grade carcinoma is used, DNA ploidy determination on the tumors themselves has not been as valuable.[55] When defined according to our criteria, only about 20% of low-grade carcinomas had aneuploid cells. The outcome among this group did not differ from that among patients with diploid tumors.

Low-grade transitional cell carcinomas must be distinguished from papillomas and high-grade cancers. They differ from papillomas primarily in their growth pattern. A uniform distribution of crowded, slightly hyperchromatic nuclei arranged on a delicate fibrovascular stalk is the hallmark of low-grade carcinoma. If papillomas and low-grade carcinomas could be compared side by side, one might see slight differences in chromatin granularity and nuclear border abnormalities as well as the smaller size of carcinoma cells and their higher nuclear:cytoplasmic ratios, but such distinctions are somewhat subtle and might escape the infrequent observer. Low-grade carcinomas are more easily distinguished from high-grade cancers. Their cells do not tend to cluster nor are their nuclei as pleomorphic. More importantly, coarsely granular, irregularly distributed chromatin is not a feature of low-grade carcinoma nor are very large nucleoli.

High-grade transitional cell carcinomas are typically nodular cancers that have already invaded the underlying tissue by the time of clinical detection. Papillary, noninvasive lesions exist and have constituted approximately 15% of high-grade lesions in at least one study.[38] Flat, noninvasive carcinomas composed of high-grade tumor cells are included in the category of carcinoma *in situ* (CIS). High-grade transitional cell carcinomas account for 25–63% of all transitional cell neoplasms, depending upon one's definition and whether or not DNA aneuploidy is considered a feature of high cytologic grade.[53] One could theorize that these cancers reflect significant deficiencies in multiple host defense mechanisms including failure to prevent abnormal cell proliferation, failure to control differentiation, and failure to inhibit the development of the multiple clones probably necessary for invasion and metastasis. One might also speculate that poor differentiation is a necessary feature for dissemination among transitional cell neoplasms since the percentage of cases with dissemination is directly proportional to the number with high-grade tumors.

Like all transitional cell neoplasms, high-grade carcinomas tend to arise at the bladder base. In contrast to other tumors, they are more likely to be multifocal and to be associated with carcinoma *in situ*, reflecting either widespread breakdown in local environmental defenses or seeding of multiple areas of mucosa by particularly virulent cancer cells. Some attempt at transitional cell differentiation is evidenced by a growth pattern of large nests bounded by thin septa, but it must be admitted that most high-grade transitional cell carcinomas cannot be distinguished from nonkeratinizing squamous carcinomas on histological grounds alone. At low magnification, pleomorphism is the hallmark of high-grade transitional cell carcinoma (Fig. 4.8). This is manifested primarily by variations in nuclear shape among adjacent cells rather than by the appearance of nuclei of significantly different size. Of equal importance is the tendency of the cells to cluster and of the nuclei to overlap. At higher magnification, the cells of high-grade carcinoma have variable nuclear:cytoplasmic ratios and may have vacuolated cytoplasm (Fig. 4.9). Nuclear chromatin is coarsely granular and irregularly distributed. Large nucleoli occur in some but not all nuclei. When high-grade areas occur in otherwise low-grade tumors, cells with nucleoli seem to aggregate at the stromal interface, as if the ability to produce messenger RNA was important for invasion.

The cells of high-grade transitional cell carcinoma are readily recognized as malignant in adequate urinary samples (Fig. 4.10). Cells may be loosely clustered or isolated. They may vary considerably in size and shape. In contrast to low-grade neoplasms, cytoplasmic vacuolization is rather common. As in the tissue, nuclear:cytoplasmic ratios vary and may not be high. There is significant variation in nuclear shape among tumor cells and nuclei tend to overlap one another within the aggregates. The chromatin is coarsely granular and irregularly distributed. Large nucleoli occur in some of the cells. Although mitoses are not generally considered to be important factors for the evaluation of malignancy in fluids, urine is a particularly hostile environment for cell growth and one would not expect to see mitoses that had not existed prior to exfoliation. Therefore, the presence of mitotic figures in urothelial cells tends to carry more diagnostic weight.

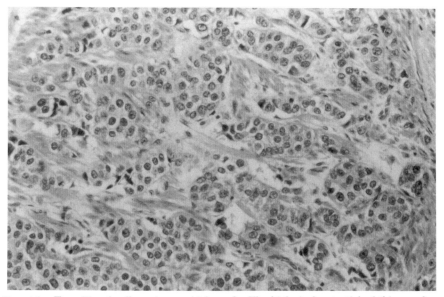

FIG. 4.8.   Transitional cell carcinoma, high grade. The biological potential of this neoplasm is indicated not only by invasion of the muscular wall but by the tendency of the nuclei to cluster. H & E, × 192.

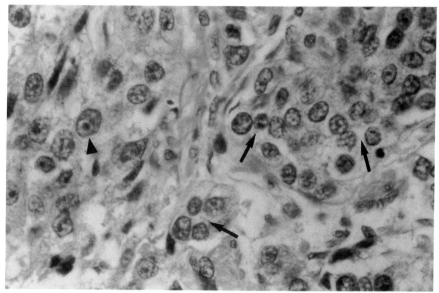

FIG. 4.9.   Higher magnification of Figure 4.8. The clustered nuclei are indicated with arrows. A few nuclei have prominent nucleoli (*arrowhead*). In addition, chromatin is coarsely granular and tends to be unevenly distributed. This neoplasm is biologically aggressive despite its apparent lack of bizarre nuclear changes. H & E, × 480.

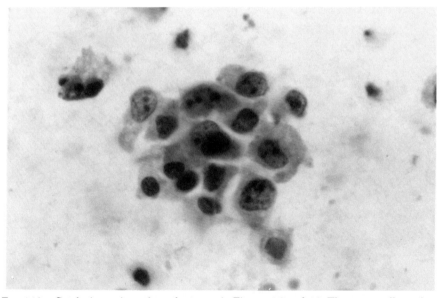

FIG. 4.10.   Cytologic specimen from the tumor in Figures 4.8 and 4.9. The tumor cells are loosely clustered and no two nuclei have the same shape. In contrast to low-grade neoplastic cells, the cytoplasm may be relatively abundant and focally vacuolated (a degenerative change). EA, × 756.

Determination of DNA ploidy has not been particularly valuable in confirming the presence of high-grade transitional cell carcinoma when the test is performed on the tumors themselves. Aneuploidy has been documented in 85–95% of all high-grade transitional cell carcinomas.[2,55,56,78] Both the number of abnormal clones and the configuration of the histogram (tetraploidy, hyperdiploidy, etc.) have been considered important by some investigators, but the significance of any particular type of abnormal DNA in an otherwise high-grade transitional cell carcinoma is unclear. Evaluation of DNA ploidy, usually by flow cytometry, is much more valuable for monitoring patients than detecting primary cancers, especially when the test is performed on urinary samples in conjunction with light microscopy.[2,56]

High-grade transitional cell carcinomas are almost always obviously malignant and the differential diagnosis rarely includes benign entities. Distinction from papillomas and low-grade carcinomas has already been mentioned and centers around the nuclear pleomorphism and more abnormal chromatin distribution of the high-grade tumors. Nonkeratinizing squamous cell carcinomas cannot be distinguished from high-grade transitional cell tumors.

SQUAMOUS CELL CARCINOMA

Urothelial neoplasms differentiating toward squamous epithelium can only be reliably recognized as such by light microscopy if they produce sufficient amounts of keratin. These tumors occur with almost equal frequency in women as men.[24] If they had arisen in the skin, where squamous epithelium is the normal standard, almost all would be considered well to moderately differentiated. In the bladder, however, neoplastic epithelium that looks like skin is distinctly abnormal, possibly reflecting a significant derangement in host influences on tumor differentiation. Pure squamous cancers of the bladder rarely occur in the absence of long-standing irritation and/or infection, often associated with structural abnormalities such as diverticula and strictures or functional problems like neurogenic bladder.[53]

Although facts are difficult to assemble, it is unlikely that squamous cell carcinomas arise from squamous metaplasia, despite the fact that squamous metaplasia is present in 25–50% of such cases. Most metaplastic lesions resemble vaginal epithelium, occur in the trigone, and apparently have little association with subsequent bladder cancer.[85] Even patients who develop keratinizing squamous metaplasia (leukoplakia) have a relatively low incidence of subsequent squamous carcinoma.[4] From a conceptual point of view, it is hard to believe that cells that have become almost terminally differentiated as keratinocytes (keratinizing squamous metaplasia) would take the genetic trouble to dedifferentiate back to a stage of reproductive function and then redifferentiate toward keratinocytes again. Theoretical approaches notwithstanding, the appearance of keratinizing squamous epithelium in the urinary bladder is a sign of abnormal behavior and the risk of cancer is not only greater than normal but is probably related to the amount of squamous epithelium present.

Histologically, squamous cell carcinomas are invasive lesions with a nodular infiltrative growth pattern (Fig. 4.11). Flat, noninvasive lesions composed of

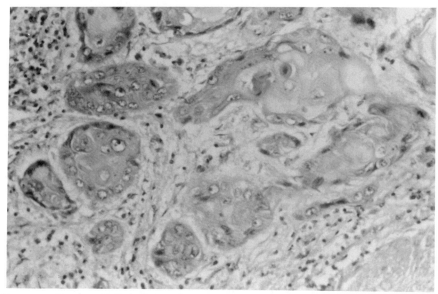

FIG. 4.11.   Squamous cell carcinoma invading the muscular wall of the urinary bladder. Despite deep invasion, the tumor nests tend to form keratin. H & E, × 192.

anaplastic squamous cells have rarely been observed and are not well characterized. Differentiation toward the surface is the rule and even deeply invasive tumors recapitulate keratinizing epithelium. At low magnification, the malignant epithelium is usually surrounded by a dense infiltrate rich in lymphocytes. Sheets and irregularly shaped nests of tumor cells are composed of a basophilic outer layer that soon evolves into the typical pavement-like arrangement of cells with acidophilic cytoplasm and distinct borders. Keratin pearls are common, as are areas of individual cell necrosis. At higher magnification, the cells have irregular nuclei with variable chromatin granularity. Many nuclei contain prominent nucleoli.

Cells exfoliated from squamous cell carcinomas are often fiber-like, reflecting changes that occur as the cells differentiate toward the surface. Their nuclei often lack the significant anaplasia seen in deeper portions of the histological specimens. Nevertheless, pure squamous cell cancers can almost always be detected in cytologic samples. Degeneration among the tumor cells is more common in squamous carcinomas than in any other type of urothelial malignancy. This may actually aide in cytologic diagnosis since degeneration tends to accentuate nuclear abnormalities and the unaltered nuclei tend to have fewer atypicalities than one might expect for a malignant neoplasm. The role of ancillary techniques such as flow cytometry in the detection, monitoring, and prognostication of squamous cell carcinomas has not been well defined, perhaps because the lesions are relatively uncommon and histologically distinctive.

MIXED CARCINOMA

As the name implies, a small percentage of urothelial neoplasms are composed of cells differentiating toward more than one type of epithelium. The most common situation mixes transitional cell with keratinizing squamous elements, but any combination can occur. Transitional cell-squamous carcinomas have often been classified as either very high-grade cancers (TCC-IV in the Friedman and Ash and Broders systems).[9,27] Mixed differentiation in the WHO scheme has been considered a form of metaplasia.[51] While the histological appearances are distinctive, it is more difficult to determine the biological significance of these tumors. Squamous differentiation is often found on the superficial portions of large transitional cell cancers, suggesting a nonspecific reaction to irritation. Almost all of the individual elements of a mixed carcinoma are associated with a poor prognosis when they occur in pure form and one might question whether mixtures make the outcome any worse. Since all of the elements usually represent high-grade cancer, malignant cells are readily apparent in urinary specimens. One might expect DNA ploidy to be abnormal since all mixtures contain high-grade transitional cells that are known to have a very high frequency of aneuploidy.

UNDIFFERENTIATED CARCINOMA

The term "undifferentiated" has been chosen to designate a rather heterogeneous group of neoplasms composed of small cells with very high nuclear:cytoplasmic ratios (Fig. 4.12). Pure forms of this tumor are rare, most reports having a large percentage of more differentiated elements.[7] At low magnification, the examiner is immediately concerned about lymphoma or small round cell sarcoma, but this problem is readily solved using appropriate immunoperoxidase reactions. Some cells with neuroendocrine differentiation are usually present, but elevated hormone levels in the circulation are uncommon. In general, these neoplasms look and act like small cell lung cancers. At higher

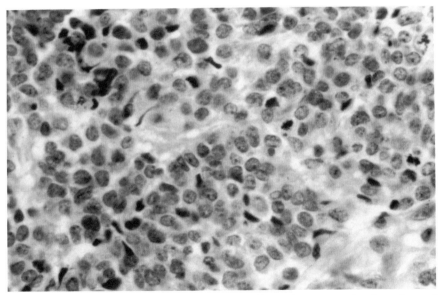

FIG. 4.12. Undifferentiated carcinoma of urinary bladder. These tumors often have the cytologic characteristics of small cell carcinomas of the lung. H & E, × 480.

magnification, the tumor cells have very scanty cytoplasm and fairly uniform nuclei that are densely packed in the tissue specimens. Intercellular cohesion occurs. Although small, the nuclei tend to be pleomorphic in the sense that no two have exactly the same shape. The chromatin is surprisingly evenly distributed and less coarsely granular than one might expect for a highly aggressive cancer. Nucleoli are not prominent.

In urinary specimens, malignant cells are numerous and loosely clustered. The cytoplasm is scanty and there are irregularities of nuclear borders. Chromatin is evenly distributed and tends to be finely granular. Nucleoli are not readily apparent. Although the nuclei tend to cluster and are larger than lymphocytes, they may be difficult to accurately classify.

ADENOCARCINOMA

Adenocarcinomas are relatively rare urothelial neoplasms that cannot be distinguished on pathological examination from similar cancers arising in the large intestine.[53] Every type of differentiation seen in the intestine has been observed in cancers arising in the bladder. Like other urothelial neoplasms, most adenocarcinomas arise at the bladder base. Adenocarcinomas arising in the dome have long been considered of urachal origin and there is no good reason to dispute this even though urachal remnants may be difficult to find in some cases and a significant percentage of urachal carcinomas are of nonglandular differentiation.[70]

All of the conceptual reasoning concerning the relationship between squamous metaplasia and squamous carcinoma can be applied to the relationship between intestinal metaplasia and adenocarcinoma (see section on "Squamous Cell Carcinoma"). The risk of cancer among patients with intestinal metaplasia seems to be proportional to the amount of urothelium that has been replaced by goblet cells so that individuals with cystitis glandularis, a condition in which goblet cells are relatively sparse, are at almost no risk for subsequent cancer. In contrast, patients with widespread intestinal metaplasia are at great risk.[53] Transitional cells have the capacity to create both intracellular and intercellular lumina.[14] In fact, normal superficial cells can secrete and store mucin, and a few mucin-containing cells can be identified in both normal and neoplastic transitional cell epithelium. When lumen formation among transitional cells is marked, some confusion as to the proper classification of the tumor usually occurs. Recognizing that small amounts of mucin can be produced by both normal and malignant transitional cells, it has been our preference to restrict the term "adenocarcinoma" to those malignancies that resemble the range of large intestinal cancers (Fig. 4.13).

Bladder adenocarcinomas occasionally occur as deeply infiltrating cancers without significant epithelial involvement.[31] In most such cases, the histological type is poorly differentiated and signet ring cells are prominent. The histogenesis of this type of infiltration is difficult to explain. The cells of bladder adenocarcinomas usually exhibit features of high-grade neoplasia and can be recognized in urinary samples. Accurate classification as adenocarcinoma is more difficult.

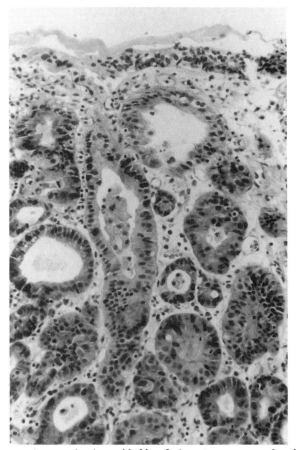

FIG. 4.13. Adenocarcinoma of urinary bladder. It is not uncommon for these lesions to be predominantly infiltrative rather than exophytic. They cannot be distinguished on light microscopic grounds from adenocarcinomas of the colon. H & E, × 150.

In rare instances, the glandular neoplasm is so well differentiated that its cells cannot be recognized as malignant when disaggregated from the tumor. The majority of bladder adenocarcinomas have aneuploid cell lines.[73]

The differential diagnosis of adenocarcinomas of the bladder is not extensive. Rarely, the neoplasm is so well differentiated that it can be recognized only by its infiltrative growth pattern. Portions of such tumors tend to have a villous pattern and the possibility of villous adenoma is the main differential consideration. As previously mentioned, adenocarcinomas of the bladder can be distinguished from similar lesions arising in the large intestine only by clinical and/or historical information. Transitional cell carcinomas with glandular lumina are composed of cells that secrete very small amounts of mucin and do not have a goblet cell appearance. Mucinous prostatic carcinomas have distinctive nuclear features and can be identified by their positive reactions for prostate-specific antigen.

CARCINOMA *IN SITU*

Despite several decades of study, carcinoma *in situ* (CIS) remains an enigma.[53] In the first place, it is difficult to define. While it may be axiomatic that all epithelial neoplasms must have an *in situ* phase, it is not at all clear when in the process of carcinogenesis this phase occurs, nor do we know how to recognize it. Most researchers and practitioners will agree that intraepithelial lesions composed of anaplastic cells that do not regress spontaneously are *in situ* carcinomas. But what about the intraepithelial lesions of lesser degrees of cellular atypia that may regress spontaneously? Are they also CIS or are they some other process—dysplasia, atypical hyperplasia? Do these lesser lesions evolve into the anaplastic ones or are they "dead-end" abnormalities that merely mark the organ as one at risk for developing cancer in the future? What about the anaplastic lesions? Are they young carcinomas detected before they could invade and metastasize or are they a special type of neoplasia with a limited potential for aggressive behavior that we can detect because it remains *in situ* for long periods of time? The answers to these questions are not known and accurate data are extremely difficult to collect. One might theorize that CIS occurs when the host has failed to prevent abnormal proliferation and control differentiation but has either managed to inhibit the development of the clonal heterogeneity necessary for dissemination or lacks some factor(s) that the neoplasm needs for aggressive behavior.

For the purpose of this discussion, carcinoma *in situ* will be defined as a flat, noninvasive urothelial lesion composed primarily of anaplastic cells that resemble those of low- and high-grade papillary and invasive carcinomas (G2 and G3 in WHO terminology) (Fig. 4.14). Replacement of the entire thickness of epithelium with anaplastic cells is not necessary for recognition of the neoplasm. A urothelial counterpart to severe dysplasia of the uterine cervix probably does not exist as a distinct biological entity.

Carcinoma *in situ* differs from other urothelial neoplasms in aspects other than its configuration. The difference in signs and symptoms has already been mentioned. In contrast to most urothelial tumors, CIS is not necessarily localized to the bladder base but occurs in multiple foci throughout the epithelium.[23,40] Most often, the *in situ* lesions have either been preceded by a papillary or invasive high-grade cancer or are found in association with one. CIS rarely accompanies papillomas. In this respect the disease could be considered part of a multifocal breakdown in local host defenses or seeding of the urothelium from a single focus of cancer. CIS occurring with or after a papillary or infiltrating neoplasm may have different significance to the patient than CIS that develops *de novo*.

Almost all thoroughly examined cystectomy specimens removed for bladder cancer have had areas of CIS, but the frequency of CIS in the bladders of individuals being followed with selected site biopsies for clinically manageable (superficial) carcinomas has been extremely low.[23,40,58] This data could be interpreted to mean that multifocal *in situ* lesions usually develop along with rather than prior to those bladder cancers that will require removal of the entire organ.

When patients develop CIS as their initial urothelial neoplasm, the long-term

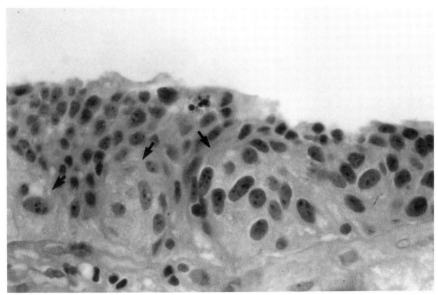

FIG. 4.14. Carcinoma *in situ* of urothelium. As in this case, it is not uncommon for the cells of CIS to undermine the adjacent normal epithelium. The demarcation between tumor and normal in this case is indicated by the *arrows*. H & E, × 480.

outlook is much better than if they had developed a papillary or invasive tumor of similar cytologic grade.[22] Death from disease is less than 20% compared to more than 50%; invasion occurs in only 34% compared to more than 80% of cases; and infiltration of the muscular wall is uncommon. This favorable outlook for a lesion composed of cells that are not phenotypically different from those comprising high-grade papillary and invasive cancers is a paradox that remains to be explained.[82] It tends to support the contention that aggressive behavior is not totally a function of tumor cell anaplasia.

Bladder biopsies from patients harboring carcinoma *in situ* are often denuded of diagnostic cells. In suspicious cases, an accurate interpretation cannot be rendered on the tissue specimens, but a clue to the process can often be obtained from the urinary sample. In the untreated case, CIS cells exfoliate in large number and appear in urine as high-grade cancerous elements that can be easily recognized by trained observers (Fig. 4.15). Urinary cytology is an essential procedure for the detection and monitoring of CIS since cystoscopy is only partially effective at localization and histology, even if tissue is taken from the lesion, may be noncontributory. The cells of carcinoma *in situ* do not differ significantly from those already described for high-grade transitional cell carcinomas, although they may occasionally be more uniform in size and exhibit less nuclear pleomorphism.

When tissue specimens are adequate, a range of neoplastic changes within urothelium may be seen in urothelial CIS. In the most common situation, the normal epithelium is almost completely replaced by cells with increased nuclear:cytoplasmic ratios and pleomorphic nuclei that have lost their normal

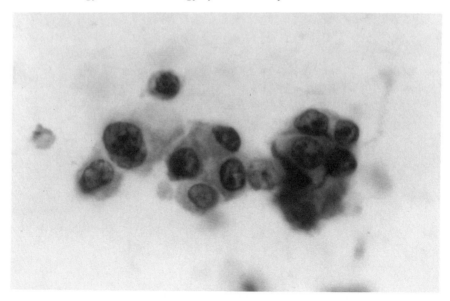

FIG. 4.15.   Urinary cytology from the lesion in Figure 4.14. The cellular features are indistinguishable from those of invasive transitional cell carcinoma. EA, × 756.

orientation (Fig. 4.14). Like other high-grade lesions, nuclear chromatin is coarsely granular and irregularly distributed. Nucleoli may be prominent in some nuclei. Mitoses are common and occur at all levels. Superficial cells may be retained, often in an attenuated form. In unusual cases, the cells may be very small with scanty cytoplasm or very large with acidophilic cytoplasm, but anaplastic nuclear features are a constant characteristic of CIS. A limited degree of maturation among neoplastic cells has been accepted in CIS, but grading has been discouraged primarily because slight maturation among epithelial cells in these lesions has not been shown to alter their biological behavior.

The cells of CIS seem to prefer an intramucosal environment. They grow by undermining the adjacent normal mucosa rather than invading the underlying tissue. Even under favorable conditions, *e.g.*, disruption of the mucosa by biopsies, the intraepithelial pattern is retained. Pathologists observing the finger-like projection of intramucosal CIS in sections taken *"en face"* should be aware of this growth preference to avoid an erroneous interpretation of dysplasia or atypia.

Both DNA aneuploidy and an increased proliferation rate are constant findings in urothelial CIS.[77] Neither finding has apparently altered the empirically observed favorable prognosis, at least in primary lesions. To confound the issue further, the antibody reactions to CIS more closely resemble those of a low-grade papillary tumor than those of a high-grade invasive cancer.[3]

POSSIBLE PRECURSORS OF UROTHELIAL NEOPLASIA

This discussion would not be complete without a reference to lesions that have long been considered premalignant and which some experts have included among the intraepithelial neoplasms. The subject is complicated and can only be summarized here.[53,60] Most pathologists and students of carcinogenesis believe that carcinomas must arise in epithelium and are created by proliferation of a single cell whose DNA has been unalterably changed by a limited number of mutational events. Until recently, the prevailing theory held that neoplasms progress through a series of graded morphological changes from slight to marked to CIS before invading the adjacent tissues. Based on this paradigm, it is only necessary for pathologists to be familiar with the characteristics of invasive cancers and to recognize intraepithelial changes of decreasing severity to identify the earliest neoplasms. In fact, most studies of chemical carcinogenesis in experimental animals seem to support this view.

This approach has not been strongly supported by many empirical observations, some of which have already been summarized in the section on "Transitional Cell Papillomas." Among intraepithelial lesions, the earliest changes observed in experimental animals tend to be subtle and difficult to adequately describe, especially since the cells in any particular area do not progress in lock-step from one degree of severity to the next. Further, long-term follow-up of these lesions in human bladders has not been possible and our knowledge of their likely growth potential has been deduced from observations of patients who already have cancer. The situation is further complicated when experts in carcinogenesis tell us that the creation of an epithelial neoplasm might take more than 100 interrelated steps and is at least potentially never irreversible. Little wonder, then, that long-time students of bladder cancer cannot agree on even basic things such as what these lesions should be called and how they should be defined.

In our view, carcinogenesis is a dynamic interaction between potential neoplastic events and host defense systems.[6,19,21,28,49,61,63,68,74,75] Most often, the host wins, cancer does not develop, and the individual dies of something else. Occasionally the neoplasm wins and the host succumbs to a cancer or a complication directly related to it. During any particular period of observation, either host or tumor may seem to have the upper hand. The phase of this interaction at which epithelial cells assume independent regulation of their growth, *i.e.*, become a neoplasm, may or may not be immediately revealed by phenotypic changes that can be reliably recognized under the light microscope.[37,60]

When epithelial cells invade the surrounding tissue or metastasize to other sites, we know they are neoplastic regardless of their resemblance to normal. When changes are confined to the epithelium, however, we must depend on two factors to recognize a neoplasm: cellular anaplasia and lack of spontaneous reversibility to normal. When one or both are missing, we cannot be certain that the lesions are neoplastic and should not label them as such. Intraepithelial lesions of lesser severity than CIS probably represent a situation where the host seems to have the upper hand, *i.e.*, has been able to control but not prevent abnormal proliferation and differentiation as well as completely inhibit the formation of the clonal heterogeneity necessary for invasion. This situation may change over time and patients with these lesions are at risk for the future development of carcinoma.[66] More progress in the area might be made if we were to concentrate more effort on determining the degree of risk for cancer that is associated with dysplastic urothelial changes.

Given this conceptual framework, urothelial lesions of lesser severity than CIS have been called dysplasia, although we would not object to equivalent terms such as atypical hyperplasia so long as the words neoplasia, carcinoma, and cancer are not included. Dysplastic lesions manifest a spectrum of morphological changes between CIS and normal. They can be distinguished on morphological grounds from reactive/regenerative/reparative states but we cannot be certain that similar epithelial changes could not be caused by noncarcinogenic events. After all, the ability of epithelium to respond to abnormal stimuli is limited and we observe tissue reactions rather than causal events in our light microscope. Our knowledge of the morphological characteristics of urothelial dysplasia has been heavily influenced by studies of experimental carcinogenesis where the development of transitional cell carcinomas could be directly observed by light microscopy.[37,66]

In dysplastic urothelium, the cells are abnormally oriented and the nuclei appear to cluster at low magnifications (Fig. 4.16).[59] This nuclear crowding and overlapping is the hallmark of dysplastic change and the diagnosis is suspect in its absence. The cytoplasmic clearing so characteristic of normal basal and intermediate urothelial cells is reduced or absent. The superficial cell layer is retained. Dysplastic lesions in humans are rarely hyperplastic. At higher magnification, nuclei are larger than normal and tend to be rounded or oblong. They often have a single sharp indentation or shallow depression in their borders. Chromatin is finely granular and evenly distributed. Nucleoli are small or absent.

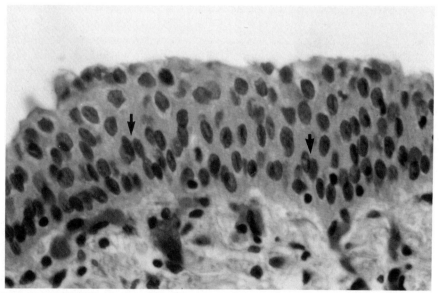

FIG. 4.16.   Urothelial dysplasia. Note the tendency for nuclear clustering (*arrows*) as well as the slight loss of nuclear polarization. H & E, × 480.

Few dysplastic cells are exfoliated into urinary samples. When present, their features are similar to those described above. The changes of urothelial dysplasia are often subtle. Fortunately, normal urothelial cells are almost always present elsewhere in the specimen for comparison.

Adjunctive tests such as those documenting blood group antigens, DNA ploidy, and antigenic composition have not usually been performed on purely dysplastic lesions and the reported results are difficult to evaluate. In many cases, photomicrographs of lesions called dysplasia reveal changes that would not fit our definition. Since the cells of dysplasia can be considered the flat phenotypic counterparts of transitional cell papillomas, one might expect similar results, *i.e.*, a high frequency of normal blood group antigens, DNA euploidy, and normal antigenic expression.

SUMMARY

Urothelial neoplasia is a complex subject that can be only partially understood by careful study of the light microscopic features of individual lesions. Despite decades of study, our knowledge concerning the interaction of neoplastic events and host responses remains rudimentary. Most information has been collected by observing cases (usually in retrospect) that have been grouped according to relatively arbitrary criteria based on the phenotypic appearances of lesions as they are viewed through the light microscope. When evaluating human disease, we are always forced to reason backwards to determine the most likely histogenesis and to project forward to assess the most likely prognosis. Both types of reasoning must be filled with conjecture since direct observations from the initial events to the end results are not possible. Under these constricting circumstances, a conceptual framework into which our often anecdotal observations can be placed is more important than we would like to admit. With this in mind, I have taken advantage of the monograph format to risk a speculative approach to the subject, at least as it applies to the significance of the pathological features.

In the past, we have accepted the view that all human hosts are essentially the same and that variations in cancer type and behavior are related almost entirely to the genetic ingenuity of the cancer cells themselves. Perhaps we should now entertain the opposite view, that carcinogenic events are ubiquitous and that cancer in any individual patient represents only what that patient will allow to grow in his or her body. We have devoted almost all of our collective research energy to examining the tumor. I believe that the pace of future progress can be significantly increased if we can think of more ways to examine the patient.

REFERENCES

1. Babu, V. R., Lutz, M. D., Miles, B. J., Farah, R. N., Weiss, L., and Van Dyke, D. L. Tumor behavior in transitional cell carcinoma of the bladder in relation to chromosomal markers and histopathology. *Cancer Res 47:* 6800–6805, 1987.
2. Badalament, R. A., Hermansen, D. K., Kimmel, M., Gay, H., Herr, H. W., Fair, W. R., Whitmore, W. F., Jr., and Melamed, M. R. The sensitivity of bladder wash flow cytometry, bladder wash cytology and voided cytology in the detection of bladder carcinoma. *Cancer 60:* 1423–1427, 1987.
3. Bander, N. H. Monoclonal antibodies in urologic oncology. *Cancer 60:* 6058–6067, 1987.

4. Benson, R. C., Jr., Swanson, S. K., and Farrow, G. M. Relationship of leukoplakia to urothelial malignancy. *J Urol 131:* 507–511, 1984.

5. Bergkvist, A., Ljungqvist, A., and Moberger, G. Classification of bladder tumours based on the cellular pattern. *Acta Chir Scand 130:* 371–378, 1965.

6. Biswas, C. Tumor cell stimulation of collagenase production by fibroblasts. *Biochem Biophys Res Commun 109:* 1026–1034, 1982.

7. Blomjous, C. E. M., Vos, W., De Voogt, H. J., Van Der Valk, P., Meijer, C. J. L. M. Small cell carcinoma of the urinary bladder: A clinicopathologic, morphometric, immunohistochemical, and ultrastructural study of 18 cases. *Cancer 64:* 1347–1357, 1989.

8. Boring, C. C., Squires, T. S., and Tong, T. Cancer statistics. *CA 41:* 19–36, 1991.

9. Broders, A. C. Epithelium of the genito-urinary organs. *Ann Surg 75:* 574–604, 1922.

10. Chowaniec, J. Aetiology: Epidemiological and experimental considerations. In *Bladder Cancer,* vol 60, edited by P. Skrabanek and A. Walsh. Geneva, UICC Technical Report Series, 1981, pp. 118–143.

11. Coon, J. S., Deitch, A. D., de Vere White, R. W., Koss, L. G., Melamed, M. R., Reeder, J. E., Weinstein, R. S., Wersto, R. P., and Wheeless, L. L. Check samples for laboratory self-assessment in DNA flow cytometry: The National Cancer Institute's Flow Cytometry Network experience. *Cancer 63:* 1592–1599, 1989.

12. Crabbe, J. G. S. Cytology of voided urine with special reference to "benign" papilloma and some of the problems encountered in the preparation of the smears. *Acta Cytol 5:* 233–240, 1961.

13. Cutler, S. J., Heney, N. M., and Friedell, G. H. Longitudinal study of patient's with bladder cancer: Factors associated with disease recurrence and progression. In *Bladder Cancer,* AUA Monographs, vol 1, edited by W. W. Bonney. Baltimore, Williams & Wilkins, 1982, pp. 35–46.

14. Delladetsima, J., Antonakopoulos, G. N., Dapolla, V., and Kittas, C. Intraepithelial lumina in urothelial bladder neoplasms: A histochemical, immunohistochemical, and electron microscopy study. *APMIS 97:* 406–412, 1989.

15. Del Senno, L., Maestri, I., Piva, R., Hanau, S., Reggiani, A., Romano, A., and Russo, G. Differential hypomethylation of the c-myc protooncogene in bladder cancers at different stages and grades. *J Urol 142:* 146 149, 1989.

16. DeMeester, L. J., Farrow, G. M., and Utz, D. C. Inverted papillomas of the urinary bladder. *Cancer 36:* 505–513, 1975.

17. Droller, M. J. Transitional cell cancer: Upper tracts and bladder. In *Campbell's Urology,* edited by P. C. Walsh, R. F. Gittes, A. D. Perlmutter, and T. A. Stamey, Ed. 5. W. B. Saunders, Philadelphia, 1986, pp. 1343–1440.

18. Dukes, C. E., and Masina, F. Classification of epithelial tumours of the bladder. *Br J Urol 21:* 273–295, 1949.

19. Dvorak, H. F. Tumors: Wounds that do not heal. *N Engl J Med 315:* 1650–1659, 1986.

20. El-Aaser, A. A. Aetiology of Bilharzial bladder cancer in Egypt. In *Bladder Cancer,* vol 60, edited by P. Skrabanek and A. Walsh. Geneva, UICC Technical Report Series, 1981, pp. 110–117.

21. Farber, E. Cancer development and its natural history: A cancer prevention perspective. *Cancer 62:* 1676–1679, 1988.

22. Farrow, G. M., and Utz, D. C. Observations on microinvasive transitional cell carcinoma of the urinary bladder. *Clin Oncol 1:* 609–615, 1982.

23. Farrow, G. M., Utz, D. C., and Rife, C. C. Morphological and clinical observations of patients with early bladder cancer treated with total cystectomy. *Cancer Res 36:* 2495–2501, 1976.

24. Faysal, M. H. Squamous cell carcinoma of the bladder. *J Urol 126:* 598–599, 1981.

25. Fradet, Y., Tardif, M., Bourget, L., and Robert, J. Clinical cancer progression in urinary bladder tumors evaluated by multiparameter flow cytometry with monoclonal antibodies. *Cancer Res 50:* 432–437, 1990.

26. Friedell, G. H., Bell, J. R., Burney, S. W., Soto, E. A., and Tiltman, A. J. Histopathology and the classification of urinary bladder carcinoma. *Urol Clin North Am 3:* 53–70, 1976.

27. Friedman, N. B., and Ash, J. E. Tumors of the urinary bladder. Atlas of tumor pathology fascicle #31a, 1st series. Washington D.C., AFIP, 1959.

28. Frost, P., and Fidler, I. J. Biology of metastasis. *Cancer 58:* 550–553, 1986.

29. Fujii, H., Cunha, G. R., and Norman, J. T. The induction of adenocarcinomatous differentiation in neoplastic bladder epithelium by an embryonic prostatic inductor. *J Urol 128:* 858–861, 1982.
30. Gibas, Z., Prout, G. R., Jr., Connolly, J. G., et al. Nonrandom chromosomal changes in transitional cell carcinoma of the bladder. *Cancer Res 44:* 1257–1264, 1984.
31. Grignon, D. J., Ro, Jy, Ayla, A. G., and Johnson, D. E. Primary signet-ring cell carcinoma of the urinary bladder. *Am J Clin Pathol 95:* 13–20, 1991.
32. Guirguis, R., Schiffmann, E., Liu, B., et al. Detection of autocrine motility factor in urine as a marker of bladder cancer. *J Natl Cancer Inst 80:* 1203–1211, 1988.
33. Heney, N. M., Ahmed, S., Flanagan, M. J., et al. Superficial bladder cancer: Progression and recurrence. *J Urol 130:* 1083–1086, 1983.
34. Hoover, R., and Cole, P. Population trends in cigarette smoking and bladder cancer. *Am J Epidemiol 94:* 409–418, 1971.
35. Huland, E., Huland, H., and Schneider, A. W. Quantitative immunocytology in the management of patients with superficial bladder carcinoma I. A marker to identify patients who do not require prophylaxis. *J Urol 144:* 637–640, 1990.
36. Illmensee, K., and Stevens, L. C. Teratomas and chimeras. *Sci Am 240:* 121–132, 1979.
37. Ito, N., Matayoshi, K., Arai, M., Frable, W., Corder, M. P., Hafermann, M. D., and Hawkins, I. R. for the National Bladder Cancer Collaborative Group. Effect of various factors on induction of urinary bladder tumors in animals by N-butyl-N-(4-hydroxybutyl)nitrosamine. *GANN 62:* 151–159, 1973.
38. Jordan, A. M., Weingarten, J., and Murphy, W. M. Transitional cell neoplasms of the urinary bladder: Can biologic potential be predicted from histologic grading? *Cancer 60:* 2766–2774, 1987.
39. Koss, L. G. Tumors of the urinary bladder. Atlas of tumor pathology fascicle #11. 2nd series. Washington, D.C., AFIP, 1975.
40. Koss, L. G. Mapping of the urinary bladder: Its impact on the concepts of bladder cancer. *Hum Pathol 10:* 533–548, 1979.
41. Kurz, K. R., Pitts, W. R., and Vaughan, E. D., Jr. The natural history of patients less than 40 years old with bladder tumor. *J Urol 137:* 395–397, 1987.
42. Lerman, R. I., Hutter, V. P., and Whitmore, W. F. Papilloma of the urinary bladder. *Cancer 25:* 333–342, 1970.
43. Limas, C., and Lange, P. A, B, H antigen detectability in normal and neoplastic urothelium: Influence of methodologic factors. *Cancer 49:* 2476–2484, 1982.
44. Liotta, L. A., and Kohn, E. Cancer invasion and metastases. *JAMA 263:* 1123–1126, 1990.
45. Lower, G. M., Jr. Concepts in causality: Chemically induced human urinary bladder cancer. *Cancer 49:* 1056–1066, 1982.
46. Lynch, C. F., Platz, C. E., Jones, M. P., and Gazzaniga, J. M. Cancer registry problems in classifying invasive bladder cancer. *J Natl Cancer Inst 83:* 429–433, 1991.
47. Melamed, M. R., and Klein, F. A. Flow cytometry of urinary bladder irrigation specimens. *Hum Pathol 15:* 302–305, 1984.
48. Messing, E. M. Clinical implications of the expression of epidermal growth factor receptors in human transitional cell carcinoma. *Cancer Res 50:* 2530–2537, 1990.
49. Moroco, J. R., Solt, D. B., and Polverini, P. J. Sequential loss of suppressor genes for three specific functions during in vivo carcinogenesis. *Lab Invest 63:* 298–306, 1990.
50. Morrison, D. A., Murphy, W. M., Ford, K. S., and Soloway, M. S. Surveillance of stage O, grade I bladder cancer by cytology alone—is it acceptable? *J Urol 132:* 672–674, 1984.
51. Mostofi, F. K., Sorbin, L. H., and Torloni, H. Histological typing of urinary bladder tumours, international classification of tumours. 10, Geneva, WHO, 1973.
52. Murphy, W. M. *Atlas of Bladder Carcinoma.* Chicago, ASCP Press, 1986.
53. Murphy, W. M. Diseases of the urinary bladder, urethra, ureters, and renal pelves. In *Urological Pathology,* edited by W. M. Murphy. Philadelphia, W. B. Saunders, 1989, pp. 64–96.
54. Murphy, W. M. Current status of urinary cytology in the evaluation of bladder neoplasms. *Hum Pathol 21:* 886–896, 1990.

55. Murphy, W. M., Chandler, R. W., and Trafford, R. M. Flow cytometry of deparaffinized nuclei compared to histological grading for the pathological evaluation of transitional cell carcinomas. *J Urol 135:* 694–697, 1986.

56. Murphy, W. M., Emerson, L. D., Chandler, R. W., Moinuddin, S. M., and Solway, M. S. Flow cytometry vs. urinary cytology in the evaluation of patients with bladder cancer. *J Urol 136:* 815–819, 1986.

57. Murphy, W. M., and Miller, A. W. Cytology in the detection and followup of urothelial tumors. In *Bladder Cancer*, edited by N. Javadpour. Baltimore, Williams & Wilkins, 1984, pp. 100–122.

58. Murphy, W. M., Nagy, G. K., Rao, M. K., Soloway, M. S., Parija, G. C., Cox, C. E., II, and Friedell, G. H. "Normal" urothelium in patients with bladder cancer. A preliminary report from the National Bladder Cancer Collaborative Group A. *Cancer 44:* 1050–1058, 1979.

59. Murphy, W. M., and Soloway, M. S. Developing carcinoma (dysplasia) of the urinary bladder. *Pathol Annu 17:* 197–217, 1982.

60. Murphy, W. M., and Soloway, M. S. Urothelial dysplasia. *J Urol 127:* 849–854, 1982.

61. Nemec, R. E., Toole, B. P., and Knudson, W. The cell surface hyaluronate binding sites of invasive human bladder carcinoma cells. *Biochem Biophys Res Commun 149:* 249–257, 1987.

62. Nemoto, R., Hattori, K., and Uchida, K. Estimation of growth fraction in situ in human bladder cancer with bromodeoxyuridine labelling. *Br J Urol 65:* 27–31, 1990.

63. Noguchi, S., Yura, Y., Sherwood, E. R., et al. Stimulation of stromal cell growth by normal rat urothelial cell-derived epidermal growth factor. *Lab Invest 62:* 538–544, 1990.

64. Okamura, K., Miyake, K., Koshikawa, T., and Asai, J. Growth fractions of transitional cell carcinomas of the bladder defined by the monoclonal antibody Ki-67. *J Urol 144:* 875–878, 1990.

65. Ooms, E. C. M., Anderson, W. A. D., Alon, S. C. L., Boon, M. E., and Veldhuizen, R. W. Analysis of the performance of pathologists in the grading of bladder tumors. *Hum Pathol 14:* 140–143, 1983.

66. Oyasu, R., Samma, S., Ozono, S., Bauer, K., Wallemark, C. B., and Homa, Y. Induction of high-grade, high-stage carcinomas in the rat urinary bladder. *Cancer 59:* 451–458, 1987.

67. Parry, W. L., and Hemstreet, G. P., III. Cancer detection by quantitative fluorescence image analysis. *J Urol 139:* 270–274, 1988.

68. Pauli, B. U., and Knudson, W. Tumor invasion: A consequence of destructive and compositional matrix alterations. *Hum Pathol 19:* 628–639, 1988.

69. Prout, G. J., Jr. Bladder carcinoma and the TNM system of classification. *J Urol 117:* 583–590, 1977.

70. Sheldon, C. A., Clayman, R. V., Gonzalez, R., et al. Malignant urachal lesions. *J Urol 131:* 1–8, 1984.

71. Smeets, W., Pauwels, R., Laarakkers, Debruyne, F., and Geraedts, J. Chromosomal analysis of bladder cancer. III. Nonrandom alterations. *Cancer Genet Cytogenet 29:* 29–41, 1987.

72. Soloway, M. S., Murphy, W. M., Johnson, D. E., et al. Summary of workshop on initial evaluation and response criteria for patients with superficial bladder cancer. *Br J Urol 66:* 380–385, 1990.

73. Song, J., Farrow, G. M., and Lieber, M. M. Primary adenocarcinoma of the bladder: Favorable prognostic significance of deoxyribonucleic acid diploidy measured by flow cytometry. *J Urol 144:* 1115–1118, 1990.

74. Studzinski, G. P., Moore, D. C., and Carter, D. L. Suppressor genes; restraint of growth or of tumor progression? *Lab Invest 63:* 279–282, 1990.

75. Tannock, I. F. Biology of tumor growth. *Hosp Practice 18:* 81–93, 1983.

76. Torti, F. M., Lum, V. L., Aston, D., Mackenzie, N., Faysel, M., Shortliffe, L. D., and Freiha, F. Superficial bladder cancer: The primacy of grade in the development of invasive disease. *J Clin Oncol 5:* 125–130, 1987.

77. Tribukait, B. Flow cytometry in surgical pathology and cytology of tumors of the genitourinary tract. In *Advances in Clinical Cytology*, vol II, edited by L. G. Koss and D. V. Coleman. New York, Masson, 1984, pp. 163–189.

78. Tribukait, B. Flow cytometry in assessing the clinical aggressiveness of genito-urinary neoplasms. *World J Urol 5:* 108–122, 1987.

79. Tsi, Y. C., Nichols, P. W., Hiti, Al, et al. Allelic losses of chromosomes 9, 11, and 17 in human bladder cancer. *Cancer Res 50:* 44–47, 1990.

80. Utz, D. C., Farrow, G. M., Rife, C. C., Segura, J. W., and Zincke, H. Carcinoma *in situ* of the bladder. *Cancer 45:* 1842–1848, 1980.

81. Viola, M. V., Fromowitz, F., Oravez, S., et al. *ras* Oncogene p21 expression is increased in premalignant lesions and high grade bladder carcinoma. *J Exp Med 161:* 1213–1218, 1985.

82. Weinstein, R. S., Miller, A. W., III, and Pauli, B. U. Carcinoma in situ: Comments on the pathobiology of a paradox. *Urol Clin North Am 7:* 523–531, 1980.

83. Wheelock, E. F., and Robinson, M. K. Biology of disease: Endogenous control of the neoplastic process. *Lab Invest 48:* 120–139, 1983.

84. Wied, G. L., Bartels, P. H., Bibbo, M., and Dytch, H. E. Image analysis in quantitative cytopathology and histopathology. *Hum Pathol 20:* 549–571, 1989.

85. Widran, J., Sanchez, R., and Gruhn, J. Squamous metaplasia of the bladder: A study of 450 patients. *J Urol 112:* 479–482, 1974.

86. Young, R. H. Unusual variants of primary bladder carcinoma and secondary tumors of the bladder. In *Pathology of the Urinary Bladder*, edited by R. H. Young. New York, Churchill Livingstone, 1989, pp. 103–138.

87. Yura, Y., Hayashi, O., Kelly, M., and Oyasu, R. Identification of epidermal growth factor as a component of the rat urinary bladder tumor-enhancing urinary fractions. *Cancer Res 49:* 1548–1553, 1989.

Chapter 5

Image Analysis and Flow Cytometry of Tumors of Prostate and Bladder; With a Comment on Molecular Biology of Urothelial Tumors

LEOPOLD G. KOSS AND BOGDAN CZERNIAK

The quest for objective information on behavior and prognosis of human cancer, hence, by implication, the optimal modes of therapy, has led to a large number of studies testing the value of measurements of various cell components. These studies ranged from a simple morphometry of cancer cells, already initiated in 1930s, to more sophisticated approaches that currently include image analysis, flow cytometry, and molecular biology.[32] Image analysis and flow cytometry are two related yet dissimilar techniques that serve to quantitate various cell components. The similarities and differences between the two techniques are shown in Table 5.1.

These two techniques have been applied to quantitation of DNA content, and, more recently, to the study of various cell components identified by molecular biological techniques, such as steroid and other receptors, and a variety of oncogenes.[15] In reference to tumors of the two organs under discussion, *i.e.*, the prostate and the bladder, both techniques have been applied for purposes of objective assessment and prognosis. A review of the work accomplished to date by us and others is the subject of this summary.

THE PROSTATE

Carcinoma of the prostate is a common disease, affecting primarily elderly males. Depending on the method of investigation, anywhere from 20–100% of males living to the age of 75 years and dying of other causes will have microscopic foci of carcinoma in their prostates.[46] Death from prostatic carcinoma is comparatively very infrequent. For 1989, the American Cancer Society projected that 103,000 males would be diagnosed as having prostate cancer and only about 28,000 would die of it.[48] As the stage of the disease is not considered in such statistics, it is likely that the annual prevalence rate of 100,000 cases includes all stages of disease, many of the carcinomas being incidental findings in prostatic chips and some discovered by the new ultrasound detection methods.[2,37] If one were to calculate a ratio of occult to clinically manifest prostatic cancer, it would likely be on the order of 10:1, assuming that there are, in the United States,

TABLE 5.1. INFORMATION PROCESSING AND DATA EXTRACTION IN FLOW CYTOMETRY AND IMAGE ANALYSIS

	Flow Cytometry	Image Analysis Cytophotometry
Sample preparation	Single particle suspension (complex)	Smear (simple)
Staining	Specific fluorochromes	Nonspecific or specific stains
Principal single parameter measurement	Histograms of fluorescence (*i.e.*, DNA)	Histograms of digitized images based on light absorption or transmission (*i.e.*, DNA, steroid receptors)
Two or more parameter measurements	Synchronous, limited (*i.e.*, DNA vs. oncogene expression)	Synchronous or sequential limited by stain
Morphologic features of cells	Very limited	Multiple feature extraction
Visual control	None (except by sorting)	Yes
Software	LIST mode histogram analysis. Cell cycle compartments (rapid)	Multifeature analysis (relatively slow)
Cell sorting	Yes	No
Control samples	Multiple options	Limited
Applicability to histology	No	Yes

about 2 million living males over the age of 75, that half of them have occult carcinoma, and that only 100,000 of them will have the diagnosis established. The ratio of occult carcinoma to death from prostatic cancer, based on the same reasoning, would be approximately 40:1. Similar conclusions have been recently reached by Gittes.[22] While these figures are probably not accurate, they strongly suggest that not all cancers of the prostate have the same behavior or clinical significance. Such observations raise serious questions as to whether small, prostatic carcinomas incidentally discovered by ultrasound[27] should be treated at par with clinically overt disease. Answering this question may have a major impact on the quality of life for a substantial segment of the society. Finding the suitable tumor parameters that would answer this question is yet another matter. While some of the parameters in cells can be measured, others, possibly more important, still remain elusive.

To address this question in the simplest possible manner, we decided to measure DNA in two synchronous studies: (1) a prospective study based on prostatic aspiration smears and fragments of prostatic chips; and (2) a retrospective study based on follow-up of patients with known disease, on whom old material in the form of aspiration smears and tissue biopsies was available. The emphasis in the prospective study was on small prostatic carcinomas, preferably stage A. In the retrospective study most tumors were in stages B, C, and D.[1]

MATERIAL AND METHODS

FLOW CYTOMETRY

Material for the prospective DNA analysis was obtained by direct aspiration of palpable prostatic nodules or by aspirating prostatic chips or prostatectomy specimens with a 24-caliber needle attached to the syringe. The diagnoses in all samples obtained by direct aspirations were confirmed by histological examination of the prostatic biopsy or prostatectomy specimens. In samples obtained from surgical material the tissue was identified and processed for histological examination to determine whether the sample pertained to cancer or to a benign process. The material was processed for flow cytometry, as previously described, using propidium iodide as fluorochrome.[34] DNA histograms were obtained initially on an Ortho ICP-22A flow cytometer and subsequently on an EPICS C flow cytometer (Coulter Electronics, Hialeah, FL), using the 488 nm line of an argonion laser, at 250 mW of output power. The results, based on a minimum of 10,000 nuclei per sample, were analyzed on a DEC 11/73 computer (Digital Equipment Corp., Maynard, MA), using a cell cycle analysis program previously described.[34] Nucleated chicken erythrocytes and normal human lymphocytes were used as controls.

IMAGE ANALYSIS

Direct prostatic smears, whether in the prospective or the retrospective study, were destained and stained with Feulgen, as previously described.[1] Quantitation of DNA was performed using a CAS 100 image analysis instrument (Cell Analysis System, Elmhurst, IL). Rat hepatocytes, provided by the manufacturer, and normal prostatic cells were used as controls.

HISTOGRAM CLASSIFICATION

Although the classification of DNA histograms is not always easy or simple,[34] the results of this study are presented by classifying the histograms as "diploid" and "nondiploid." This histogram classification is less controversial than a more precise analysis. In general there was reasonable concordance between the two modes of measurement, although occasionally image analysis disclosed aneuploid cells in the absence of abnormalities on the histograms obtained by flow cytometry, as previously noted.[36] In such cases the more abnormal of the two histograms was judged to be valid. Examples of histograms obtained by the two methods on the same patients are shown in Figures 5.1 and 5.2.

RESULTS

PROSPECTIVE STUDY

The results are presented in Tables 5.2 through 5.7. The study is based on 652 samples with adequate DNA histograms (Table 5.2). The following comments are in order.

BENIGN PROSTATIC HYPERTROPHY

Five hundred twenty (98%) of the cases studied were either diploid or had a slight increase in the S-phase cells, not exceeding 6%. Eleven cases (2%) disclosed aneuploid pattern of DNA, including four cases with a tetraploid type of histogram (Table 5.3). Several of these cases were restudied histologically by step sections and no evidence of carcinoma was observed. Whether these patients are

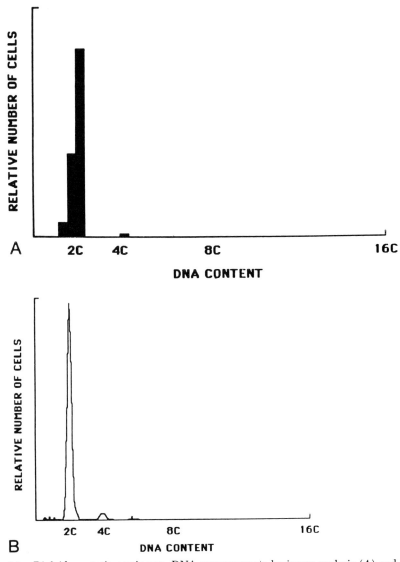

FIG. 5.1.   Diploid prostatic carcinoma. DNA measurements by image analysis (*A*) and by flow cytometry (*B*). (Courtesy of Dr. James Amberson.)

candidates for a future development of prostate cancer cannot be stated at this time.

PROSTATIC CARCINOMA

The analysis pertains to 82 fully evaluated cases of prostatic carcinoma (Table 5.4). The distribution of cell cycle compartments in diploid and nondiploid carcinomas is shown in Table 5.5. It may be noted that the proportion of cells in the diploid compartment is the same for diploid carcinomas and for benign

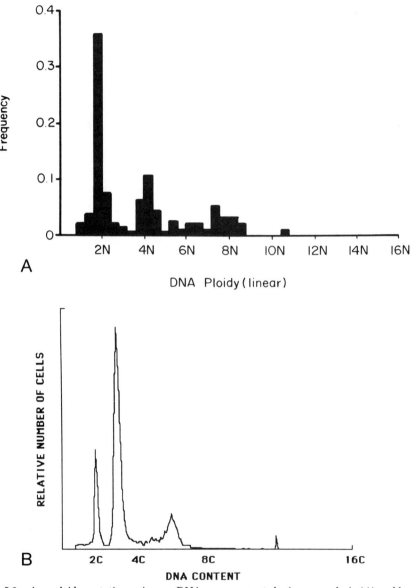

FIG. 5.2.   Aneuploid prostatic carcinoma. DNA measurements by image analysis (*A*) and by flow cytometry (*B*). (Courtesy of Dr. James Amberson.)

prostatic hypertrophy. As may be seen from Table 5.6, most diploid carcinomas were still confined to the prostate. There was, however, a clear difference in behavior: none of the 34 patients with stage A carcinoma showed evidence of disease after 3 to 5 years of follow-up. On the other hand, 22 of 24 patients with diploid carcinomas in stage B of disease had clinical evidence of residual disease or recurrence. In 14 of the 18 patients with carcinomas classified as nondiploid

TABLE 5.2. PROSTATE: PROSPECTIVE STUDY OF DNA CONTENT, MATERIAL

Material	n
Adequate DNA histograms (patients)	
Benign prostatic hypertrophy	531
Documented carcinoma	101
Total	632
Inadequate DNA histograms	20
Grand total	652

TABLE 5.3. PROSTATE: PROSPECTIVE STUDY OF DNA CONTENT, BENIGN PROSTATIC HYPERTROPHY

DNA Histograms	n
Diploid	520
Nondiploid	11[a] (2%)
	531

[a] No cancer found in extensive studies of chips.

TABLE 5.4. PROSTATE: PROSPECTIVE STUDY OF DNA CONTENT, PROSTATIC CARCINOMA (FULLY EVALUATED CASES)

Type	n
Diploid	64
Nondiploid	18
Total	82

TABLE 5.5. PROSTATE: PROSPECTIVE STUDY OF DNA CONTENT, CELL CYCLE COMPARTMENTS

	Diploid Compartment	>Diploid
Benign prostatic hypertrophy (50 diploid cases)	92.0 ± 5.6^a	7.2 ± 3.8
Prostatic carcinoma diploid ($n = 64$)	92.15 ± 4.8	7.8 ± 4.3
Nondiploid (18)	64.80 ± 22.7	33.6 ± 21.5

[a] Mean and standard error.

TABLE 5.6. PROSTATE: PROSPECTIVE STUDY, CORRELATION OF DNA PLOIDY WITH STAGES OF PROSTATIC CARCINOMA[a]

	n	Intraprostatic		Disseminated	
		A	B	C	D
Diploid	64	34 (0)	24 (22)	6	
Nondiploid	18		5 (5)	6 (2)	7 (7)
Total	82				

[a] Numbers in parentheses are patients with clinical evidence of disease.

TABLE 5.7. PROSTATE: RETROSPECTIVE STUDY, CORRELATION OF DNA PLOIDY WITH
STAGES OF PROSTATIC CARCINOMA[a]

		Intraprostatic		Disseminated	
	n	A	B	C	D
Diploid	17	1	6	1	9
Nondiploid	51	0	13	7	31
Total	68				

[a] Modified from Amberson, J. B., and Koss, L. G. Measurements of DNA as a prognostic factor in prostatic carcinoma. In *Prognostic Cytometry and Cytopathology of Prostate Cancer*, edited by J. P. Karr, D. S. Coffey, and W. Gardner, Jr. New York, Elsevier, 1988, pp. 281–286.

in stages B, C, and D of disease, there was evidence of persisting or recurring disease.

RETROSPECTIVE STUDY

This study conducted by Dr. James Amberson at the New York Hospital-Cornell was concluded after an evaluation of 68 cases of prostatic carcinoma. The DNA ploidy was determined on prostatic aspiration smears by image analysis. The summary is provided in Table 5.7. It may be noted that there were only 16 diploid carcinomas (23%) in stages B, C, and D of disease, the bulk of tumors in advanced stages being nondiploid. By combining the results from the prospective and retrospective studies, it is evident that the proportion of diploid tumors decreases and nondiploid tumors increases with advancing stages of prostatic carcinoma (Tables 5.8 and 5.9).

COMMENT

The results of the studies summarized above clearly suggest that most stage A prostatic carcinomas with DNA content in the diploid range constitute little danger to the patient. This is most likely applicable to incidentally discovered small prostatic cancers. There is also evidence, however, that some of the diploid tumors may progress beyond stage A. Once they have reached stage B or higher, their behavior may change to some extent. Still, there is evidence from several retrospective studies[20,25,38,39,43,50] that even in these advanced stages the behavior of diploid carcinomas is less aggressive than that of aneuploid tumors. Auer and Zetterberg[3] and Forsslund and Zetterberg[21] studied retrospectively the DNA distribution in prostatic aspiration smears of two groups of patients with prostatic carcinoma: those whose disease progressed rapidly and those who have remained free of disease for 10 years or more. Nearly all tumors in the progressive group were nondiploid, whereas most tumors in the "cured" group were in the diploid range. Tribukait[52,53] has also documented that comparatively few carcinomas in stages C and D are diploid, whereas most stage A carcinomas are in that category. One is loath to make recommendations of clinical significance based on a laboratory study, but there appears to be excellent evidence that measuring the DNA content of prostatic carcinomas may be a very important laboratory procedure that may help in deciding the optimal treatment options (or the

TABLE 5.8. PROSTATIC CARCINOMA: COMBINED DNA PLOIDY DATA FROM THE PROSPECTIVE AND RETROSPECTIVE STUDIES

		Stage			
	n	A	B	C	D
Diploid	71	35	30	7	9
Nondiploid	69	0	18	13	38
Total	150	35	48	20	47

TABLE 5.9. PROPORTION OF DIPLOID PROSTATIC CARCINOMAS IN STAGES A, B, C, AND D[a]

Stage	%
A	100
B	62.5
C	53.8
D	19.1

[a] Prospective and retrospective study.

nontreatment option) in patients, particularly those, ever-increasing in number, whose stage A tumors are incidentally discovered. There is a very strong suggestive evidence that a no-treatment option should be seriously considered in patients with small, incidentally discovered diploid tumors. Clinical follow-up will readily disclose progression of these tumors. Should this occur, a new therapeutic option can be considered.

UROTHELIAL TUMORS OF THE BLADDER

Pioneering flow cytometric studies of DNA content of urothelial tumors, notably by Tribukait,[52,53] have allowed excellent correlation between tumor grade and ploidy patterns. In general, well-differentiated, Grade I papillary tumors have a DNA content in the diploid range. Grade III tumors and flat carcinomas *in situ* have a highly aneuploid pattern of DNA distribution, strongly suggesting that these two lesions are related.[31] This observation confirms the clinical data on the origin of most invasive carcinomas of the urinary bladder from carcinoma *in situ*, suggested by the observations of Brawn[9] and by Kaye and Lange,[26] and in bladder with papillary tumors by Koss[29,30] and by Koss and Czerniak.[33] The intermediate group of tumors, graded as II, is quite heterogeneous: some of the tumors are in the diploid range and others are aneuploid. The correlation of ploidy patterns with stage of the disease[53] also confirms that aneuploid tumors are much more likely to invade muscle and beyond, whereas diploid tumors rarely progress beyond the lamina propria of the bladder.

Several other parameters of bladder tumors could be correlated with ploidy (Table 5.10). The density of the nuclear pores is greater in aneuploid than in diploid tumors.[17] The expression of a monoclonal antibody known as epitectin is higher in aneuploid than in diploid tumors.[16] The expression of blood group antigens, while not nearly as well correlated, also appears to be correlated with ploidy, with diploid tumors usually expressing blood group antigens and the

TABLE 5.10. CHARACTERISTICS OF TWO GROUPS OF BLADDER CANCER

Feature	Low-grade Papillary Carcinomas	High-grade Papillary and Invasive Carcinomas
Epithelial abnormality of origin	Hyperplasia	Flat carcinoma *in situ* and related abnormalities ("dysplasia")
Invasive potential	Low	High
DNA ploidy pattern	Predominantly diploid	Predominantly aneuploid
Density of nuclear pores	Normal	Increased
Expression of Ca antigen (Epitectin)	As in normal urothelium	Increased
Blood group isoantigen expression	Usually present	Usually absent

aneuploid tumors failing in this regard.[55] It is of incidental interest that cytology of the urinary sediment generally follows the ploidy patterns. It has been documented that diploid tumors generally do not shed cells recognizable as abnormal, whereas the accuracy is high for aneuploid tumors.[19,35]

Monitoring of bladder tumors by flow cytometric analysis of cells in bladder washings has been advocated chiefly by Melamed and his group.[5,28,40–42,47,49] Aneuploid patterns of DNA were thought to indicate a residual or recurrent bladder tumor. The technique was successfully utilized for monitoring of patients treated with bacillus Calmette-Guérin for carcinoma *in situ*.[4] However, a large number of histograms that failed to reveal an aneuploid peak but had an elevation of hyperdiploid cells, arbitrarily set at 15% or more, also suggested a recurrence.[40,41] These observations were repeatedly challenged, notably by deVere White *et al.*[18] and by Koss *et al.*[36] deVere White notably pointed out that aneuploid histograms and histograms with elevation of the hyperdiploid cells may also occur in a variety of non-neoplastic disorders and that this criterion led to a substantial false-positive rate. Koss *et al.* pointed out that image analysis of the cells in the urinary sediment frequently disclosed aneuploid DNA patterns that were not observed by flow cytometry and that a combination of image analysis and conventional cytology was a more reliable predictor of recurrence than flow cytometry.

The study of bladder washings led to the formation of a "network" of five laboratories, sponsored by the National Cancer Institute, to study the general utility of flow cytometric analysis of bladder washings as a clinical tool. The results of a 3-year cooperation were somewhat mixed. On the one hand, a broad approximation of similar results could be obtained on tissue sections and "cell cocktails," provided by Dr. John Coon and co-workers.[13] On the other hand, significant inter- and intralaboratory differences in histogram construction and interpretation were observed.[56] Further, in spite of assurances to the contrary, the clinical procedure to secure bladder washing samples in outpatients is neither easy nor painless to the patient and, except for some academic centers, the method has not received a wide clinical following. The possibility must be considered that the development of specific monoclonal antibodies may facilitate the recognition of tumor cells. There has been, so far, no significant evidence that this approach will be of clinical value.

There are several commercial entities that offer monitoring of urinary sediment for patients with bladder symptoms.[23] In the absence of published persuasive data, the value of these procedures must be considered questionable.

MOLECULAR BIOLOGY OF UROTHELIAL TUMORS

The evidence summarized above strongly suggests that DNA ploidy of urothelial bladder tumors is a marker of their morphology and behavior. This fact does not shed light on the mechanisms responsible for the differences between the diploid and aneuploid categories. In fact, it has been shown by *in situ* hybridization that chromosomal abnormalities do occur in the diploid tumors; hence, even these tumors are fundamentally aneuploid.[24] Means are now available to look further into the makeup of these tumors at the level of molecular genetics.

Cellular genes with potential oncogenic activity have been first identified by their homology to transforming retroviral oncogenes.[6] The first human cellular oncogene was discovered in a bladder cancer cell line, T24.[10] The mutation and/ or overexpression of this prototype gene can lead to malignant transformation in experimental systems. The transforming gene of the T24 line, later found to be a cellular counterpart of the viral Ha-*ras* gene,[10] belongs to the *ras* gene family consisting three members (Ha-, Ki-, and N-*ras*).[7] These genes are encoding a group of closely related 21,000-dalton proteins (p21). The *ras* p21 is capable of binding guanine nucleotides with high affinity and has guanosine triphosphatase (GTPase) activity.[7] The p21 molecule is anchored to the cytoplasmic surface of the cell membrane and it has been postulated that it may serve as a transducer molecule for signals affecting cell proliferation and differentiation.

Two mechanisms have been proposed for the ability of *ras* genes to transform cells. One involves a single nucleotide mutation in the coding sequence (most frequently in codons 12 or 61).[7,8] This results in an aminoacid substitution and a change of the gene product, affecting the GTP binding domain, and reducing GTPase activity.[51] The second possible mechanism involves overexpression of the *ras* gene products. Recently, it has been documented that a point adenine-guanine (A-G) mutation in the last intron at position 2719 of cellular Ha-*ras* gene in T24 cells is responsible for a significant increase in p21 expression and transforming efficiency.[12] Subsequently, a sequence of nucleotides situated around the intron D position 2719 was shown to play a regulatory role in the formation of Ha-*ras* mRNA.[44] Such sites initiate a multistep splicing process of elimination of introns (noncoding sequences of a gene) from the mRNA. Such sites are usually located at the exon-intron boundary. Because of an unusual position of the Ha-*ras* splicing site (away from the customary position at the exon-intron boundary), the mRNA is unstable and does not result in production of p21 but instead encodes another protein of 19,000 daltons (p19). This protein possibly acts as an antioncogene and protects the cell from the effects of the oncogene.[11] This mechanism of protection is abolished by an A-G mutation in position 2719, resulting in uninhibited expression of the Ha-*ras* gene product, as observed in the human bladder cancer cell line T24.[12] It was thought that if this overexpressed *ras* gene product were to be modified by a mutation of the exon in either position 12 or 61, the synchronous exon-intron mutation may conceivably correlate with aggressive behavior of human bladder tumors.

To verify this hypothesis, the DNA was extracted from 67 prospectively collected urinary bladder tumors. The appropriate fragments of Ha-*ras* gene were amplified by the polymerase chain reaction (Fig. 5.3) with the use of appropriate primers (Table 5.11), and screened for mutation at codons 12 and 61 and at position 2719 of the last intron.[12,54] The results were subsequently related to *ras*-p21 levels measured by a novel technique in which the immunohistochemically visualized protein was quantitated by computer-assisted image analysis.[15] The mutations and p21 levels were related to such prognostic factors as histological grade and DNA ploidy. The fragments of the Ha-*ras* gene amplified by the polymerase chain reaction (PCR) were analyzed for the following substitutions, using dot blotting technique, with ^{32}P-labeled oligonucleotide probes specific for: GLY, SER, CYS, ARG, VAL, ALS, ASP and ALA at codon 12 and for ARG, GLN, HIS, GLU, LEU, PRO, and LYS at codon 61.[54]

A G-T substitution at codon 12 was evident in 30 tumors (Fig. 5.4). It resulted in the substitution of the aminoacid valine at position 12, instead of glycine in the gene product.[14] No other codon 12 or codon 61 substitutions were seen. It is of interest that the hybridization signal varied in intensity from case to case reflecting the heterogenity of tumor cells in reference to the G-T mutation.[45] The

AMPLIFICATION OF HUMAN *c*-Ha-*ras* GENE FRAGMENTS BY POLYMERASE CHAIN REACTION

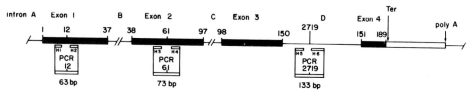

FIG. 5.3.   Fragments of human c-Ha-*ras* gene amplified by the polymerase chain reaction. Primers are designated as indicated in Table 5.11. Three fragments of c-Ha-*ras* gene containing codons 12 and 61 and nucleotide 2719 of intron D were amplified. The fragments were 63, 73, and 133 bp in length, respectively.

TABLE 5.11.   LIST FOR PRIMERS USED FOR AMPLIFICATION OF HUMAN C-HA-*RAS* GENE FRAGMENTS

Primer	Sequence	Length of Fragment	Gene Fragment
H1	5'-GAC GGA ATA TAA GCT GGT GG-3'	63 bp[a]	Codon 12
H2	5'-TGG ATG GTC AGC GCA CTC TT-3'		
H3	5'-AGA CGT GCC TGT TGG ACA TC-3'	73 bp	Codon 61
H4	5'-CGC ATG TAC TGG TCC CGC AT-3'		
H5	5'GGG CAG CCG CTC TGG CTC TA-3'	133 bp	Intron D, position 2719
H6	5'CAG ACC CCG GCC CTC GCC TCC CTC ACT GCC CTG CCG TCC CGG GTC[b] AC-3'		

A

[a] Base pairs.

[b] Indicates A to T mismatch.

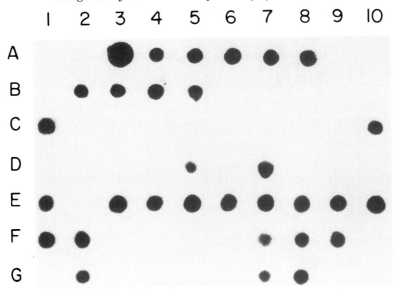

Fig. 5.4. Dot blot hybridization with a codon 12 valine-specific oligonucleotide probe of a PCR-amplified fragment of the Ha-*ras* gene. *1A*, no DNA; *2A*, human placenta; *3A*, T24. The remaining samples represent 67 bladder tumors, with 30 showing a positive reaction.

TABLE 5.12. CODON 12 VALINE FOR GLYCINE SUBSTITUTION OF HA-*RAS* GENE IN RELATION TO DNA PLOIDY AND HISTOLOGICAL GRADING IN BLADDER CANCER

		Histological Grade[a]		
	n	I	II	III
Diploid[b]				
Nonmutated (Gly)	20	11	8	1
Mutated (Val)	8		7	1
Aneuploid				
Nonmutated (Gly)	17 (3)[c]	1	8 (1)	8 (2)
Mutated (Val)	22 (13)		6 (1)[d]	16 (12)[d]

[a] WHO histological grade.

[b] Gly, glycine; Val, valine.

[c] Number of invasive tumors is in parentheses.

[d] Seven of the tumors (two Grade II and five Grade III) had a synchronous codon 12 and intron mutation in position 2719; six were invasive.

rate of mutations at codon 12 was higher in the aneuploid tumors than in the diploid tumors (Table 5.12). There were also higher rates of codon 12 mutation in Grade II and Grade III tumor in comparison to Grade I tumors. No relation between codon 12 mutation alone and invasion was found.

The amplification of the last intron containing a nucleotide at position 2719 was performed with a reverse primer containing an A-T mismatch at position 2723 (Table 5.11) to facilitate the creation of a *BStEII* restriction site in the amplified fragment (Fig. 5.5). In order to increase the sensitivity of detection a ^{32}P-labeled forward primer was added during the extension step of periultimate

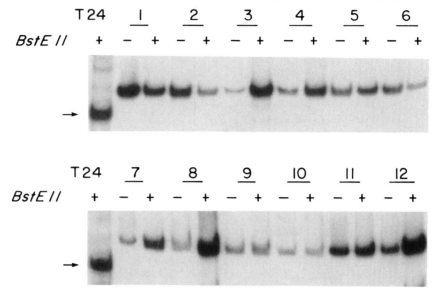

FIG. 5.5. A fragment of the gene between positions 2633 and 2766 was amplified. In order to generate a *BstEII* restriction site dependent on the presence of a G residue at position 2719, a mismatch was introduced in the downstream reverse primer, *i.e.*, in the position corresponding to nucleotide 2723 an A was replaced by a T residue (Table 5.11). The amplified fragments were labeled at the 5′ end with ³²P and is cut (*arrow*) when exposed to the *BstEII* enzyme, thus confirming the presence of an A to G substitution at position 2719 of Ha-*ras* gene.

PCR cycle. Then an A-G mutation at position 2719 was identified on polyacrylamide gels by the presence of a *BStEII* restriction fragment.[12] In seven cases an A-G intron D mutation was identified. All of the cases with intron D mutation also had a substitution at codon 12. These seven tumors, which expressed approximately 10 times higher levels of *ras*-p21, were Grade II and III aneuploid tumors and six of them were invasive.

This study documents for the first time that synchronous alterations of coding and regulatory sequences of the same gene can be associated with aggressive clinical behavior of human tumors. However, it must be noted that the synchronous exon and intron D mutations of the Ha-*ras* gene were identified in only about 40% of invasive carcinomas of the urinary bladder. Hence, other biological mechanisms accounting for invasive behavior of aneuploid bladder tumors must be anticipated. It must also be noted that this study provides only a circumstantial evidence for the association between synchronous exon/intron mutations of the H-*ras* gene and a highly aggressive variant of urinary bladder carcinoma. If this is proved to be correct by further analysis of a representative number of urinary bladder cancer, one can envision that it may serve as a novel molecular marker identifying a subset of urinary bladder carcinomas with particularly aggressive clinical behavior. Furthermore, it can be anticipated that with the use of PCR the entire test can be performed on cells in voided urine, thus providing a convenient way to test and monitor the patients with urothelial tumors.

EPILOGUE

The analysis of total DNA content (DNA ploidy) in human tumors is only a very rough measure of their biological behavior and aggressive potential. In the work described above, it has been shown that prostate and bladder tumors with DNA content in the diploid range behave differently from aneuploid tumors. In general, the diploid range tumors of these two organs are less aggressive than aneuploid tumors. It may be speculated at this time that in the diploid range tumors some of the regulatory genes are still in place and/or that a significant number of the transforming genes have not been turned on.

On the other hand, the reasons for the aggressive behavior of aneuploid tumors remains largely unknown. A glimpse at a modification of the coding and regulatory sequence in the last intron of the Ha-*ras* gene in bladder tumors suggests that synchronous single nucleotide substitutions of coding and regulatory elements of the gene correlate with invasion in some of these tumors. Clearly, additional insights are still needed to determine other genetic changes leading to invasion. Such work is currently in progress.

ACKNOWLEDGMENTS

This work was supported in part by grants 1R01 CA35745, 1U01 CA41025, 1R01 CA32345, 5R01 CA34790 from the National Cancer Institute to Leopold G. Koss, M.D. We thank Gary Cohen, M.D., Ph.D., and Fritz Herz, Ph.D., for their contribution to this study.

REFERENCES

1. Amberson, J. B., and Koss, L. G. Measurements of DNA as a prognostic factor in prostatic carcinoma. In *Prognostic Cytometry and Cytopathology of Prostate Cancer*, edited by J. P. Karr, D. S. Coffey, and W. Gardner, Jr. New York, Elsevier, 1988, pp. 281–286.
2. Angell, A., and Resnick, M. I. Prostatic ultrasound for the early detection of prostate cancer. *Cancer Treat. Res. 46:* 1–13, 1989.
3. Auer, G., and Zetterberg, A. The prognostic significance of nuclear DNA content in malignant tumors of breast, prostate, and cartilage. In *Advances in Clinical Cytology*, edited by L. G. Koss and D. V. Coleman. Vol. 2. New York, Masson, 1984, pp. 123–134.
4. Badalament, R. A., Gay, H., and Whitmore, W. F., Jr., et al. Monitoring intravesical bacillus Calmette-Guerin treatment of superficial bladder carcinoma by serial cytometry. *Cancer 58:* 2751–2757, 1986.
5. Badalament, R. A., Hermansen, D. K., and Kimmel, M., et al. The sensitivity of bladder wash flow cytometry, bladder wash cytology, and voided cytology in the detection of bladder carcinoma. *Cancer 60:* 1423–1427, 1987.
6. Barbacid, M. *ras* Genes. *Annu. Rev. Biochem. 56:* 779–827, 1987.
7. Bos, J. F. *ras* Oncogene in human cancer. A review. *Cancer 49:* 4682–4689, 1989.
8. Bos, J. L., Fearon, E. R., Hamilton, S. R., Verlaan-de Vries M., van Boom, J. H., Eb, A. J., and Vogelstein, B. Prevalence of *ras* gene mutations in human colorectal cancers. *Nature (Lond.) 327:* 293–297, 1987.
9. Brawn, P. N. The origin of invasive carcinoma of the bladder. *Cancer 50:* 515–519, 1982.
10. Capon, D. J., Chen, E. Y., Levinson, A. D., Seeburg, P. H., and Goeddel, D. V. Complete nucleotide sequences of the T24 human bladder carcinoma oncogene and its normal homologue. *Nature (Lond.) 302:* 33–37, 1983.

11. Cohen, J. B., Broz, S. D., and Levinson, A. D. Expression of the Ha-*ras* protooncogene is controlled by alternative splicing. *Cell 85:* 461–472, 1989.

12. Cohen, J. B., and Levinson, A. D. A point mutation in the last intron responsible for increased expression and transforming activity of the c-Ha-*ras* oncogene. *Nature (Lond.) 334:* 119–124, 1988.

13. Coon, J. S., Deitch, A. D., deVere White, W. R., Koss, L. G., Melamed, M. R., Reeder, J. E., Weinstein, R. S., Wersto, R. P., and Wheeless, L. L. Interinstitutional variability in DNA flow cytometric analysis of tumors: The National Cancer Institute's flow cytometry network experience. *Cancer 61:* 126–130, 1988.

14. Czerniak, B., Deitch, D., Simmons, H., Etkind, P., Herz, F., and Koss, L. G. Ha-*ras* gene codon 12 mutation and DNA ploidy in urinary bladder carcinoma. *Br. J. Cancer 62:* 762–763, 1990.

15. Czerniak, B., Herz, F., Wersto, R. P., Alster, P., Puszkin, E., Schwartz, E., and Koss, L. G. Quantitation of oncogene products by computer assisted image analysis and flow cytometry. *J. Histochem. Cytochem. 38:* 463–466, 1990.

16. Czerniak, B., and Koss, L. G. Expression of Ca antigen on human urinary bladder tumors. *Cancer 55:* 2380–2383, 1985.

17. Czerniak, B., Koss, L. G., and Sherman, A. B. Nuclear pores and DNA ploidy in human bladder carcinomas. *Cancer Res. 44:* 3752–3756, 1984.

18. deVere White, R. W., Olsson, C. A., and Deitch, A. D. Flow cytometry: Role in monitoring transitional cell carcinoma of bladder. *Urology 8:* 15–20, 1986.

19. Farrow, G. M. Urine cytology in the detection of bladder cancer: A critical approach. *J. Occupational Med. 32:* 817–821, 1990.

20. Fordham, M. V. P., Burge, A. H., Matthews, J., Williams, G., and Cooke, T. Prostatic carcinoma cell DNA content measured by flow cytometry and its relation to clinical outcome. *Br. J. Surg. 73:* 400–403, 1986.

21. Forsslund, G., and Zetterberg, A. Ploidy level determinations in high-grade and low-grade malignant variants of prostatic carcinoma. *Cancer Res. 50:* 4281–4285, 1990.

22. Gittes, R. F. Carcinoma of the prostate. *N. Engl. J. Med. 324:* 236–245, 1991.

23. Hemstreet, G. P. III, Hurst, R. E., Bass, R. A., and Rao, J. Y. Quantitative fluorescence image analysis in bladder cancer screening. *J. Occupational Med. 32:* 822–828, 1990.

24. Hopman, A. H. N., Ramaekers, F. C. S., Raap, A. K., Beck, J. L., Devilee, P., Vander Ploeg, M. and Vooijs, G. P. In situ hybridization as a tool to study numerical chromosome aberrations in solid bladder tumors. *Histochemistry 89:* 307–316, 1988.

25. Jones, E. C., McNeal, J., Bruchovsky, N., and de Jong, G. DNA content in prostatic adeno-carcinoma. A flow cytometry study of the predictive value of aneuploidy for tumor volume, percentage gleason grade 4 and 5, and lymph node metastases. *Cancer 66:* 752–757, 1990.

26. Kaye, K. W., and Lange, P. H. Mode of presentation of invasive bladder cancer: Reassessment of the problem. *J. Urol. 128:* 31–33, 1982.

27. Kenny, G. M., and Hutchinson, W. B. Transrectal ultrasound study of prostate. *Urology 32:* 401–402, 1988.

28. Klein, F. A., Herr, H. W., Whitmore, W. F., Jr., Sogani, P. C., and Melamed, M. R. An evaluation of automated flow cytometry (FCM) in detection of carcinoma in situ of the urinary bladder. *Cancer 50:* 1003–1005, 1982.

29. Koss, L. G. Mapping of the urinary bladder: Its impact on concepts of bladder cancer. *Hum. Pathol. 10:* 533–548, 1979.

30. Koss, L. G. Tumors of the urinary bladder. *Atlas of Tumor Pathology*, Second Series, Fascicle 11. Washington, D. C., Armed Forces Institute of Pathology, 1974. (Suppl 1985.)

31. Koss, L. G. Precursor lesions of invasive bladder cancer. *Eur. Urol. 14:* 4–6, 1988.

32. Koss, L. G. Image Cytophotometry and flow cytometry. In *Diagnostic Flow Cytometry*, edited by J. S. Coon and R. S. Weinstein. Baltimore, Williams & Wilkins, 1991, pp. 147–163.

33. Koss, L. G., and Czerniak, B. Biology and management of urinary bladder cancer. *N. Engl. J. Med. 324:* 125–126, 1991.

34. Koss, L. G., Czerniak, B., Herz, F., and Wersto, R. P. Flow cytometric measurements of DNA

and other cell components in human tumors. A critical appraisal. *Hum. Pathol. 20:* 528–548, 1989.

35. Koss, L. G., Deitch, D., Ramanathan, R., and Sherman, A. B. Diagnostic value of cytology of voided urine. *Acta Cytol. 29:* 810–816, 1985.

36. Koss, L. G., Wersto, R. P., Simmons, D. A., Deitch, D., Herz, F., and Freed, S. Z. Predictive value of DNA measurements in bladder washings. Comparison of flow cytometry, image cytophotometry, and cytology in patients with a past history of urothelial tumors. *Cancer 64:* 916–924, 1989.

37. Lee, F., Siders, D. B., Torp-Pedersen, S. T., Kirscht, J. L., McHugh, T. A., and Mitchell, A. E. Prostate cancer: transrectal ultrasound and pathology comparison. A preliminary study of outer gland (Peripheral and Central Zones) and inner gland (Transition Zone) cancer. *Cancer 67:* 1132–1142, 1991.

38. Lee, S. E., Currin, S. M., Paulson, D. F., and Walther, P. J. Flow cytometric determination of ploidy in prostatic adenocarcinoma: A comparison with seminal vesicle involvement and histopathological grading as a predictor of clinical recurrence. *J. Urol. 140:* 769–774, 1988.

39. McIntire, T. L., Murphy, W. M., Coon, J. S., Chandler, R. W., Schwartz, D., Conway, S., and Weinstein, R. S. The prognostic value of DNA ploidy combined with histologic substaging for incidental carcinoma of the prostate gland. *Am. J. Clin. Pathol. 89:* 370–373, 1988.

40. Melamed, M. R. Flow cytometry detection and evaluation of bladder tumors. *J. Occupational Med. 32:* 829–833, 1990.

41. Melamed, M. R., and Klein, F. A. Flow cytometry of urinary bladder irrigation specimens. *Hum. Pathol. 15:* 302–305, 1984.

42. Melamed, M. R., Traganos, F., Sharpless, T., and Darzynkiewicz, Z. Urinary cytology automation: Preliminary studies with acridine orange stain and flow-through cytofluorometry. *Invest Urol. 13:* 333–338, 1976.

43. Montgomery, B. T., Nativ, O., Blute, M. L., Farrow, G. M., Myers, R. P., Zincke, H., Therneau, T. M., and Lieber, M. M. Stage B prostate adenocarcinoma. Flow cytometric nuclear DNA ploidy analysis. *Arch. Surg. 125:* 327–331, 1990.

44. Mount, S. M. A catalogue of splice junction sequences. *Nucl. Acid Res. 10:* 459–472, 1982.

45. Mulder, M. P., Keijzer, W., Verkerk, A., Boot, A. J., Prins, M. E., Splinter, T. A., and Bos, J. L. Activated *ras* genes in human seminoma: evidence for tumor heterogeneity. *Oncogene 4:* 1345–1351, 1989.

46. Peterson, R. O. *Urologic Pathology.* Philadelphia, J. B. Lippincott Company, 1986, pp. 613–638.

47. Ring, K. S., Karp, F. S., Olsson, C. A., O'Toole, K., Bixon, R., and Benson, M. C. Flow cytometric analysis of localized adenocarcinoma of the prostate: The use of archival DNA analysis in conjunction with pathological grading to predict clinical outcome following radical retropubic prostatectomy. *Prostate 17:* 155–164, 1990.

48. Silverberg, E., and Lubera, J. A. American Cancer Society Cancer Statistics. *CA 39:* 3–32, 1989.

49. Stenkvist, B., and Olding-Stenkvist, E. Cytological and DNA characteristics of hyperplasia/ inflammation and cancer of the prostate. *Eur. J. Cancer 26:* 261–267, 1990.

50. Stephenson, R. A., James, B. C., Gay, H., Fair, W. R., Whitmore, W. F., Jr., and Melamed, M. R. Flow cytometry of prostate cancer: relationship of DNA content to survival. *Cancer Res. 47:* 2504–2507, 1987.

51. Taparowsky, E., Suard, Y., Fasano, O., Shimizu, K., Goldfarb, M., and Wigler, M. Activation of the T24 bladder carcinoma transforming gene is linked to a single amino acid change. *Nature (Lond.) 300:* 762–765, 1982.

52. Tribukait, B. Flow cytometry in assessing the clinical aggressiveness of genito-urinary neoplasms. *World J. Urol. 5:* 108–122, 1987.

53. Tribukait, B. Flow cytometry in surgical pathology and cytology of tumors of the genito-urinary tract. In *Advances in Clinical Cytology,* edited by L. G. Koss and D. V. Coleman. Vol. 2. New York, Mason Publishing, 1984, pp. 163–189.

54. Verlaan-de Vries, M., Bogaard, M. E., van den Elst, H., van Boom, J. H., van der Eb, A. J., and

Boss, J. L. A dot-blot screening procedure for mutated *ras* oncogenes using synthetic oligo-deoxynucleotides. *Gene 50:* 313–320, 1986.
55. Weinstein, R. S., Alroy, J., Farrow, G. M., Miller, A. W. III, and Davidsohn, I. Blood group isoantigen detection in carcinoma in situ of the urinary bladder. *Cancer 43:* 661, 1979.
56. Wheeless, L. L., Coon, J. S., Cox, C., Deitch, A. D., deVere White, R. W., Koss, L. G., Melamed, M. R., O'Connell, M. J., Reeder, J. E., Weinstein, R. S., and Wersto, R. P. Measurement variability in DNA flow cytometry of replicate samples. *Cytometry 10:* 731–738, 1989.

Chapter 6

The Prostate—Overview: Recent Insights and Speculations

WILLIAM A. GARDNER, JR. AND BETSY D. BENNETT

The prostate gland in the "normal" adult male is a relatively small organ, measuring approximately 4 cm in maximum dimension and weighing about 20 grams. It may be truthfully said, however, that gram for gram there is not a tissue in the body that causes more mischief and about which so little is known. This lack of information applies not only to the function of the prostate, but extends even to its anatomy and histology, areas in which fundamental knowledge is still unfolding. This Chapter is intended to indicate the dimensions of the potential impact of prostate disease on the practice of pathology, to review some recent observations of basic histopathology, especially as noted in the young adult prostate, to emphasize an often neglected aspect of prostate disease, *i.e.*, prostatitis, and finally, to speculate regarding possible roles of the prostate gland in the acquired immunodeficiency syndrome.

Evidence of the increasing importance of the prostate gland to pathologists is seen in the number of recent texts and monographs devoted solely or in part to the histopathology of this organ.[13,31,59] The most common surgical procedure performed on United States males is done for prostatic hyperplasia and results in total medical costs exceeding 1 billion dollars per year.[19] Assuming an average of five microscopic slides per case of benign prostatic hyperplasia, it is estimated that in 1991 United States pathologists examined and rendered a diagnosis on five stacks of microscopic slides, each of which would reach the height of the Sears Tower.

With 122,000 new cases identified in 1991, prostate cancer is likely to have surpassed lung cancer as the most commonly diagnosed malignancy in United States males. An estimated 32,000 deaths from prostate cancer in 1991 made it the second leading cause of cancer deaths in men. Moreover, it has been calculated that at the present time at least 10 million United States males harbor a latent or "incidental" prostate cancer. These data were put into perspective at a recent NIH conference on prostate cancer. "In summary, in the average lifetime one half of all men will harbor latent prostate cancer, one out of eleven will be clinically diagnosed with prostate cancer, and one third of these patients will die from the cancer."[22] A comparable statement for the year 2000 will be even more dramatic because of the increasing incidence of prostate cancer combined with the aging of the United States population; *i.e.*, it is projected that the death rate from prostate cancer will increase by 50% in the next 15 years.[19]

Such figures call for improved screening programs that will allow earlier diagnosis and treatment of lesions determined to have potential clinical significance. "National Prostate Cancer Awareness Week," which emphasizes screening programs for prostate cancer (sponsored by a drug company that manufactures a chemotherapeutic agent used in treatment of this disease), is one measure of societal awareness of this subject. Screening programs for prostate cancer are controversial, however, with a major area of concern being the appropriateness and effectiveness of therapy subsequent to case identification. The principle problem in this area lies in our current relative inability to discriminate between prostate cancers that have potential clinical significance and those that do not. Nonetheless, there is increasing use of serum prostate-specific antigen in conjunction with digital rectal examination[20,21] and ultrasonography as screening procedures in at least a subset of the male population. The number of prostate cancers that will be recognized initially by one or a combination of these methods can only be estimated. Although debate will continue as to the cost-benefit aspects of screening programs and questions will remain about proper therapy, there is no doubt that with improving ultrasonographic resolution and technology and with refinement of laboratory methods there will be an inevitable increase in the number of prostate specimens passing under the microscope of the surgical pathologist.

EPIDEMIOLOGY

Although the most clearly established risk factor for prostate cancer is, as noted above, growing old, other influences have been implicated. A striking geographic difference in incidence of prostate cancer has been recognized for decades. Worldwide, one of the highest incidence rates occurs in the United States in the black population, while the lowest incidence of clinical prostate cancer is found in Asia. These findings are in contrast with the almost uniform prevalence worldwide of the small latent or incidental carcinomas found at autopsy. This difference led Donn and Muir[30] to conclude that factors initiating development of latent carcinomas of the prostate are evenly distributed across areas of both high and low incidence of clinical prostate cancer. This observation might imply that the initiating event in prostate carcinogenesis is a relatively universal occurrence and, further, that the subsequent "hits" required for progression to clinical disease represent environmental influences. These influences then would be responsible for the striking geographical variation in clinical incidence.

Speculation about the nature of these environmental agents has produced an extraordinarily lengthy list of influences that have been found to be "associated" in some way with prostate cancer. These include dietary factors (principally fats and carotenoids), occupational exposures (especially cadmium), hormonal status, infectious diseases (especially sexually transmitted ones), and a variety of sexual practices.[18,52] In evaluating the influence of sexual activity on development of prostate cancer, Rotkin[90] found that the greatest difference between patients and controls occurred during late adolescence and the early twenties. He further examined the relationships of many risk variables relating to aspects of sexuality and concluded that "limitation upon sexuality activity at any time of life may increase risks."

For many of the putative environmental influences on prostate cancer, conclusions are either inconsistent or ambiguous. For example, Hsing, *et al.*,[52] in summarizing the findings of 10 studies related to consumption of vitamin A and β-carotene, noted that five studies showed increased risk, four reduced risk, and one concluded that there was no association. A second example concerns the possible relationship between vasectomy and prostate cancer as noted in companion articles in a recent issue of the *American Journal of Epidemiology*. Rosenberg *et al.*,[89] in a hospital-based case study, found an unexpected association between history of vasectomy and prostate cancer; *i.e.*, vasectomy had occurred in 10% of 220 cases of prostate cancer and in 3.3% of the control group. In a similar study, Mettlin *et al.*[69] also found significantly increased risk with a history of vasectomy, although the relative risk was less. Moreover, in the latter study there seemed to be an association between the length of time since vasectomy and the degree of risk. Neither of these reports, however, suggested a plausible hypothesis as to how vasectomy might be causally related to prostate cancer. In a companion paper, Guess[45] put the statistical and epidemiological variables of these papers into perspective. Despite this commentary, these papers generated sufficient interest and alarm that the American Urological Association thought it necessary to respond.[51] This response cited the inherent weakness of hypothesis-generating papers and concluded that the studies did not contain sufficient evidence to influence the clinical practice of vasectomy. A similar lack of consistently validated association exists for most of the other risk factors.

One notable exception that could and should influence clinical practice and subsequently the practice of pathology is familial risk. In studies of Mormon geneological records in Utah, Cannon *et al.*[17] found a familial aggregation of prostate cancers. This work has been substantiated by Meikle *et al.*[67] showing a several-fold higher relative risk among brothers of prostate cancer patients. Elsewhere, family history as a significant risk factor for prostate cancer was substantiated when Steinberg *et al.*,[98] in Baltimore, found that men with a father or brother with prostate cancer were twice as likely to develop the disease as were men with no affected relatives. They also noted an apparent increased risk with *increased numbers* of affected family members, *i.e.*, a man with two or three first-degree relatives with prostate cancer had a 5- to 11-fold increased risk of developing the disease. As this information becomes more widely distributed in the population at large and more a part of the practice of clinical urology, we can expect our surgical pathology laboratories to see the consequences thereof.

MICROSCOPIC ANATOMY

The fundamental characteristics of the gross and microscopic anatomy of the prostate are well known and described in numerous textbooks. Despite these widespread general descriptions, however, it is evident that much about the basic anatomy, histology, and associated developmental changes of the prostate remains to be described. The concept of prostatic anatomy has evolved from five lobes to four anatomic zones[48] and will no doubt undergo further alteration as new methods of investigation are developed and refined. Changing concepts of microscopic anatomy and development seem to occur at somewhat faster rates. These changes have been due in part to developments in immunohistochemistry and in part to increasing use of whole-mount histological sections. The latter allows comparisons with clinical imaging[70] as well as within differing regions at multiple levels within the same gland. These concepts include discovery and description of neuroendocrine cells within the prostate and a more complete description of fetal prostatic growth and development. Recent histological studies of the prostate have provided new insights into physiology and pathophysiology by demonstrating, for example, the presence of sperm within prostatic glandular lumina and illustrating atrophic and proliferative changes (previously thought to be characteristic of aging) in the prostates of young adults.

The Endocrine Prostate

An example of the recent developments in the knowledge of basic prostatic histology is the increasing recognition (largely through the work of di Sant'Agnese[28,29]) of the extraordinary variety of endocrine-paracrine cells that normally inhabit the prostate. These cells have been identified with a combination of the Grimelius stain, which targets chromagranin A, and immunohistochemical stains using a variety of antibodies. With these techniques, neuroendocrine cells have been shown to be distributed irregularly throughout the glandular and ductal epithelium of the normal, hyperplastic, and neoplastic prostate as well as the urothelium of the prostatic urethra. Many of these cells have been found to contain serotonin. In addition, immunoreactivity for bombesin (gastrin-releasing peptide), somatostatin, thyroid-stimulating hormone, and calcitonin occurs regularly in small populations of neuroendocrine cells.[3,28,29] Other less frequent neuroendocrine products demonstrated within prostatic cells include the α subunit of human chorionic gonadotropin, adrenocorticotropic hormone, leu-enkephalin, β-endorphin, and glucagon.[3,28,29,32] Given these findings, it is not surprising that a spectrum from focal to dominant neuroendocrine differentiation may be seen in prostatic carcinomas. This phenomenon may be reflected by the presence of neurosecretory products such as chromogranin A in the plasma of patients with prostate cancer. Recent studies by Kadmon et al.[56] have suggested that monitoring of such products may have prognostic and therapeutic implications.

Prostatic Development

A recent study of fetal prostates at various stages of development[106] demonstrated that prostatic epithelial secretion in the fetus with no endocrine or urogenital congenital anomalies occurs somewhat later than previously described. Furthermore, the appearance of periodic acid-Schiff (PAS)-positive secretory products is asynchronous, both within the gland as a whole and within a specific duct-gland complex. This asychrony persists into adulthood and can be demonstrated in young adults, as was shown in a subsequent study of prostates from men in the third decade (Fig. 6.1).[37] In 43% of these cases, focal glands or entire segments of prostate could be identified in which a prepubertal unstimulated appearance was maintained. This finding suggests that prostatic segments previously given the diagnosis of lobular atrophy may actually represent lobular hypoplasia.

Spermatozoa in the Prostate

Retrograde ejaculation of spermatozoa into the prostate was recently demonstrated in an autopsy study of 100 prostates obtained in the course of medicolegal autopsies. Sperm were present in 9% of the prostates examined with no specific anatomic region of the prostate showing a predilection for their accumulation.[77]

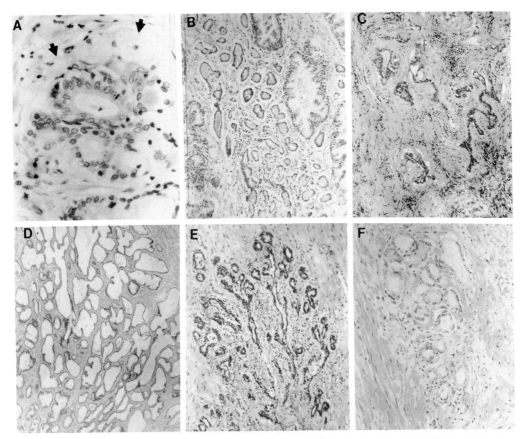

FIG. 6.1. Patterns of epithelial proliferative (*A*, *B*, and *F*) and atrophic (*C* to *E*) dysplasia of prostate gland. (*A*) Budding hyperplasia of single-layered prostatic acini (*arrows*) in 20-year-old man. H&E, reduced from ×600. (*B*) Infiltrative pattern of small acinar carcinoma in 22-year-old man. H&E, reduced from ×150. (*C*) Sclerotic atrophy of stroma and glandular epithelium in 28-year-old man. H&E, reduced from ×150. (*D*) Subcapsular segment of dilated acini with flattened epithelium in 28-year-old man. H&E, reduced from ×60. (*E*) Subcapsular segment of "atrophic" acini and ducts resembling prepubertal unstimulated prostate in 29-year-old man. H&E, reduced from ×150. (*F*) Nodular atypical hyperplasia of acini in 26-year-old man. H&E, reduced from ×240.

Later animal studies in dogs (J. Strandberg, personal communication) and monkeys also showed the routine presence of sperm within the prostate.[78]

Demonstration of intraprostatic spermatozoa raises several interesting possibilities regarding various aspects of prostatic physiology. First, the sperm themselves may serve as etiological agents for lesions within the prostate. Sperm were demonstrated within corpora amylacea, for example, and may be postulated to serve as a nidus for accumulation of prostatic secretions. "Nonspecific" granulomatous prostatitis, at least in some cases, may represent a reaction to the presence of sperm. This mechanism is a well-documented cause of granulomatous inflammation in the epididymis.[41,43] In the above studies, sperm were frequently found admixed with an inflammatory infiltrate and occasionally fragments of sperm were identified within macrophages, *i.e.*, spermiophages (Fig. 6.2). Animal and human tissue culture experiments have demonstrated that penetration of sperm into somatic cells may occur and can produce changes similar to those induced by a variety of carcinogens.[6,47] Other animal studies suggest an even stronger relationship between the introduction of sperm into the prostate and the development of carcinoma.[99] The carcinogenic potential associated with sperm may be related to the presence of substances such as polyamines (*e.g.*, spermine and spermidine) in seminal fluid. Fletcher *et al.*[33] have recently shown that these proteins can induce aneuploidy in cervical epithelium in tissue cultures. Second, the presence of sperm within glandular lumina in the prostate lends support to the concept of urethral reflux into the prostate in the absence of distal obstruction and to the role of urinary reflux in the development of prostatitis and possibly prostate carcinoma. Third, presence of sperm within the prostate supports the possibility of a local immune response playing a role in the development of antibodies to spermatozoa.[92]

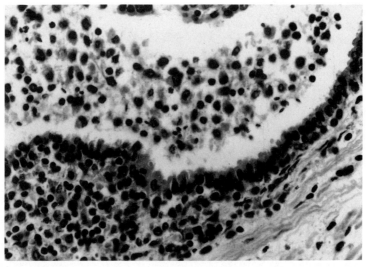

FIG. 6.2. Prostatic gland containing numerous intact sperm heads, macrophages with intracellular sperm fragments (spermiophages) and occasional neutrophils. Note adjacent chronic inflammatory infiltrate. H&E, ×400.

YOUNG ADULT PROSTATES

Atrophic and proliferative lesions in prostatic epithelium have been assumed to represent changes naturally associated with aging. This assumption is biased by the fact that until recently most histopathological studies of the prostate were performed on tissue obtained at surgery or at autopsy of hospitalized males, most of whom were middle-aged or elderly and who had major underlying health problems. Recent studies on tissue obtained from males under the age of 40 indicate that many of the changes previously thought to be characteristic of older males have their inception much earlier.[36–38] These include a variety of epithelial proliferative abnormalities encompassing the spectrum of ductal hyperplasia, atypical glandular hyperplasia, and infiltrating adenocarcinoma. (Fig. 6.1). Inflammatory and atrophic lesions, also usually considered to be age-related phenomena, have been found in two-thirds to three-fourths of prostates from males under the age of 40.[9] The concept of abnormally proliferative epithelium in the prostates of young adults is supported by a recent study of Malinin *et al.*, [63] who regularly identified aneuploid epithelial nuclei in histologically "normal" prostates from males 13–38 years of age. Other authors have recognized incidental prostate adenocarcinoma in young patients; for example, Davis and Weigel[25] found prostatic adenocarcinoma in patients (aged 25 and 36) who underwent total prostatovesiculectomy for refractory prostatitis.

Excessive epithelial proliferation similar to the above has also been noted in pubertal prostates. This has led to the speculation[38] that the hormonal changes associated with puberty may in fact represent the initiating event in the development of prostate carcinoma; *i.e.*, the differential sensitivity within the gland would suggest that some foci would be exquisitely sensitive to the hormonal stimuli of puberty and that these might represent the foci for abnormal proliferation and subsequent development of clinical carcinoma. This notion would be consistent with the epidemiological data presented above, *i.e.*, the relatively uniform worldwide occurrence of latent prostate carcinoma and the postulated similar distribution of the initiating events. A possible role of long-standing inflammatory events as promoters for clinical carcinoma is discussed below under "Prostatitis."

CRYSTALLOIDS

These characteristic and enigmatic structures have a strong association with prostatic adenocarcinoma as noted in multiple studies.[7,9,35,54,87] In conventional biopsy and routine histological sections, the structures occur in about 10% of prostate cancers.[54,87] Using whole organ sections of prostate, several studies have demonstrated them in approximately two-thirds of cancers.[35,87] Furusata *et al.*[35] noted the crystalloids primarily at the periphery of prostatic carcinomas, and in their study of latent prostate cancers found them to be associated more strongly with small tumors than with large ones. On this basis, the authors concluded that crystalloids may be related to early development of prostate carcinoma. This assertion would, however, not be supported by the observation, albeit infrequent, of crystalloids within metastatic foci.[7] Crystalloids have also been seen in a small percentage of cases of nodular hyperplasia. In the latter setting, as well as in the study of young adult prostates described above, the crystalloids are found in the setting of coexistent atypical glandular proliferation.[10,86]

Although these structures have been only recently recognized in the pathology literature, Sir Henry Thompson,[101] in his classic text on diseases of the prostate in 1860, illustrated some similar prostatic elements. His noncommittal commentary on their composition, *i.e.*, "crystals of some earthy carbonate," is still applicable. The term "crystalloids" is the current designation for such structures and this term would seem to be appropriate as they do not display the characteristic fibrillar or prismatic lattice configuration of true crystals. The structures are readily recognizable at low power, staining brightly eosinophilic with the approximate tinctorial qualities of red cells. They have a variety of geometric shapes—rhomboidal, hexagonal, triangular, and needle-like (Fig. 6.3). Their sharp angulations readily differentiate them from corpora amylacea, although they may occasionally be seen within a corpus apparently serving as nidus for its formation. Neither conventional histochemical stains nor immunostains have been successful in identifying the composition of these structures. Ultrastructural and x-ray analytical studies have been equally unrewarding, and their chemical composition and biological origin remain unknown.[86]

The presence of numerous crystalloids within the prostate gives rise to a finely stippled echo pattern on high-resolution transrectal ultrasonography. This sonographic finding in the periphery of the prostate is felt to be a strong suggestion of malignancy and an indication for biopsy.[46] Histologically, crystalloids are most

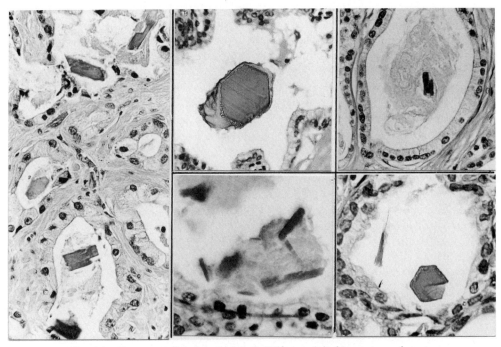

FIG. 6.3.   Representative shapes of crystalloids in acini of prostate carcinoma.

helpful in biopsies in which crush or cautery artifact renders adjacent glandular epithelium nondiagnostic. In this case, their presence is sufficient evidence to justify examination of multiple-step sections or rebiopsy of the lesion.[7,54,86,87]

REACTION TO BACILLUS CALMETTE-GUERIN (BCG)

The intravesicular instillation of BCG, a live but attenuated strain of *Myco-bacterium bovis*, is standard for both prophylaxis and therapy of superficial transitional cell carcinomas of the urinary bladder.[47] The organism is occasionally capable of invasion and, with disseminated infection, even fatal complications have been reported.[4,26] Although disseminated disease is rare, local spread of the organism occurs on a regular basis. BCG traverses the prostatic ducts, enters the acini and, in virtually 100% of patients followed with biopsy, produces a granulomatous prostatitis. The granulomata demonstrate a full histological spectrum, ranging from vaguely nodular collections of histiocytes with relatively few giant cells to full-blown caseating granulomata. Caseating granulomas are most commonly seen in the first 3 months after instillation of BCG (Fig. 6.4*A*). Epithelioid, sarcoid-like granulomata may also occur (Fig. 6.4*B*) and in some cases giant cells may be sectioned in a plane so as to produce an acinus-like appearance. Acid-fast stains frequently demonstrate the organisms. Live organisms can, however,

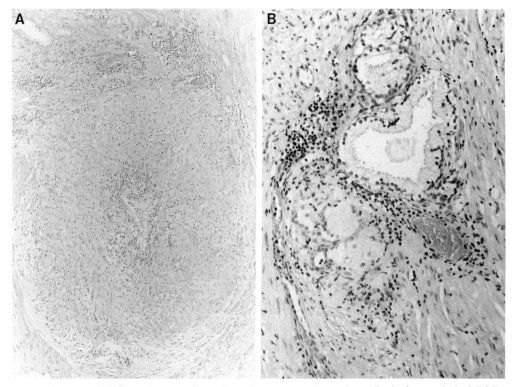

FIG. 6.4. (*A*) Caseating granuloma from the prostate of a patient who had recently had BCG instilled into the bladder for treatment of transitional cell carcinoma. H&E, ×100. (*B*) Epithelioid granuloma (etiology unknown) adjacent to a small blood vessel (contrast with *A*). H&E, ×400.

be recovered from the bladder up to a year later, so it is not surprising that granulomas may also be found in the prostate more than a year after BCG therapy.[73]

As the granulomata resolve, the ensuing fibrosis may produce a palpable nodule that is hypoechoic on ultrasonography, suggesting carcinoma.[102] Fortunately the granulomatous prostatitis produced by BCG does not cause the diagnostic difficulties seen in the more diffuse types of granulomatous prostatitis. In the latter situation, sheets of "infiltrating" macrophages may be present.[34] The individual cells are frequently surrounded by a clear zone further mimicking epithelial cells and may resemble a diffusely infiltrating, poorly differentiated adenocarcinoma. This histological appearance of diffuse granulomatous prostatitis is one of the more frequent causes of misdiagnosis of prostate carcinoma. The application of immunocytochemical stains may prove useful in resolving this differential diagnosis. Presti and Weidner[84] have demonstrated the utility of antilysozyme in the identification of histiocytes within prostate stroma. In their study, antilysozyme appeared to be more useful than antikeratins for this purpose, since no staining with antilysozyme was seen in prostatic epithelial cells but some antikeratin staining was present in cells, presumably macrophages, within the prostatic stroma.

PROSTATITIS

There will be nearly 1 million office visits to urologists for prostatitis in 1992 and the etiology of most cases will never be fully established. Most of the literature on the pathology of prostatitis has been derived from surgical specimens (hyperplasias, carcinomas) from hospitalized, older patients. Indeed, for decades, infiltration of the prostate by lymphocytes and plasma cells, especially in areas of glandular atrophy, has been considered part of the normal aging process. Nielson and Christensen[79] examined 233 biopsies of hyperplasia and found that two-thirds contained chronic inflammatory changes. Mostofi and Sesterhenn[72] noted a chronic inflammatory infiltrate or granulomatous prostatitis in 80% of 700 prostates containing carcinomas. McClinton et al.[65] more recently found that most of the lymphocytes in both hyperplasia and carcinoma were T-lymphocytes, which did not differ with respect to their CD3 positivity. Fifteen to 20% of these lymphocytes expressed the IL-2 receptor, indicating recent activation.

BACTERIAL AND ABACTERIAL PROSTATITIS

Most cases of clinical prostatitis are of unknown etiology, *i.e.*, no bacteria, fungus, parasite, or virus can be shown to be the causative agent. When bacterial prostatitis occurs, the agents involved are the same as those causing urinary tract infections, with *Escherichia coli* being most commonly identified.[76,83] The frequency of *E. coli* infection in the genitourinary tract has been at least partially explained by the demonstration of a specific glycolipid receptor for the pili-fimbria of *E. coli* in urothelial cells (including prostatic urethra) of both human and nonhuman primates.[27]

Organisms (ureaplasma, for example) go in and out of vogue as potential causes of acute and chronic nonbacterial prostatitis.[15,66,68,81] It is generally considered that the prostate is a reservoir for the transmission of *Trichomonas vaginalis*, but the role of this organism in the etiology of prostatitis remains controversial.[39,83] *T. vaginalis* may be demonstrated by immunoperoxidase techniques within intraepithelial vacuoles in the prostate, but these have been seen only rarely.[39]

Chlamydia trachomatis has long been speculated to be a pathogen for a variety of genitourinary infections including nonbacterial prostatitis.[14,24,44,93,95,104] Using immunoperoxidase techniques with monoclonal antibodies, Shurbaji[93] demonstrated chlamydial antigens in 5 of 16 cases of histologically proven prostatitis, the majority of which were cases of chronic nonbacterial prostatitis. More recently, Abdelatif et al.[1,2] used *in situ* hybridization on formalin-fixed, paraffin-embedded material to demonstrate chlamydial bodies in 7 of 23 transurethral resection specimens with histological evidence of chronic prostatitis. Inclusions were found in epithelial cells and also within intraluminal histiocytes. The frequency with which this organism is the etiological agent of abacterial prostatitis is yet to be established.[1,2,93,94]

Other causes of nonbacterial prostatitis have been proposed and supported by a variety of evidence. Miller,[71] for example, has identified a group of patients for whom he suggests the term "stress prostatitis" as an appropriate label, because the most satisfactory therapy has been stress management. This suggestion is supported by the presence of adrenergic, cholinergic, and vasoactive intestinal polypeptide secreting fibers in the prostate. Miller observed that the prostate has the same autonomic innervation as other organs known to be stress targets (stomach, colon, bronchi, blood vessels). Stress may thus be a potent factor in the development, prolongation, and perturbation of symptoms of what is generally called chronic prostatitis.[42] Gaitenbeck et al.,[40] in reviewing the well-recognized clinical connection between stress and symptoms of chronic prostatitis, noted that in rats, prostatic hemoperfusion is sensitive to stress factors. In their experiments (10 days of standardized stress stimuli of restricted confinement in small cages and low temperatures), all rats developed extensive diffuse inflammatory histopathological changes both within the acini and the stroma. In contrast, no inflammatory changes were present in any other genital organs nor in control animals.

EXPERIMENTAL PROSTATITIS

In experimental animals, the incidence of prostatitis is noted to increase with age. Naslund et al.[75] also demonstrated the effects of genetic background on development of prostatitis, noting substantially different degrees of prostatic inflammation in different strains of rats of a similar age and subjected to similar environmental influences. These investigators and others have demonstrated that the administration of estradiol to rats results in increased incidence and severity of chronic abacterial prostatitis.[74,88]

Earlier work by Naslund and Coffey[74] also demonstrated the role of hormonal influence in development of prostatitis by showing that in rats neonatal *hormonal surges* appear to permanently mark or "imprint" the prostate and determine its subsequent growth and pathophysiology even into adulthood. They found that neonatal treatment with hormones could alter the course of prostatitis in adult rats.

"NORMAL PROSTATITIS"

We have recently examined 150 prostates from forensic autopsies on males ranging in age from 16–42. In this study, approximately three-fourths of the total subjects demonstrated acute and/or chronic prostatitis. There was some variability in occurrence among age groups, but in all groups the majority of subjects were affected. The most common pattern of involvement was a mixed acute and chronic prostatitis as defined by the presence of polymorphonuclear and chronic inflammatory infiltrates within or immediately adjacent to prostatic glands. Stromal macrophages and lymphocytes alone were not considered to represent prostatitis.[8,9]

Several etiologies may be suggested to explain the observation of a microscopic prostatitis in presumably healthy males. The frequency of this finding suggests that it may be related to physiological changes. The following physiological phenomenon could contribute to the development of prostatitis: (1) In persistent foci of unstimulated (hypoplastic) prostate it may be assumed, based on the microscopic appearance of the epithelium, that there is abnormal epithelial secretion. Abnormal amount or composition of prostatic secretions may predispose to inflammation. In recent studies unstimulated areas commonly contained polymorphonuclear leukocytes within ductal and glandular lumina[8,37] and could represent one reason for "physiological" prostatitis. (2) As the normal spherical corpora amylacea are juxtaposed, angulated edges are produced that occasionally abrade the epithelium and extend into the adjacent stroma. In many cases such stromal corpora elicit a granulomatous inflammatory reaction (Fig. 6.5). (3) The

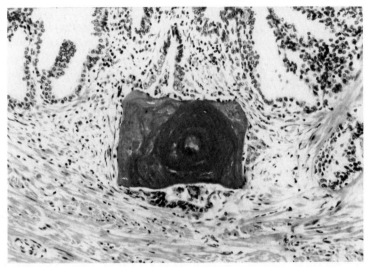

FIG. 6.5.   Large rectangular corpus amylaceum, which has eroded through prostatic epithelium. Note adjacent mild chronic inflammatory infiltrate. A giant cell is present in the glandular lumen just below the corpus. H&E, ×400.

physiological phenomenon of sperm within the prostate may elicit a histiocytic response with production of so-called spermiophages and chronic inflammation.[77]

CONSEQUENCES OF PROSTATITIS

Many of the sequelae of prostatic inflammation are predictable and similar to responses to injury in other sites. Fibrosis occurs and is usually associated with development of atrophic and irregularly angulated glands and ducts. The long-term effects of scarring on adjacent prostatic parenchyma are largely unknown. In other sites, scarring is commonly associated with abnormal epithelial proliferation, *e.g.*, scar cancers in the lung, thyroid, etc. In the prostate, epithelial changes are also noted. Glandular epithelium adjacent to areas of inflammation may, for example, undergo focal squamous metaplasia. Other changes frequently seen in prostatic epithelium adjacent to foci of inflammation are increased cytoplasmic basophilia and enlargement of nuclei with development of prominent nucleoli—changes considered dysplastic in other settings. These histological changes were noted by Stiens *et al.*[100] to be most severe in epithelial nuclei within areas of granulomatous prostatitis. These authors found other evidence to support the histological suggestion of increased nuclear activity by comparing thymidine-labeling indices for prostatic epithelium in areas of inflammation to that in areas of hyperplasia. They found a markedly higher labeling index in glands adjacent to foci diagnosed as "chronic nonspecific prostatitis."

The possible consequences of years or even decades of exposure of prostatic epithelium to the metabolic products of chronic inflammatory cells is unknown. Many theoretical relationships between inflammation and the initiation of stromal hyperplasia have been proposed.[96] One of these proposes an IgE-mediated response that results in histamine/heparin release from mast cells in the prostatic stroma and suggests mechanisms whereby this release could induce stromal proliferation. Other products, including reactive oxygen species, could influence the nucleic acid messages within the epithelium. There is evidence that reactive oxygen is responsible for the stimulation of colonic epithelial proliferative activity associated with inflammatory bowel disease.[23] Lewis and Adams[62] concluded that reactive oxygen intermediates secreted by macrophages may produce DNA lesions in nearby cells comparable to those of ionizing radiation. The effect of chronic localized release of reactive oxygen species in the prostate is unknown. Prostatitis with its myriad of local biochemical and metabolic influences over many years could serve as a promoting influence for prostate carcinogenesis. Studies remain to be done to determine if there is a geographic variation in histological prostatitis that corresponds with the geographic variation in prostate carcinogenesis.

AIDS AND THE PROSTATE

Virtually every molecule of the human immunodeficiency virus (HIV) has been identified. Researchers have an exquisite understanding of some of its more intimate molecular secrets. We know the molecules specifically involved in binding receptors, amino acid sequences of the proteins, and even some three-dimensional molecular configurations. We have some understanding of its evolutionary biology,[50] yet we know remarkably little about the natural history of the sexually transmitted disease state produced by this organism. We know even less about risk factors other than sexual practices or about its association with other sexually transmitted diseases.[55,58,97] In this regard, a hypothetical connection may be drawn between the existence of prostatitis and the pathogenesis of acquired immunodeficiency syndrome.

The hypothesis is that a major risk factor for the sexual transmission of HIV is the presence of an inflammatory reaction within the prostate. The presence of large numbers of HIV-positive white blood cells within the lumina of prostatic glands would provide these cells with ready access to seminal fluid. The admixture of the white cells with luminal sperm could also account for detection of viral proteins within sperm themselves.[64] The presence of the CD4 receptor on the sperm membrane[5] in combination with prolonged exposure to HIV-positive white cells within the prostate could explain the transmission of this agent to a cell that would not otherwise be expected to have been exposed to the virus in high enough titer to become infected. Thus, the prostate, by providing the 3 million white cells present in the "average" ejaculate,[80] could serve as an anatomical reservoir or incubator (or in the case of sperm, perhaps a percolator) for the human immunodeficiency virus.

As part of the test of this hypothesis, other origins of these infected white blood cells must be considered and ruled out if possible. Potential additional sites of origin include the testis, epididymis, vas deferens, and seminal vesicles (Fig. 6.6). The testes are frequently examined, both at autopsy and postsurgically. Microscopically it is unusual to see inflammatory cells in any portion of the testis, and it is especially rare to find such cells within the lumen of testicular tubules. Microscopic sections of epididymis similarly show only spermatozoa within the lumen. Occasional sperm granulomata with associated stromal inflammation may be present, but significant inflammation, especially within the lumen, is rare. Further, we know that after vasectomy, the "normal" inflammatory cells in the ejaculate persist; thus, their origin in the ejaculate must be elsewhere. A third possible site for harboring ejaculatory leukocytes and thus the cells responsible for HIV transmission is the seminal vesicle. A number of studies undertaken to define the histopathology and tabulate the prevalence of chronic seminal vesiculitis have instead shown that this condition is almost nonexistent.[12,16,57,105] In these studies, a total of 3 of 500 cases showed inflammatory changes within seminal vesicles. In two of these there was significant inflammation in adjacent organs that had apparently spread to the seminal vesicles. The histology, then, of the seminal vesicle with its characteristic lipofuscin pigment and enlarged so-called epithelial monster cells is characteristically without inflammatory infiltrate or luminal exudate. In contrast to these sites, white cells in the lumina of the prostate are almost a normal finding. As described previously, they are present in three-fourths of prostates of presumably healthy males between the ages of 16 and 42.[9] Such cells could thus account for the infectious component of HIV-positive semen.

This hypothesis would explain several clinical observations. (1) Some HIV-positive patients seem not to transmit the virus to their partners, while others have a high rate of transmission.[53,82] (2) The intermittent HIV positivity of semen

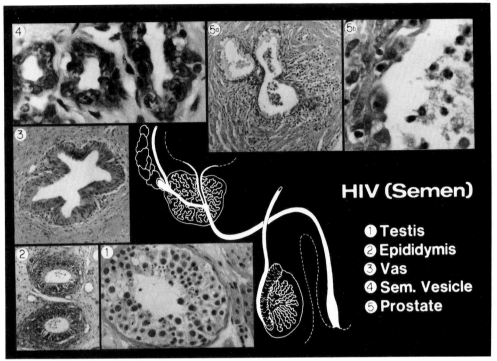

FIG. 6.6. Potential sources of seminal fluid lymphocytes in patients with AIDS. Inflammatory infiltrate is rare in the lumen of the male reproductive tract except in the prostate.

observed in HIV-seropositive patients could reflect a characteristic waxing and waning of chronic prostatitis. (3) The several 100-fold variation in the number of infected cells observed in semen of various individuals could be explained by the presence of prostatitis in some of these patients and not in others.[61] Weissman,[103] in discussing the relationship between sperm positivity for CD4 and HIV, noted "one of the most important questions to be answered is: What cells represent the reservoir for HIV infection?". He called for special attention to be paid to organs involved in the function of the hematopoietic and lymphoid systems as well as the skin and nervous system. An NIH request for grant applications, however, states that "local factors that may play a permissive role or hinder transmission of the virus through the genitourinary tract have not been defined nor has there been a clear definition of the specific origin in the genitourinary tract where the virus resides and/or replicates."[85] Osmond *et al.*[82] further point out that the question of under what conditions can a seropositive individual transmit HIV has been largely unanswered.

Additional unanswered questions relating to this hypothesis have to do with the relationship of inflammatory foci to the onset of clinical AIDS.[91] The mechanism by which an individual converts from being merely seropositive to having the acquired immunodeficiency syndrome has not been fully examined. Yet one of the metabolic products of chronic inflammatory cells, namely hydrogen peroxide, has been shown to be one of the most potent stimulators of HIV replication.[60] Thus it is possible that exacerbation of acute and/or chronic inflammation in a site such as the prostate might play a role in the clinical evolution of an individual from seropositivity to the disease state of acquired immunodeficiency syndrome.

Strategies for prevention and intervention against human immunodeficiency virus must take into account the natural history of the infection.[11] Thus far, such strategies have emphasized the development of vaccines, antiviral chemotherapies, immunostimulants, etc. The above hypotheses would seem to be readily testable and if validated could suggest interventional strategies to influence the prostatic component of the ejaculate, thus affecting the transmission of the virus and potentially its activation/replication.

The above discussion proposes novel hypotheses concerning the transmission and replication of human immunodeficiency virus and the clinical disease it produces. The dimensions of this tragedy (estimated to reach more than 3 million persons in the western hemispheres by the mid-1990s) would seem to warrant, if not invite, hypotheses albeit that most will prove to be false. Speculations about the prostate gland have been fueled by the principles noted above, *i.e.*, the extraordinary frequency of disease at this site and a very incomplete knowledge of the organ's structure and function.

REFERENCES

1. Abdelatif, O. M. A., Chandler, F. W., and McGuire, B. S. *Chlamydia trachomatis* in chronic abacterial prostatitis: Demonstration by colorimetric *in situ* hybridization. *Hum. Pathol. 22:* 1, 41–44, 1991.
2. Abdelatif, O. M. A., Chandler, F. W., and McGuire, B. S. *Chlamydia trachomatis* in chronic abacterial prostatitis. Letter to the Editor. *Hum. Pathol. 22:* 625, 1991.
3. Abrahamsson, P. A., Falkmer, S., Falt, K., and Grimelius, L. The course of neuroendocrine differentiation in prostatic carcinomas. An immunohistochemical study testing chromogranin A as an "endocrine marker." *Path. Res. Pract.* 185, 373–380, 1989.
4. Armstrong, R. W. Complications after intravesical instillation of Bacillus Calmette-Guerin: Rhabdomyolysis and metastatic infection. *J. Urol. 45:* 1264–1266, 1991.
5. Ashida, E. R., and Scofield, E. R. Lymphocyte major histocompatibility complex-encoded class II structures may act as sperm receptors. *Proc. Nath. Acad. Sci. USA* 84, 3395–3399, 1987.
6. Bendich, A., Borenfreund, E., and Witkin, S. S. Information transfer and sperm uptake by mammalian somatic ells. *Prog. Nucl. Acid Res. Mol. Biol. 17:* 43–75, 1976.
7. Bennett, B. D. Prostatic crystalloids: A photo-essay. *JAMA 260:* 2287, 1988.
8. Bennett, B. D., Richardson, P. H., and Gardner, W. A. Histopathology and cytology of prostatitis. In *Prostate Diseases*, edited by H. Lepor and R. K. Lawson. Philadelphia, W. B. Saunders, (In Press).
9. Bennett, B. D., Culberson, D. E., Petty, C. S., and Gardner, W. A. Histopathology of prostatitis. *J. Urol. 143:* 4, 265A, 1990.
10. Bennett, B., and Gardner, W. A., Jr. Crystalloids in prostatic hyperplasia. *Prostate 1:* 31–35, 1980.
11. Bolognesi, D. P. Prospects for prevention of and early intervention of HIV. *JAMA 261:* 20, 3007–3013, 1989.
12. Bostrom, K. Chronic inflammation of human male accessory sex glands and its effect on the morphology of the spermatozoa. *Scand. J. Urol. Nephrol. 5:* 133–140, 1971.
13. Bostwick, D. G., editor. *Pathology of the Prostate.* New York, Churchill Livingstone, 1990.
14. Bruce, A. W., and Reid, G. Prostatitis associated with chlamydia trachomatis in 6 patients. *J. Urol. 142:* 1006–1007, 1989.

15. Brunner, H., Weidner, W., and Schiefer, H. Quantitative studies on the role of ureaplasma urealyticum in non-gonococcal urethritis and chronic prostatitis. *Yale J. Biol. Med. 56:* 545–550, 1983.

16. Calams, J. A. A histopathologic search for chronic seminal vesiculitis. *J. Urol. 74:* 5, 638–645, 1955.

17. Cannon, L., Bishop, D., Spolneck, M., Hunt, S., Lyon, J., and Smart, C. Genetic epidemiology of prostate cancer in the Utah Mormon genealogy. *Cancer Survey 1:* 47–69, 1983.

18. Carter, B. S., Carter, H. B., and Isaacs, J. T. Epidemiologic evidence regarding predisposing factors to prostate cancer. *Prostate 16:* 187–197, 1990.

19. Carter, H. B., and Coffey, D. S. The prostate: An increasing medical problem. *Prostate 16:* 39–48, 1990.

20. Catalona, W. J., Coffey, D. S., and Karr, J. P., editors. *Clinical Aspects of Prostate Cancer. Assessment of New Diagnostic and Management Problems.* New York, Elsevier, 1989, pp. 201–206.

21. Catalona, W. J., Smith, D. S., Ratliff, T. L., Dodds, K. M., Coplen, D. E., Yuan, J. J., Petros, J. A., and Andriole, G. L. Measurement of prostate-specific antigen in serum as a screening test for prostate cancer. *N. Engl. J. Med. 324:* 1156–1161, 1991.

22. Chiarodo, A. National Cancer Institute roundtable on prostate cancer: Future research directions. Meeting Report. *Cancer Res. 51:* 2498–2505, 1991.

23. Craven, P. A., Pfanstiel, J., and DeRubertis, F. R. Role of reactive oxygen in bile salt stimulation of colonic epithelial proliferation. *J. Clin. Invest. 77:* 850–859, 1986.

24. Crum, C., Mitao, M., Winkler, B., Reumann, W., Boon, M. E., and Richart, R. M. Localizing chlamydial infection in cervical biopsies with the immunoperoxidase technique. *Int. J. Gynecol. Pathol. 3:* 19–197, 1984.

25. Davis, B. E., and Weigel, J. W. Adenocarcinoma of the prostate discovered in 2 young patients following total prostatovesiculectomy for refractory prostatitis. *J. Urol. 144:* 744–745, 1990.

26. Deresiewicz, R. L., Stone, R. M., and Aster, J. C. Fatal disseminated mycobacterial infection following intravesical bacillus Calmette-Guerin. *J. Urol. 144:* 1331–1334, 1990.

27. Dilworth, J. P., Neal, D. E., Jr., Fussell, E. N., and Roberts, J. A. Experimental prostatitis in nonhuman primates: I. Bacterial adherence in the urethra. *Prostate 17:* 227–231, 1990.

28. di Sant'Agnese, P. A. Prostatic endocrine-paracrine cells and neuroendocrine differentiation in prostatic carcinoma. In *Progress in Reproductive and Urinary Tract Pathology*, edited by I. Damjanov, A. H. Cohen, S. E. Mills, and R. H. Young. New York, Field & Wood, 1990, pp. 87–108.

29. di Sant'Agnese, P. A., and de Mesy-Jensen, K. L. Neuroendocrine differentiation in prostatic carcinoma. *Hum. Pathol. 18:* 8 849–856, 1987.

30. Donn, A. S., and Muir, C. S. Prostatic cancer: Some epidemiological features. *Bull Cancer (Paris) 72:* 381–390, 1985.

31. Epstein, J. I. *Prostate Biopsy Interpretation.* New York, Raven Press, 1989.

32. Fetissof, F., Arbeille, B., Guilloteau, D., and Lanson, Y. Glycoprotein hormone chain immuno-reactive endocrine cells in prostate and cloacal-derived tissues. *Arch. Pathol. Lab. Med. 111:* 836–840, 1987.

33. Fletcher, S., Neill, W. A., and Norval, M. Seminal polyamines as agents of cervical carcinoma: Production of aneuploidy in squamous epithelium. *J. Clin. Pathol. 44:* 410–415, 1991.

34. Fox, H. Nodular histiocytic prostatitis. *J. Urol. 96:* 372–374, 1966.

35. Furusata, M., Kato, H., Takahashi, H., Wakui, S., Tokuda, T., Kawashima, Y., Aizawa, S., and Mostofi, F. K. Crystalloids in latent prostatic carcinoma. *Prostate 15:* 259–262, 1989.

36. Gardner, W. A. Pathology paradigms. In *Current Concepts and Approaches to the Study of Prostate Cancer*, edited by D. Coffey, N. Bruchovsky, W. Gardner, M. Resnick, and J. Karr. New York, Alan R. Liss, Inc., 1987, pp. 693–702.

37. Gardner, W. A., and Culberson, D. E. Atrophy and proliferation in the young adult prostate. *J. Urol. 137:* 53–56, 1987.

38. Gardner, W. A., and Culberson, D. E. *The Proto-Biology of Prostate Cancer. A Multidisciplinary Analysis of Controversies in the Management of Prostate Cancer*, edited by D. S. Coffey, M. Resnick, F. A. Dorr, and J. P. Karr. New York, Plenum Press, 1988, pp. 35–39.

39. Gardner, W. A., Culberson, D. E., and Bennett, B. D. Trichomonal vaginalis in the prostate gland. *Arch. Pathol. Lab. Med. 110:* 432, 1986.

40. Gatenbeck, L., Aronsson, A., Dahlgren, S., Johansson, B., and Stromberg, L. Stress stimuli-induced histopathological changes in the prostate: An experimental study in the rat. *Prostate 11:* 69–76, 1987.

41. Glassy, J. F., and Mostofi, F. K. Spermatic granulomas of the epididymis. *Am. J. Clin. Pathol. 26:* 1303–1313, 1956.

42. Goldstein, A. M. B., and Padma-Nathan, H. Stress prostatitis. Letter to the editor. *Urology 33:* 449, 1989.

43. Goodson, J. M., and Fruchtman, B. Spermatic granulomas of the epididymis. *Urology 5:* 278–280, 1975.

44. Grant, J. B. F., and Costello, C. B., Sequeua, J. L., and Blacklock, N. J. The role of Chlamydia trachomatis in epididymitis. *Br. J. Urol. 60:* 355–359, 1987.

45. Guess, H. A. Invited commentary: Vasectomy and prostate cancer. *Am. J. Epidemiol. 132:* 1062–1065, 1990.

46. Hamper, U. M., Sheth, S., Walsh, P. C., and Epstein, J. I. Bright echogenic foci in early prostatic carcinoma: Sonographic and pathologic correlation. *Radiology 176:* 339–343, 1990.

47. Higgins, P. J., Borenfreund, E., and Wahiman, M. A. In vitro consequences of sperm. Somatic cell interactions. *Eur. J. Cancer 16:* 1047–1055, 1980.

48. Hill, G. S. *Uropathology. Vol. II.* New York, Churchill Livingstone, 1989, pp. 1165–1180.

49. Hillyard, R. W., Jr., Ladaga, L., and Schellhammer, P. F. Superficial transitional cell carcinoma of the bladder associated with mucosal involvement of the prostatic urethera: Results of treatment with intravesical bacillus Calmette-Guerin. *J. Urol. 139:* 290–293, 1988.

50. Ho, D. D., Pomerantz, R. J., and Kaplan, J. C. Pathologenesis of infection with human immunodeficiency virus. *N. Engl. J. Med. 317:* 5, 278–286, 1987.

51. Howards, S. S. American Urological Association response to articles concerning the relationship of vasectomy and prostate cancer. *AUA Today 4:* 3, 1991.

52. Hsing, A. W., Comstock, G. W., Abbey, H., and Polk, B. F. Serologic precursors of cancer. Retinol, carotenoids, and tocopherol and risk of prostate cancer. *J. Natl. Cancer Inst. 82:* 941–946, 1990.

53. Hube, R. V. Genital tract inflammation linked to AIDS transmission. *AUA Today 3:* 4, 1990.

54. Jensen, P. E., Gardner, W. A., Jr., and Piserchia, P. V. Prostatic cystalloids: Association with adenocarcinoma. *Prostate 1:* 25–30, 1980.

55. Jessamine, P. G., Plummer, F. A., Ndinya-Achola, J. O., Wainberg, M. A., Wamola, I., D'Costa, L. J., Cameron, D. W., Simonsen, J. N., Plourde, P., and Ronald, A. R. Human immunodeficiency virus, genital ulcers and the male foreskin: Synergism in HIV-1 transmission. *Scand. J. Infect. Dis.(Suppl.) 69:* 181–186, 1990.

56. Kadmon, D., Thompson, T. C., Lynch, G. R., and Scardino, P. T. Elevated plasma chromogranin A concentrations in prostatic carcinoma. *J. Urol. 146:* 358–361, 1991.

57. Karolyi, P., Szentirmay, Z., and Krasznai, G. Cytophotomatric investigations in atypical epithelial cells of the human seminal vesicle. *Int. Urol. Nephrol. 24:* 399–402, 1989.

58. Kingsley, L. A., Kaslow, R., Rinaldo, C. R., Detre, K., Odaka, N., VanRaden, M., Detels, R., Polk, B. F., Chmiel, J., Kelsey, S. F., Ostrow, D., and Visscher, B. Risk factors for seroconversion to human immunodeficiency virus among male homosexuals. *Lancet 1:* 345–348, 1987.

59. Kovi, J. *Surgical Pathology of Prostate and Seminal Vesicles.* Boca Raton, FL, CRC Press, 1989.

60. Legrand-Poels, S., Vaira, D., Pincemail, J., Van De Vorst, A., and Piette, J. Activation of human immunodeficiency virus type 1 by oxidative stress. *AIDS Res. Hum. Retroviruses 6:* 12, 1389–1397, 1990.

61. Levy, J. A. The transmission of AIDS: The case of the infected cell. *JAMA 259:* 20, 3037–3038, 1988.

62. Lewis, J. G., and Adams, D. O. Induction of 5, 6-ring-saturated thymine bases in NIH-3T3 cells by phorbol ester-stimulated macrophages: Role of reactive oxygen intermediates. *Cancer Res. 45:* 1270–1275, 1985.

63. Malinin, T. I., Horneck, F. J., Block, N. L., and Malinin, G. I. Aneuploidy of glandular epithelial cells in histologically normal prostate glands. *Experentia 44:* 247–249, 1988.

64. Marx, J. L. Do sperm spread the AIDS virus? *Science 245:* 30, 1989.
65. McClinton, S., Miller, I. D., and Eremin, O. An immunohistochemical characterisation of the inflammatory cell infiltrate in benign and malignant prostatic disease. *Br. J. Cancer 61:* 400–403, 1990.
66. McCormack, W. C. Epidemiology of *Mycoplasma hominis. Sex. Trasm. Dis. 10:* 261–262, 1983.
67. Meikle, W., Smith, J., and West, D. Familial factors affecting prostate cancer risk and plasma steroid levels. *Prostate 6:* 121–128, 1985.
68. Meseguer, M. A., Martinez-Ferre, M., de Rafael, L., Galvez, M., and Baquero, F. Differential counts of ureaplasma urealyticum in male urologic patients. *J. Infect. Dis. 149:* 657, 1984.
69. Mettlin, C., Natarajan, N., and Huben, R. A brief original contribution vasectomy and prostate cancer risk. *Am. J. Epidemiol. 132:* 1056–1061, 1990.
70. Miller, G. J. Diagnostic correlations in prostate. In *Pathology and Pathobiology of Urinary Bladder and Prostate*, Baltimore, Williams & Wilkins, (In Press).
71. Miller, H. C. Stress prostatitis. *Urology 32:* 507–510, 1988.
72. Mostofi, F. K., and Sesterhenn. Plenary lecture: Lymphocytic infiltrate in relationship to urologic tumors. *National Cancer Institute Monograph 49:* 133–141, 1976.
73. Mukamel, E., Konichezky, M., Engelstein, D., Cytron, S., Bramovici, A., and Servadio, C. Clinical and pathological findings in prostates following intravesical bacillus Calmette-Guerin instillations. *J. Urol. 144:* 1399–1400, 1990.
74. Naslund, M. J., and Coffey, D. S. The differential effects of neonatal androgen, estrogen and progesterone on adult rat prostate growth. *J. Urol. 136:* 1136–1140, 1986.
75. Naslund, M. J., Strandberg, J. D., and Coffey, D. S. The role of androgens and estrogens in the pathogenesis of experimental nonbacterial prostatitis. *J. Urol. 140:* 1049–1053, 1988.
76. Neal, D. E., Dilworth, J. P., Kaack, M. B., Didier, P., and Roberts, J. A. Experimental prostatitis in nonhuman primates: II. Ascending acute prostatitis. *Prostate 17:* 233–239, 1990.
77. Nelson, G., Culberson, D. E., and Gardner, W. A. Intraprostatic spermatozoa. *Hum. Pathol. 19:* 4, 541–544, 1988.
78. Nelson, G. A., Scimeca, J. M., Abee, C. A., and Gardner, W. A. Intraprostatic spermatozoa in the squirrel monkey. *Prostate 12:* 321–324, 1988.
79. Nielsen, M. L., and Christensen, P. Inflammatory changes in the hyperplastic prostate. *Scand. J. Urol. Nephrol. 6:* 6–10, 1972.
80. Olsen, G. P., and Shields, J. W. Seminal lymphocytes, plasma and AIDS. *Nature (Lond.) 309:* 10, 116–117, 1984.
81. Oriel, J. D. Role of genital mycoplasmas in nongonococcal urethritis and prostatitis. *Sex. Trasm. Dis. 10:* 263–270, 1983.
82. Osmond, D., Bacchetti, P., Chaisson, R. W., Kelly, T., Stempel, R., Carlson, J., and Moss, A. R. Time of exposure and risk of HIV infection in homosexual partners of men with AIDS. *Am. J. Pub. Health 78:* 8, 944–948, 1988.
83. Paulson, D. F., editor. *Prostatic Disorders.* Philadelphia, Lea & Febiger, 1989, pp. 71–106.
84. Presti, B., and Weidner, N. Granulomatous prostatitis and poorly differentiated carcinoma. Their distinction with the use of immunohistochemical methods. *Am. J. Clin. Pathol. 95:* 330–334, 1991.
85. RFA Announcement 88-DK-02. Genitourinary tract manifestations of the Human immunodeficiency virus (HIV). National Institutes of Health, Bethesda, Md, 1987.
86. Ro, J. Y., Ayala, A. G., Ordonez, N. G., Cartwright, J., and MacKay, B. Intraluminal crystalloids in prostatic adenocarcinoma. *Cancer 57:* 2397–2407, 1986.
87. Ro, J. Y., Grignon, D. J., Troncoso, P., and Ayala, A. G. Intraluminal crystalloids in whole-organ sections of prostate. *Prostate 13:* 233–239, 1988.
88. Robinette, C. L. Sex-hormone-induced inflammation and fibromuscular proliferation in the rat lateral prostate. *Prostate 12:* 271–286, 1988.
89. Rosenberg, L., Palmer, J. R., Zauber, A. G., Warshauer, M. E., Stolley, P. D., and Shapiro, S. Vasectomy and the risk of prostate cancer. *Am. J. Epidemiol. 132:* 1051–1055, 1990.
90. Rotkin, I. D. Studies in the epidemiology of prostatic cancer: Expanded sampling. *Cancer Treatment Reports 61:* 173–180, 1977.

91. Roy, S., and Wainberg, M. A. Role of the mononuclear phagocyte system in the development of acquired immunodeficiency syndrome (AIDS). *J. Leukocyte Biol. 43:* 91–97, 1988.
92. Rumke, P. The origin of immunoglobulins in semen. *Clin. Exp. Immunol. 17:* 287–297, 1974.
93. Shurbaji, M. D. *Chlamydia trachomatis* in chronic abacterial prostatitis. *Hum. Pathol. 22:* 625, 1991.
94. Shurbaji, M. S., Dumler, J. S., Gage, W. R., Pettis, G. L., Gupta, P. K., and Kuhadja, F. P. Immunochemical detection of chlamydia antigens in association with cystitis. *Am. J. Clin. Pathol. 93:* 363–366, 1990.
95. Shurbaji, M. S., Gupta, P. K., and Myers, J. Immunohistochemical demonstration of chlamydial antigens in association with prostatitis. *Mod. Pathol. 1:* 348–351, 1988.
96. Smith, C. J., and Gardner, W. A. Inflammation—Proliferation: Possible relationships in the prostate. In *Current Concepts and Approaches to the Study of Prostate Cancer,* edited by D. Coffey, N. Bruchovsky, W. Gardner, M. Resnick, and J. Karr. New York, Alan R. Liss, Inc., 1987, pp. 317–325.
97. Stamm, W. E., Handsfield, H., Rompalo, A. M., Ashley, R. L., Roberts, P. L., and Corey, L. The association between genital ulcer disease and acquisition of HIV infection in homosexual men. *JAMA 260:* 10, 1429–1433, 1988.
98. Steinberg, G. D., Carter, B. S., Beaty, T. H., Childs, B., and Walsh, P. C. Family history and the risk of prostate cancer. *Prostate 17:* 337–347, 1990.
99. Stein-Werblowsky, R. On the etiology of cancer of the prostate. *Eur. Urol. 4:* 370–373, 1978.
100. Stiens, R., Helpap, B., and Bruhl, P. The proliferation of prostatic epithelium in chronic prostatitis. *Urol. Res.* 21–24, 1975.
101. Thompson, Sir Henry. *Diseases of the Prostate.* London, Churchill, 1860.
102. Torres, G. M., Kaude, J. V., and Drylie, D. Bacille-Calmette-Guerin vaccine-induced granulomatous prostatitis: Another hopoechoic nonneoplastic lesion. *AJR 155:* 195–196, 1990.
103. Weissman, I. Approaches to an understanding of pathogenetic mechanisms in AIDS. *Rev. Inf. Dis. 20:* 385–398, 1988.
104. Winkler, B., Gallo, L., Reumann, W., Richart, R. M., Mitao, M., and Crum, C. P. Chlamydial endometritis. A histological and immunohistochemical analysis. *Am. J. Surg. Pathol. 8:* 771–770, 1984.
105. Wittstok, G., and Korchner, I. Zur biomorphose der samenblasen unter besonderer berucksichtigung der chronischen spermatocystitis. *Virch. Archiv. Path. Anat. 341:* 12–20, 1970.
106. Xia, T., Blackburn, W. R., and Gardner, W. A. Fetal prostate growth and development. *Pediatr. Pathol. 10:* 527–537, 1990.

Chapter 7

Controversies in Prostate Pathology: Dysplasia and Carcinoma *In Situ*

JONATHAN I. EPSTEIN

INTRODUCTION

Within this manuscript a framework for understanding the broad topic of atypical hyperplastic lesions within the prostate will be presented. A brief yet critical summary of some of the most frequently quoted older references on this topic will provide an understanding as to why atypical hyperplasia of the prostate has been, until recently, one of the most confusing topics within the field of prostate pathology. Although this Chapter will emphasize prostatic lesions with cytologic atypia, a concise yet comprehensive discussion of the most common atypical prostatic lesion that resembles carcinoma yet lacks cytologic atypia will also be provided.

SUMMARY OF OLDER LITERATURE: PROBLEMS WITH TERMINOLOGY

Earlier studies dealing with atypical lesions within the prostate suffered from three major deficiencies: (1) the analysis of lesions with diverse histology as one entity[23]; (2) the use of vague and nonreproducible definitions[20,36]; and (3) the inclusion of lesions as atypical hyperplasia that currently would be regarded as infiltrating carcinoma.[7,8,35,44] Throughout this article I will use the term "atypical hyperplasia of the prostate" in the broad sense to denote lesions that resemble in some manner carcinoma of the prostate. Atypical lesions of the prostate can be subclassified into two major categories: (1) lesions that lack cytologic atypia and resemble adenocarcinoma of the prostate in their architectural appearance; and (2) lesions that cytologically resemble adenocarcinoma of the prostate that may or may not have accompanying architectural abnormalities. As will be discussed later, this distinction is critical since lesions without cytologic atypia do not appear to be as strongly linked with carcinoma as those lesions of atypical hyperplasia with cytologic atypia.

One of the most frequently cited authors on atypical hyperplasia of the prostate is Kastendieck.[23] His work was one of the first to provide an extremely detailed attempt to correlate lesions of atypical hyperplasia on the prostate to carcinoma.

However, it is difficult to compare current studies with that of Kastendieck since lesions with and without cytologic atypia were lumped together and considered under the broad category of atypical hyperplasia. Although Kastendieck makes reference to different forms of atypical hyperplasia, in his detailed analysis of the relationship of atypical hyperplasia to carcinoma the various forms of atypical hyperplasia are not analyzed separately. The other author that is frequently quoted in this area is Helpap.[20] In particular, he is often quoted on his use of radioactively labeled thymidine to compare the proliferation rates of atypical hyperplasia to carcinoma. Similar to Kastendieck, Helpap considered as one entity lesions with minimal cytologic atypia that resemble low-grade adenocarcinoma and lesions with cytologic atypia. Furthermore, no criteria were provided as to how those lesions considered as atypical hyperplasia were distinguished from those of low-grade adenocarcinoma. The distinction between those lesions with cytologic atypia and carcinoma were similarly not defined in a manner that could be duplicated by other authors.

Another problem with earlier studies on atypical hyperplasia has been the changing diagnostic criteria for adenocarcinoma of the prostate, which in large part has been driven by clinical factors. Prior to the early 1980s, radical prostatectomies were associated with significant morbidity and were infrequently performed for clinically confined adenocarcinoma of the prostate. Following the pioneering work by Dr. Patrick Walsh on the nerve-sparing modified radical retropubic prostatectomy, the numbers of radical prostatectomies performed around the country have greatly increased.[27,48,49] This increase in the number of radical prostatectomies performed has had several consequences in terms of our pathological criteria for diagnosing adenocarcinoma of the prostate. Pathologists have had a greater number of prostatic specimens, which lack the artifacts seen in autopsy prostates, to study prostate cancer and related lesions. More importantly, knowing that a diagnosis of adenocarcinoma could lead to radical prostatectomy, where the accuracy of the diagnosis could be verified or challenged, has led to more stringent diagnostic criteria as to what constitutes carcinoma on biopsy material. Newer developments, such as the use of immunohistochemistry with basal cell specific antibodies, have further refined our diagnostic acumen in the distinction of carcinoma from mimickers of cancer, such as adenosis. In many of the older articles dealing with atypical hyperplasia of the prostate, lesions that were depicted as being precursor lesions to adenocarcinoma would currently be regarded by most experts as infiltrating adenocarcinoma.[7,8,35,44]

LESIONS THAT ARCHITECTURALLY RESEMBLE CARCINOMA YET LACK CYTOLOGIC ATYPIA

Adenosis, as we define it, is probably the most common lesion misdiagnosed as low-grade adenocarcinoma of the prostate.[14] Before discussing the diagnostic criteria and clinical implications of adenosis, it is necessary first to clarify some of the confusion related to this topic due to differences in terminology. The most confounding works on this topic are two manuscripts by Brawn,[7,8] who used the term adenosis in the broad sense to describe glandular prostatic lesions that lacked cytologic atypia. Under this all-encompassing definition, Brawn's adenosis included many lesions that most authorities would currently regard as low-grade adenocarcinoma as well as examples of basal cell hyperplasia and atrophic glands.

We use the term adenosis to describe a lesion that mimics adenocarcinoma, yet differs from low-grade adenocarcinoma in several crucial aspects. Other synonyms that have been used to describe adenosis include small alveolar proliferation, small glandular hyperplasia, atypical adenomatous hyperplasia, atypical glandular hyperplasia, and adenomatous hyperplasia. Because different authors may use the same term to denote different histological lesions, one must pay critical attention to the terminology used in describing atypical lesions within the prostate.

Adenosis at low magnification is composed of numerous crowded small, pale-staining glands that resemble a nodule of low-grade adenocarcinoma of the prostate. Yet even at scanning magnification, there are certain differences between adenosis and low-grade adenocarcinoma that can begin to suggest the diagnosis of adenosis (Table 7.1). Whereas both adenosis and low-grade adeno-carcinoma consist of glands that are relatively noninfiltrative, in adenosis the glands tend to be more circumscribed and in particular often have a lobular configuration (Fig. 7.1A). In contrast, low-grade adenocarcinoma tends to be at least minimally infiltrative at the edge of the nodules (Fig. 7.1B). Even more importantly, the glands in low-grade adenocarcinoma are not lobular but are arranged in a haphazard array with glands often appearing to infiltrate into the stroma at right angles to each other.

Another critical difference between adenosis and low-grade adenocarcinoma seen at low power is the relationship of the small glands suspicious for carcinoma to surrounding, more recognizable benign glands. In adenosis, there is a gradual transition between the small glands suspicious for carcinoma and adjacent more recognizably benign glands; some of the features seen in the benign glands include branching, larger and more irregular shapes, and papillary infoldings (Fig. 7.2A). In contrast, glands of low-grade adenocarcinoma stand out in sharp contrast to

TABLE 7.1. HISTOLOGICAL DIFFERENCES BETWEEN ADENOSIS AND LOW-GRADE ADENOCARCINOMAS

Adenosis	Low-Grade Carcinoma
1. Lobular and fairly circumscribed growth pattern (Fig. 7.1A)	1. Glands infiltrate out into surrounding stroma in different directions (Fig. 7.1B)
2. Small glands suspicious for cancer merge with benign appearing glands (Fig. 7.2A)	2. Small glands stand out in contrast to surrounding benign glands (Fig. 7.2B)
3. Pale to clear cytoplasm (Fig. 7.3A)	3. May have amphophilic cytoplasm (Fig. 7.3B)
4. Small nuclei with occasional prominent nucleoli (Fig. 7.3A and B)	4. Nuclei may be enlarged with huge nucleoli (Fig. 7.4B)
5. Crystalloids rare	5. Crystalloids frequent
6. Intraluminal mucin not visible on H&E	6. Blue-tinged mucin may be seen within glands on H&E
7. Basal cells often identifiable in some glands (Fig. 7.3A and B)	7. Basal cells absent, though fibroblasts may mimic basal cells (Fig. 7.4B)
8. Basal cell antibodies show patchy immunoreactivity (Fig. 7.5A)	8. Negative immunostaining with basal cell antibodies (Fig. 7.5B)

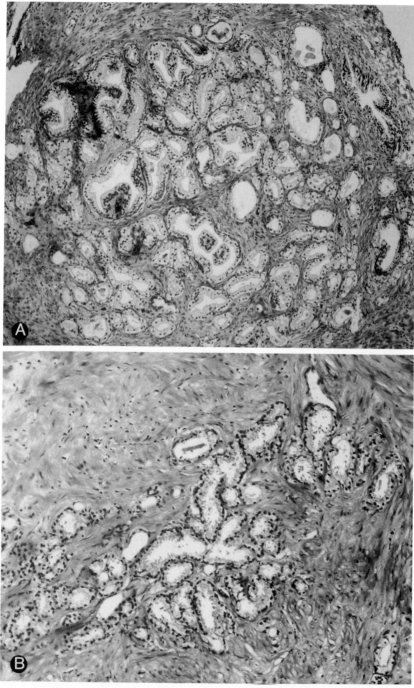

FIG. 7.1.   (*A*) Characteristic lobular growth pattern of adenosis. Note admixed among small glands suspicious for carcinoma there are larger more benign appearing glands with papillary projections, which were otherwise identical to the smaller glands. × 50. (*B*) Small focus of low-grade adenocarcinoma in which glands infiltrate into the stroma in different directions rather than the lobular pattern seen with adenosis. × 125.

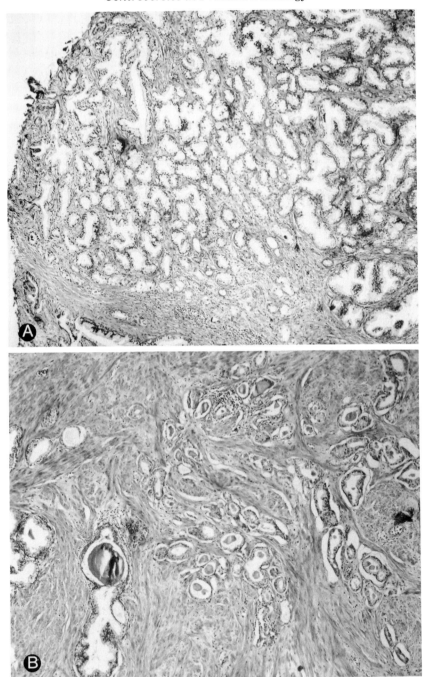

FIG. 7.2. (*A*) Adenosis in which small glands suspicious for carcinoma (left) merge with cytologically similar larger, branching more benign appearing glands (right). × 55. (*B*) Nodule of low-grade adenocarcinoma, which infiltrates haphazardly into the stroma, and stands out in contrast to the surrounding benign glands (lower left). × 55.

surrounding benign glands (Fig. 7.2B). Whereas one should be able to say with confidence when assessing a focus of adenocarcinoma of the prostate which are the benign glands and which are malignant, in adenosis this distinction cannot be made.

At higher magnification the cells of adenosis have pale-to-clear cytoplasm. Nucleoli are usually indistinct, although occassionally they may be fairly prominent (Fig. 7.3A). Although some adenocarcinomas have minimal nuclear atypia and pale-clear cytoplasm, others have more amphophilic cytoplasm and/or more prominant nucleoli (Fig. 7.3B). One of the key distinguishing features between carcinoma and benign glandular proliferations mimicking carcinoma is the lack of a basal cell layer in all adenocarcinomas of the prostate.[46] However, the use of basal cells as a diagnostic criteria in adenosis is difficult for several reasons. First, basal cells visible by light microscopy are only present in a minority of the glands of adenosis within a given nodule. In addition, the distinction of a flattened basal cell layer from closely apposed fibroblasts can be extremely difficult.

Work by Nagle et al.,[38,39] Brawer et al.,[6] Gown and Vogel,[17] and Wernert et al.[50] has led to the discovery that certain keratin antibodies selectively stain basal cells within the prostate. While some of these antibodies are privately owned and utilized for research purposes, the antibody keratin 903 (Enzo Biochemical) is commercially available and has been used by us and others for diagnostic purposes.[5,6,19] Within a nodule of adenosis, between 10 and 100% of the glands will show some staining of basal cells with keratin 903.[19] On average, approximately two-thirds of the glands within a nodule of adenosis will show some decoration of the basal cell layer. This staining may be difficult to interpret since within a given gland it is often patchy and consists of a flattened attenuated rim of immunoreactivity located beneath the secretory cell layer (Fig. 7.4A). This staining also tends to be sensitive to various lengths of formalin fixation and must be titrated accordingly. All carcinomas studied to date fixed in formalin have been negative. However, when interpreting stains for keratin 903, as with all immunoperoxidase stains, one must be aware of interpreting entrapped positive-staining benign glands (Fig. 7.4B). We have not found this to be a significant problem since entrapped benign glands tend to stain uniformly and intensely and stand out in contrast to the patchy staining in adenosis. Furthermore, the morphology of the entrapped benign glands usually stand out as well from the glands of adenosis.

Adenosis tends to be located centrally within the gland, such that it is most commonly seen in transurethral resection specimens. In transurethral resection specimens, one usually has an entire nodule of adenosis to evaluate, where it would be highly unlikely for the entire focus to show no immunoreactivity with keratin 903. Consequently, the lack of keratin 903 staining in a nodule of glands in which one is deciding between adenosis and low-grade adenocarcinoma is highly supportive of the diagnosis of adenocarcinoma. Infrequently, adenosis may be seen on needle biopsy. Because keratin staining of adenosis is often patchy and may be present in only a minority of the glands within a nodule, the lack of basal cell staining on a needle biopsy with more limited tissue is not as definitive.

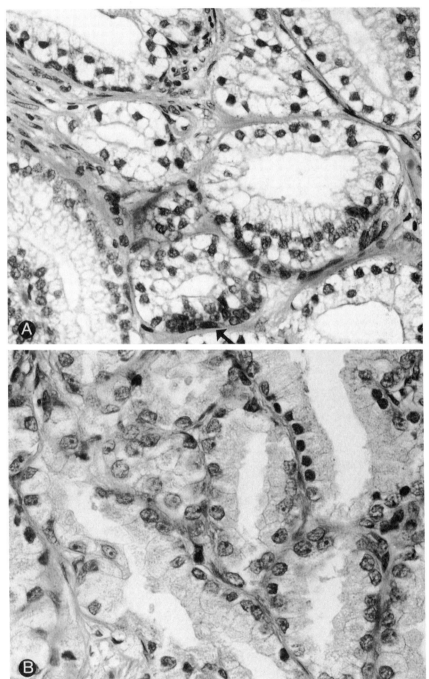

FIG. 7.3. (*A*) Higher magnification of adenosis showing glands with pale-to-clear cytoplasm and minimal nuclear atypia. Although some glands show no identifiable basal cell layer, in others, a well-defined basal cell layer (*arrow*) can be identified. Note plumper appearance of basal cell as compared to stromal fibroblasts. × 370. (*B*) High magnification of low-grade adenocarcinoma. Although some nuclei appear small and uniform, others show nuclear enlargement with more prominent nucleoli than may be seen in adenosis. Basal cells are not identified. × 580.

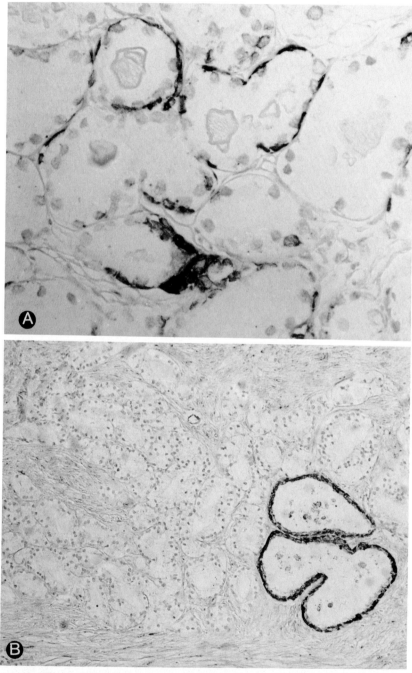

FIG. 7.4. (*A*) Keratin 903 staining of adenosis showing thin rim of immunoreactivity corresponding to flattened basal cells. Note that not all glands show immunoreactivity, yet those showing no immunoreactivity are otherwise identical to glands containing the basal cells. Consequently, the entire nodule should be considered as benign. × 400 (*B*) Focus of low-grade adenocarcinoma showing a lack of immunoreactivity with keratin 903. Note intense uniform staining of adjacent benign glands, easily recognizable by their morphology and staining as entrapped benign glands. × 130.

The positive staining of glands suspicious for adenosis on needle biopsy, however, is diagnostic of adenosis and rules out carcinoma.

The relationship of adenosis to carcinoma is still controversial. Most of the studies suggesting a link between adenosis and adenocarcinoma of the prostate are ones that were mentioned earlier in which adenosis was considered under the broad category of atypical hyperplasia. Based on these studies, any association between adenosis and carcinoma most likely resulted not from adenosis, but from other cytologically atypical lesions that appear more closely linked to carcinoma. Some of the evidence touted as linking adenosis with carcinoma is the supposed topographical relationship between adenosis and carcinoma. The study most often cited showing this phenomenon is that from Kastendieck.[23] Kastendieck uses the broad definition of atypical hyperplasia, which includes adenosis as well as lesions that have significant cytologic atypia. The coincidence of atypical hyperplasia and carcinoma of the prostate in the same location, based on his photographs, appears to be attributed to lesions of atypical hyperplasia, which have significant nuclear atypia rather than to adenosis.

The other evidence that has been proposed linking adenosis to carcinoma is the purported increased proliferation rate in adenosis based on thymidine labeling studies.[20] Helpap,[20] however, groups adenosis with other cytologically atypical lesions and does not provide well-defined criteria for separating adenosis from carcinoma. Consequently, this increase in thymidine labeling cannot be attributed to adenosis and may represent increased proliferation in other forms of atypical hyperplasia or even carcinoma.

The third line of reasoning that has been raised to argue an association between adenosis and carcinoma is the suggestion that there is an increased risk of adenosis progressing to carcinoma. The major work that has been quoted showing this is that of Brawn.[7,8] Brawn, however, provides a broad definition of adenosis to include any epithelial lesion in the prostate which lacks significant cytologic atypia. Consequently, many of his illustrations demonstrate infiltrative glandular proliferations, which most authorities would regard as low-grade carcinoma. In part, it appears that Brawn's definition of adenosis is based on a philosophical viewpoint that prostatic lesions without significant cytologic atypia do not pose a significant threat to the patient and therefore should not be called carcinoma. Consequently, even though some of the lesions that Brawn illustrates share many features with more recognizable carcinomas, such as an infiltrative haphazard growth pattern and lack of a basal cell layer, because of their low biological malignancy he would prefer to diagnose these lesions as adenosis. While this viewpoint is understandable, it must be recognized that in every organ system there is a spectrum from low-grade lesions to high-grade lesions. If these low-grade lesions share critical morphological features with higher grade adenocarcinomas, they are still regarded as carcinoma, albeit with a low malignant potential. More recent studies of these small, low-grade prostatic adenocarcinomas, which Brawn would term adenosis, have demonstrated an increased long-term risk of progression, further justifying their acceptance as adenocarcinomas of the prostate.[2,13,16,45] Brawn's reported increased risk of progression with adenosis versus ordinary hyperplasia most likely is attributable to his inclusion of low-grade carcinomas in his study. There has been no conclusive evidence showing that adenosis, as we define it, carries with it an increased risk of progressing to carcinoma.

Another line of reasoning supporting the link of adenosis to carcinoma is what some authors describe as a histological continuity between an area of adenosis merging in with carcinoma. McNeal,[29] in some of his earlier studies, demonstrated what he thought were areas of adenosis blending in with areas of carcinoma. It appears that the distinction between adenosis and carcinoma in these areas was based on the visibility of the basal cell layer. However, it is now recognized that in H&E-stained sections basal cells in adenosis are often inconspicuous, yet are visible using basal cell-specific antibodies such as keratin 903. In a nodule in which it appears that adenosis is merging in with carcinoma, using basal cell-specific antibodies often shows the entire nodule to contain basal cells. Of the 100 or so cases of adenosis that this author has seen, in only one case was there a possibility that areas of adenosis merged in with areas of low-grade adenocarcinoma. In this case, areas of adenosis with patchy basal cell layers merged in with areas of small glands with similar cytologic features, yet had an apparent lack of basal cells. Given the rarity of this association, it either may be an anecdotal true event or may represent a collision between areas of adenosis and low-grade carcinoma or an example of adenosis that lacked significant areas of basal cells.

The final argument used by authors suggesting a relationship between adenosis and carcinoma is the apparent lack of basal cells in adenosis.[3] This argument, however, takes into account only the finding of basal cells by conventional H&E light microscopy. Using stains for keratin 903, nodules of adenosis invariably contain a patchy basal cell layer in some of the glands, which is evidence for their benign nature rather than relating them to carcinoma. The fact that the basal cell layer is patchy in adenosis is not that significant, since even obviously benign glands may have a patchy basal cell layer.[19] The only definitive way to prove adenosis has an association with carcinoma would be to follow patients with a diagnosis of adenosis to assess their risk of progression. In order for such a study to be valid, first the distinction of adenosis from carcinoma must be rigid, supported by the use of objective criteria such as basal cell-specific antibodies. Secondly, the follow-up must be of sufficient length to assess the risk of progression. It has been shown that with low-grade adenocarcinoma of the prostate, the mean time to progression is between 7 and 10 years.[2,16] A study of patients with adenosis should have a similar follow-up so that the relative risks of progression with adenosis and low-grade adenocarcinoma can be compared. Until such studies are performed and show otherwise, there currently does not appear to be strong evidence that patients with adenosis have an increased risk of adenocarcinoma, either at the time of diagnosis or in the future.

LESIONS WITH CYTOLOGIC ATYPIA

Within the last few years, studies have generally distinguished among the various forms of atypical hyperplasia within the prostate. In particular, there has been greater concentration on studying atypical lesions within the prostate that have nuclear atypia, in which there may or may not be accompanying architectural abnormalities. Despite the relatively recent nature of this literature, numerous synonyms abound for these cytologically atypical lesions. Each term has its own proponent and whose argument as to which is the best term sometimes appears out of proportion to the importance of the issue. In 1986, articles by Oyasu *et al.*[41] and McNeal and Bostwick[32] described atypical lesions within the prostate characterized by glands that maintain their normal architectural patterns yet had nuclear atypia. Severe atypia was based on glands having nuclei that were greater than 50% larger than normal nuclei.[42] Nuclear prominence was a separate factor assessed. McNeal and Bostwick, during the same year, also published an article on an atypical lesion of the prostate, which they termed "intraductal dysplasia." Intraductal dysplasia was subcategorized into three grades. Grade 1 was characterized by increased nuclear size with increased variability of nuclear size, along with irregular focal crowding and multilayering. Grade 2 had similar features to Grade 1 and with hyperchromatism and occasional small prominent nucleoli (Fig. 7.5). The hallmark of Grade 3 intraductal dysplasia was the finding of numerous large prominent nucleoli (Fig. 7.6). (The relationship between intraductal dysplasia and carcinoma will be discussed in subsequent sections.) Over the ensuing years, the diagnostic criteria proposed by McNeal and Bostwick have generally been adopted as the accepted method of grading cytologically atypical lesions within the prostate. However, various criticisms of the term intraductal dysplasia were raised and other nomenclature became championed.

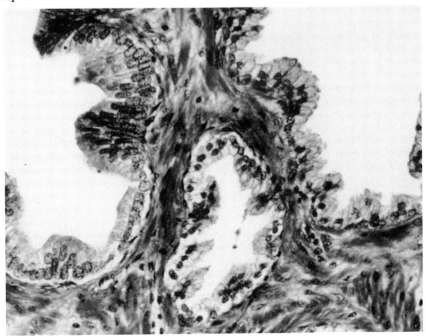

FIG. 7.5. Moderate dysplasia (left) showing the lack of frequent prominent nucleoli seen in severe dysplasia. × 175.

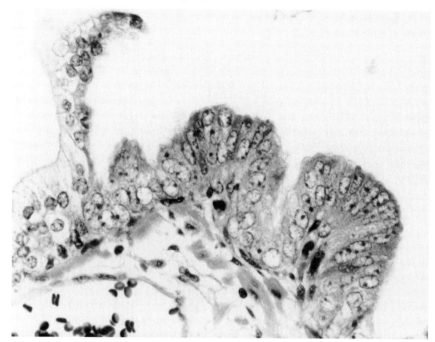

FIG. 7.6. Intraductal severe dysplasia (PIN3) showing large vesicular nuclei with prominent nucleoli that have lost their basilar orientation and have become crowded and overlapping. Note within the single gland the abrupt transition between benign-appearing nuclei and dysplastic nuclei. × 220.

Some authors have almost a visceral dislike for the term "dysplasia" to describe cytologically atypical lesions. The opposition for the term dysplasia is that it is often used to describe abnormalities in embryogenesis, such as "dysplastic kidney." Others note that the atypical lesions within the prostate often do not occur within large ducts but within acini. Kovi *et al.*[24] proposed the term "large acinar atypical hyperplasia" to address these concerns. In a slight variation on their earlier terminology, Mostofi *et al.*[37] recently proposed the term "hyperplasia with malignant change." This term was selected by virtue of its being less specific as to where the atypical nuclear features may be found as well as emphasizing what they feel is the premalignant nature of this lesion.

The other term introduced to describe the same lesion initially referred to an intraductal dysplasia is "prostatic intraepithelial neoplasia" (PIN).[4] This term was introduced as a parallel to that seen within the uterine cervix. While this nomenclature has some advantages, given that it is relatively recent and has not been used by different authors to denote different lesions, it is also not without deficiencies. Within the uterine cervix, the continuum between cervical intraepithelial neoplasia (CIN)1, CIN2, CIN3, and invasive squamous carcinoma is a well-studied phenomenon in which the risks of progressing from one step to the other has been clearly elucidated. In contrast, as will be discussed shortly, our understanding of the natural history of cytologically atypical lesions within the prostate is not nearly so well defined. By using "PIN," the potential harm is that the lesion's relationship to carcinoma will generally be assumed to parallel that seen within CIN of the cervix because of their similar terminology.

While not belittling the importance of terminology, we must rise above terminology in order to devote more energy to understanding these lesion's biological behavior. Anecdotally, I have seen manuscripts or presentations in this field totally disregarded solely because they disagreed vehemently with the term being used. Whenever describing these cytologically atypical lesions within the prostate, I use the term intraductal dysplasia as defined by McNeal and Bostwick,[32] with PIN listed in quotations as a synonym or vice versa. Since McNeal and Bostwick's publication in 1986, their method of characterizing and grading intraductal dysplasia (PIN) has been used in multiple studies on the topic. Accordingly, our foundation of knowledge on the relationship between intraductal dysplasia and carcinoma of the prostate is primarily based on studies using these definitions.

HISTOLOGICAL APPEARANCE OF INTRADUCTAL DYSPLASIA (PIN)

Although intraductal dysplasia is characterized by nuclear atypia, there are often accompanying architectural abnormalities.[14] At low magnification, severe dysplasia is characterized by glands that are separated by a modest amount of stroma and have a normal overall architectural pattern. These glands resemble benign glands in that they branch, are large, and have papillary and undulating luminal surfaces. However, at low magnification, glands with moderate or severe dysplasia tend to have a basophilic appearance (Fig. 7.7). This basophilic appearance is due to a combination of features including enlarged nuclei, hyperchromatism, overlapping of the nuclei, and epithelial hyperplasia. The earliest form of intraductal severe dysplasia (PIN3) is characterized by an increase in nuclear size with prominent nucleoli, without significant epithelial hyperplasia. Often the basal cell layer is still visible and the demarcation between dysplastic and normal nuclei is often abrupt (Fig. 7.6). With more pronounced forms of severe dysplasia, nuclei become more piled up and develop micropapillary projections (Fig. 7.8). These micropapillary projections are similar to those seen with micropapillary intraductal carcinoma of the breast, in that they are composed of tall epithelial buds lacking fibrovascular cores.

An interesting phenomenon in intraductal dysplasia is that within these epithelial projections, the nuclei toward the center of the gland tend to have a more bland cytologic appearance compared to the nuclei peripherally located up against the basement membrane. The grade of dysplasia is assigned based on assessment of the nuclei peripherally located up against the basement membrane, rather than the more bland-appearing nuclei toward the center of the gland. With further epithelial hyperplasia, more complex architectural patterns appear, such as Roman bridge and cribriform formation (Fig. 7.9). In a given gland it may be difficult to determine whether one is dealing with intraductal severe dysplasia with a cribriforming pattern or cribriforming infiltrating carcinoma. In general, this maturation of nuclei with more bland-appearing nuclei appearing within the center of the gland tends to be more prominent in cribriforming

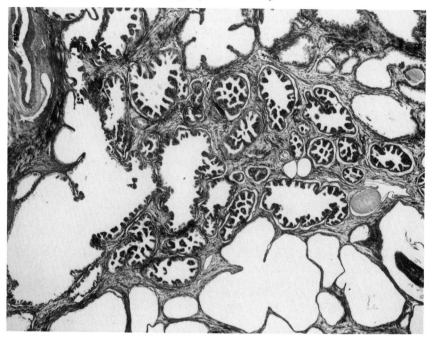

FIG. 7.7.   Intraductal severe dysplasia with preservation of normal architectural pattern of the prostate. Basophilic appearance of the dysplastic glands is due to piling up of the nuclei and the high nuclei-to-cytoplasmic ratio in these glands. × 30.

intraductal dysplasia as compared to cribriforming infiltrating carcinoma. The finding of a basal cell layer within the cribriforming glands is additional evidence that one is dealing with a dysplastic gland rather than an infiltrating cribriforming nest. (This topic is discussed further in the section on the significance of finding dysplasia on biopsy.)

RELATIONSHIP OF INTRADUCTAL DYSPLASIA (PIN) TO CARCINOMA OF THE PROSTATE

Much of the indirect evidence associating intraductal dysplasia (PIN) with carcinoma of the prostate has come from studies examining differences between prostate glands with carcinoma and prostate glands without carcinoma. The three major studies assessing these differences are from McNeal and Bostwick,[32] Kovi *et al.*,[24] and Troncoso *et al.*[47] In McNeal and Bostwick's study, autopsy specimens were utilized; both a mixture of radical prostatectomy specimens and autopsy specimens were examined in the work of Kovi *et al.*; and Troncoso *et al.* utilized cystoprostatectomy specimens performed for transitional cell carcinoma of the bladder for their study population. All three studies documented an increased incidence of higher grade dysplasia in malignant glands versus benign glands, as well as an overall higher incidence of dysplasia in organs harboring carcinoma. Furthermore, the size of the dysplastic foci as well as the number of dysplastic foci were increased in prostates with carcinoma as compared to those

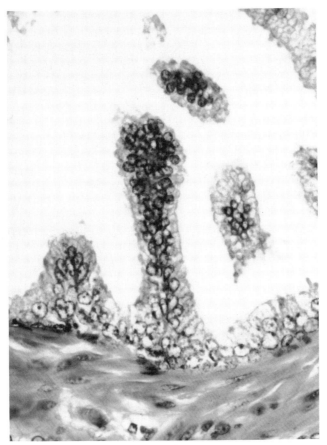

FIG. 7.8. Intraductal severe dysplasia with micropapillary tufts. Note the classic features of severe dysplasia are present in nuclei located peripherally toward the basement membrane. Nuclei toward the center of the gland have a more benign cytologic appearance. × 350.

without carcinoma. It was also noted that, with increasing amounts of dysplasia, there was a greater number of multifocal carcinomas. All of these findings would be expected if intraductal dysplasia was a precursor lesion to carcinoma of the prostate. Troncoso *et al.* also noted an increase of intraductal dysplasia in the peripheral zone of the prostate, correlating with the predilection for most adenocarcinomas of the prostate to originate in this region.

PIN1

The exact incidence of mild dysplasia (PIN1) in prostates with and without carcinoma is difficult to determine from the literature. Studies by McNeal and Bostwick[32] and Troncoso *et al.*[47] report only the dominant grade of dysplasia or the worst grade of dysplasia, so that cases with mild dysplasia (PIN1) were often obscured by higher grades of dysplasia. Nonetheless, in McNeal and Bostwick's study, mild dysplasia was the predominant grade in 35% of benign prostates. In the study by Kovi *et al.*, 22% of benign prostates had PIN1 and 40% of prostates

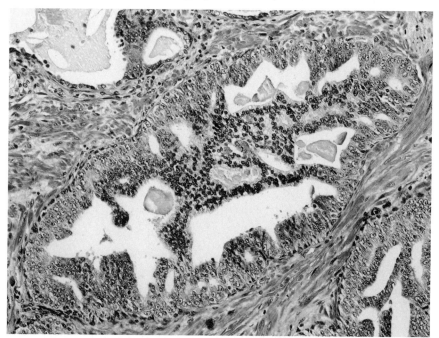

FIG. 7.9.   Cribriform gland of severe dysplasia. Note more benign-appearing nuclei toward center of the gland with classic cytologic features of severe dysplasia present in nuclei peripherally located up against the basement membrane. ×180.

with carcinoma had PIN1. There are additional explanations why these studies underrepresented the incidence of mild dysplasia (PIN1) in benign prostates. Most of these studies utilized autopsy specimens in which subtle and focal degrees of mild dysplasia would not be identifiable. In the study by Kovi *et al.*, radical prostatectomies performed for clinical adenocarcinoma of the prostate were also evaluated in which more advanced tumor could obscure focal mild dysplasia.

Histological identification of the mildest forms of atypia in almost any organ system is extremely subjective and carries with it the least clinical significance. For example, we often do not note in surgical pathology the presence of mild squamous atypia in the oral cavity and larynx because of its almost ubiquitous presence. In urological pathology, the presence of mild urothelial atypia is similarly subjective and difficult to distinguish from mild reactive atypia due to inflammation or instrumentation. Again, urologists ignore the reporting of mild urothelial atypia whether it be on cytology or in histological sections. In a subsequent work by McNeal,[30] the following quotation summarizes his consideration of PIN1: "There is not a sharp line of demarcation between grade 1 dysplasia and mild degrees of deviation from normal histology." For this reason, we do not comment on mild dysplasia in the prostate. When reading articles concerning dysplasia in the prostate, it is important to cull out data that includes mild dysplasia (PIN1) from data regarding higher grade dysplasia, such as moderate dysplasia (PIN2) or severe dysplasia (PIN3). Even in the 1986 study by McNeal and Bostwick,[32] dysplasia's relation to age and multicentric carcinoma, and data on dysplasia's extent may have been obscured since cases with mild dysplasia were often considered together with higher grades of dysplasia.

MODERATE INTRADUCTAL DYSPLASIA (PIN2)

As with mild intraductal dysplasia, it is difficult to determine the incidence of moderate dysplasia (PIN2) in glands with and without carcinoma since several of the larger studies have only reported the worst grade of dysplasia in a gland (Table 7.2). Consequently, glands with both severe dysplasia and moderate dysplasia would not be recorded as showing moderate dysplasia. McNeal and Bostwick[32] found that in 22% of prostates without malignancy studied at autopsy, moderate intraductal dysplasia was the worst grade. In over 66% of comparable prostates from cystoprostatectomy specimens studied by Troncoso *et al.,*[47] moderate dysplasia was the worst grade found. In the study by Kovi *et al.,*[24] 11% of prostates lacking malignancy had moderate dysplasia.

These widely differing incidences of moderate dysplasia in benign prostates may be multifactorial. First, whereas McNeal and Bostwick utilized autopsy specimens, Kovi *et al.* used both radical prostatectomy and autopsy specimens and Troncoso *et al.* used cystoprostatectomy specimens performed for transitional cell carcinoma of the bladder. Autopsy specimens have inherent problems, with poor tissue preservation making identification of rare foci of dysplasia difficult to identify, particularly those foci with lesser degrees of atypia. There may also be differences in diagnostic criteria among authors as to where to draw the boundary between mild, moderate, and severe dysplasia. As with all grading systems, there will be cases in which the distinction between grades will be subjective and may differ among observers. There may also be real differences in the characteristics of dysplasia in glands studied at autopsy versus radical prostatectomy specimens versus patients with transitional cell carcinoma of the bladder.

Other differences in patient characteristics exist. In the study by Kovi *et al.,* the autopsy specimens were collected from black men from Washington, D. C., and Nigeria; racial differences could account for some of the differences in their observations and in those of others. In addition, tissue sampling methods varied among the studies. Whole-mount sections were prepared in some studies in which thicker sections of the prostate were processed to prevent curling. With single sections of whole mounts, less of the prostate may be examined histologically as

TABLE 7.2. INCIDENCE OF MODERATE DYSPLASIA (PIN 2) IN BENIGN PROSTATES

Authors	Incidence in Benign Glands (%)	Type of Specimen
McNeal and Bostwick[32]	22 (worst grade)	Autopsy
Kovi *et al.*[24]	11	Autopsy + RP[a]
Troncoso *et al.*[47]	68 (worst grade)	Cysto[b]

[a] Radical prostatectomy for prostate carcinoma.
[b] Cystoprostatectomy for transitional cell carcinoma of bladder.

compared to conventional processing of 2–3 mm thick slices of tissue. In the study by McNeal and Bostwick, the most anterior sections showing predominantly nodular hyperplasia or fibromuscular tissue were discarded and an average of only 10 blocks per case was examined. In the study by Troncoso *et al.*, the first 20 of 100 cases were subtotally submitted for histological examination. All of these differences could contribute to the different incidences of moderate dysplasia (PIN2) among the various studies.

There is no data reporting the incidence of moderate dysplasia in prostates with cancer that is not also confounded by the incidence of mild or severe dysplasia. Both studies by McNeal and Bostwick and Troncoso *et al.* record their data as the worst dysplasia and the most prevalent dysplasia found in a prostate. Since in glands with cancer the worst dysplasia was often severe dysplasia and the most common dysplasia was often mild dysplasia, cases that also had moderate dysplasia would not be recorded.

SEVERE DYSPLASIA (PIN3)

The most intently investigated form of dysplasia has been that of severe dysplasia (PIN3). Severe dysplasia shows the greatest discrepancy in its incidence between glands with and without carcinoma (Table 7.3). McNeal and Bostwick[32] in their autopsy study found that 33% of glands harboring carcinoma contained severe dysplasia as compared to only 4% of benign glands. Kovi *et al.*[24] in their study of radical prostatectomy specimens performed for carcinoma of the prostate and autopsy specimens found a similar 33% incidence of severe dysplasia in glands with carcinoma, yet 15% of benign glands also had severe dysplasia. Troncoso *et al.*,[47] in their study of cystoprostatectomy specimens performed for transitional cell carcinoma of the bladder, found a much higher incidence (72%) of glands with carcinoma containing severe dysplasia. Similar to Kovi *et al.*, Troncoso *et al.* reported 18% of benign glands had severe dysplasia. In studies from our institution on radical prostatectomy specimens performed for both stage B (palpable) and stage A (incidental) adenocarcinoma of the prostate, all glands contained some foci of severe dysplasia, in addition to carcinoma. The same potential explanations for the differences between the various reported incidences

TABLE 7.3. INCIDENCE OF SEVERE DYSPLASIA (PIN3) IN PROSTATE GLANDS WITH AND WITHOUT CANCER

Authors	Incidence in Benign Glands (%)	Incidence in Malignant Glands (%)	Type of Specimen
McNeal and Bostwick[32]	4	33	Autopsy
Kovi *et al.*[24]	15	33	Autopsy + RP[a]
Troncoso *et al.*[47]	18	72	Cysto[b]
Quinn *et al.*[43]		100	RP (stage B)
Epstein *et al.*[15]		100	RP (stage A)

[a] Radical prostatectomy for prostate cancer.
[b] Cystoprostatectomy for transitional cell carcinoma of bladder.

of moderate dysplasia (PIN2) in benign and malignant glands discussed above also apply for differences in the reported incidences of severe dysplasia (PIN3).

Based on the above studies, it appears that between 15 and 18% of glands without carcinoma may have foci of severe dysplasia. The incidences of severe dysplasia in prostates with carcinoma differ to a greater extent, ranging from approximately 33% in autopsy studies to 72% in surgical specimens performed for transitional cell carcinoma to 100% in radical prostatectomy specimens performed for carcinoma of the prostate.

Because of recent studies demonstrating significant differences between stage A (incidental) carcinoma and stage B (palpable) carcinoma, we felt it was important to evaluate the relationship of dysplasia to carcinoma separately in these two patient populations.[15,43] By utilizing radical prostatectomy specimens, fixation problems inherent with autopsy specimens would be negated to minimize missing focal dysplastic lesions that could be obscured by autolysis.

We recently reported our findings relating intraductal dysplasia to stage B adenocarcinomas of the prostate.[43] As with earlier studies, our data supported a close relationship between the finding of intraductal dysplasia and some forms of adenocarcinoma of the prostate. In each of the cases, the dominant peripherally located tumor nodule had associated severe dysplasia (PIN3). The glands of severe dysplasia were either located intermingled amongst the glands of carcinoma or adjacent to the carcinoma (Fig. 7.10). In 30% of the dominant tumor nodules there were large amounts of severe dysplasia, occupying between 10 and

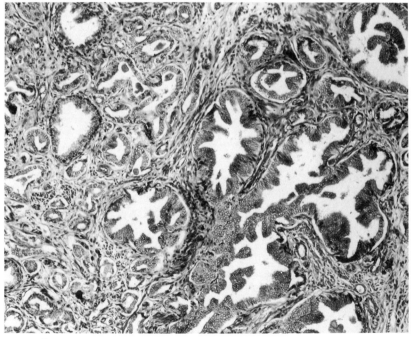

FIG. 7.10. Multiple glands of severe dysplasia (right) intimately intermingled with small glands of infiltrating adenocarcinoma. × 90.

25% of the tumor nodule, intermingled among the infiltrating cancer. In 19% of the dominant tumor nodules, there was extensive severe dysplasia, ranging in diameter from 5 to 15 mm, adjacent to the infiltrating tumor (Fig. 7.11). This consistent finding of severe dysplasia associated with peripherally located infiltrating carcinoma is strong associational evidence linking dysplasia as a potential precursor lesion to these carcinomas.

There are several arguments that this phenomenon does not merely represent an extension of carcinoma into adjacent glands. First, it is not uncommon to find identical glands of severe dysplasia away from the infiltrating carcinoma. Second, the various complex architectural patterns seen with intraductal dysplasia, such as micropapillary tufts and cribriform formation, would seem to be less likely a manifestation of intraductular extension from an invasive carcinoma rather than primary intraductal growth. Similarly, the finding of scattered cells with intraductal dysplasia interspersed among normal epithelium would be harder to explain as an extension of carcinoma into ducts versus primary dysplastic change. Another piece of evidence that argues against intraductal dysplasia merely being a manifestation of intraductal growth of carcinoma into ducts is the finding of large areas of severe dysplasia with associated microinvasive carcinoma.[43] In these foci, there are numerous dysplastic glands that upon careful examination show several small infiltrating glands apparently budding off from the dysplastic glands (Fig. 7.12).

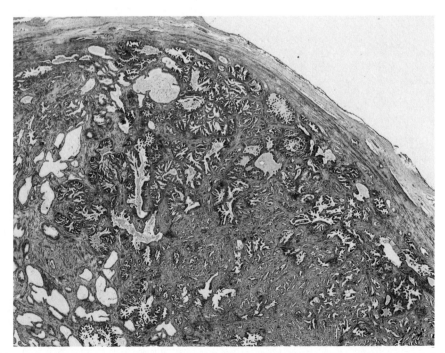

FIG. 7.11. Radical prostatectomy specimen showing dominant tumor nodule surrounded by extensive glands of severe dysplasia. × 12.

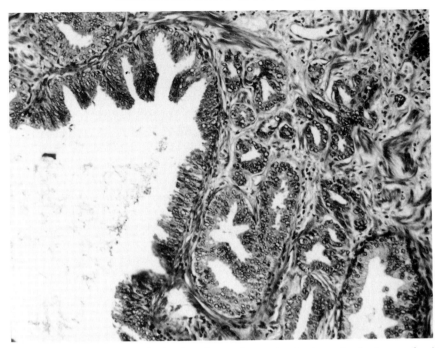

FIG. 7.12.   Severe dysplasia with microinvasive carcinoma showing large glands of severe dysplasia with several cytologically similar small glands of infiltrating carcinoma appearing to bud off from the dysplastic glands. × 145.

We also found, as have others, that with increasing amounts of severe dysplasia there are a greater number of multifocal carcinomas per gland.[43] With extensive severe dysplasia, 21 multifocal carcinomas on average per gland were identified in contrast to only 6 to 7 multifocal cancers per gland with intermediate or minimal amounts of dysplasia. This finding is additional indirect evidence that severe dysplasia is a precursor lesion to some carcinomas of the prostate.

An interesting and somewhat unexpected finding in our study on stage B carcinomas related to these multifocal cancers.[43] When we examined these multifocal cancers, which were cancers distinct from the dominant tumor nodule, 66% had adjacent severe dysplasia. When we subcategorized these multifocal cancers by location and grade of the carcinoma, we found that centrally located intermediate grade multifocal carcinoma as well as peripherally located low or intermediate grade carcinomas were associated with adjacent dysplasia in 80% of the cases. In contrast, only 39% of low-grade centrally located adenocarcinomas had adjacent dysplasia. This difference was statistically significant. These low-grade centrally located adenocarcinomas tend to be the tumors that are incidentally found in transurethral resections of the prostate performed for presumed prostatic hyperplasia. This finding raised the question as to whether low-grade incidentally found carcinomas may not be linked with severe dysplasia as closely as peripherally located palpable carcinomas. Further evidence in support of this concept is that severe dysplasia is much more frequently seen in the periphery of the gland than in the central region, even accounting for the greater area of the peripheral region.[43]

We pursued this question in a study of radical prostatectomies performed for stage A carcinoma.[15] While all of our cases of radical prostatectomies performed for stage A carcinoma contained some severe dysplasia, the extent of severe dysplasia was much less than that seen in our stage B carcinomas. Only 10% of radical prostatectomies performed for stage A carcinoma had extensive dysplasia versus 33% of stage B carcinomas. In addition, at least some of the severe dysplasia was adjacent to or intermingled with the infiltrating stage B carcinomas. In contrast, 45% of the stage A radical prostatectomy specimens had severe dysplasia as isolated foci only, where all of the foci of severe dysplasia were in areas away from carcinoma. This weaker association of severe dysplasia to incidental centrally located low-grade carcinomas is also supported by the histological differences of dysplasia as compared to these carcinomas. Centrally located low-grade adenocarcinomas tend to have bland cytologic features often lacking nuclear enlargement or nucleoli in contrast to severe dysplasia. This finding differs from peripherally located intermediate grade carcinomas in which the cytologic features of severe dysplasia are often identical to that of infiltrating carcinoma.

SIGNIFICANCE OF DYSPLASIA ON BIOPSY MATERIAL

As mentioned earlier, the finding of mild dysplasia (PIN1) is common in entirely benign prostates, and subjective and difficult to distinguish from normal or slightly reactive epithelium. Consequently, we do not comment on mild dysplasia (PIN1) on biopsy material.

When discussing the significance of higher grade dysplasia (moderate or severe dysplasia) on biopsy material, it is important to distinguish between dysplasia found on needle biopsy and dysplasia found on transurethral resection. In our study of radical prostatectomy specimens performed for stage B (palpable) carcinoma of the prostate,[43] we found that all peripherally located dominant tumor nodules had some associated severe dysplasia. We also found that in these areas of severe dysplasia adjacent to carcinoma there were often glands with moderate dysplasia as well. In addition, as noted earlier, areas of dysplastic foci both adjacent to and in the middle of the nodule could be fairly large. Consequently, in the face of a palpable lesion there is a possibility of obtaining only high-grade (severe or moderate) dysplasia on needle biopsy, where the infiltrating carcinoma was not sampled. We therefore recommend that in the face of a palpable nodule where only high-grade dysplasia is identified on biopsy, that another biopsy be taken of the patient since the likelihood is that the infiltrating carcinoma was missed on the initial biopsy. Of 20 men with high-grade dysplasia (PIN2–3) on needle biopsy that we have seen, 60% were shown on either simultaneous or subsequent biopsy to also have adenocarcinomas (Fig. 7.13).

If high-grade dysplasia (PIN2 or PIN3) is identified on a needle biopsy performed for a hypoechoic lesion seen on transrectal ultrasound without a

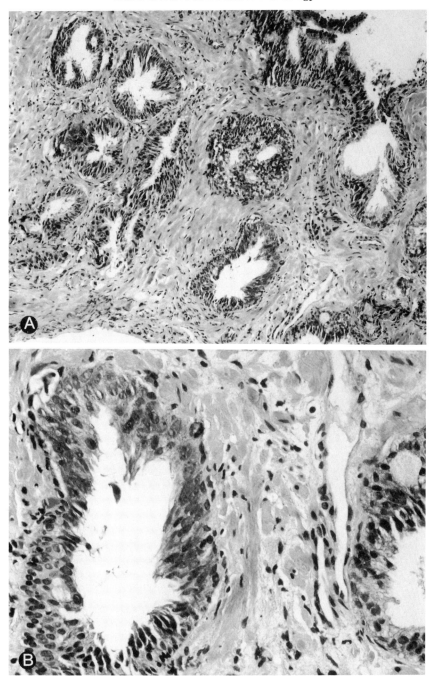

FIG. 7.13. (*A*) Focus of high-grade dysplasia on needle biopsy. Note more basophilic appearance of dysplastic glands compared to benign glands (right). × 125. (*B*) Higher magnification of dysplastic gland (left) showing enlarged stratified nuclei with hyperchromatism and some prominent nucleoli. Subsequent needle biopsy from this patient showed infiltrating adenocarcinoma. × 400.

palpable lesion, the situation is not quite as clear. We have demonstrated, as have others, that high-grade dysplasia may appear as a hypoechoic lesion even if there is no infiltrating carcinoma.[18] It would be unlikely, however, to have a large area of severe dysplasia presenting as a hypoechoic lesion without any infiltrating carcinoma at that site. Nonetheless, the potential for severe dysplasia to be the sole cause for a hypoechoic lesion exists; another biopsy of the patient should therefore be taken in order to try to identify infiltrating tumor and, if not found, closely followed with repeat biopsy in the future.

The finding of severe dysplasia or moderate dysplasia on transurethral resection is not as indicative of an accompanying infiltrating tumor. In our study on radical prostatectomy specimens performed for stage A carcinoma,[16] we found that finding severe dysplasia on transurethral resection was proportionate to the extent of severe dysplasia in the radical prostatectomy specimen, as one might expect (Fig. 7.14). However, we found that the extent of severe dysplasia in the transurethral resection specimen showed no correlation with the amount of carcinoma within the radical prostatectomy specimen. It therefore follows that finding severe dysplasia on transurethral resection was not proportionate to the amount of tumor within a radical prostatectomy specimen. Furthermore, it was not uncommon to find severe dysplasia on transurethral resection as isolated foci separate from prostatic chips that contained carcinoma. For example, in one of

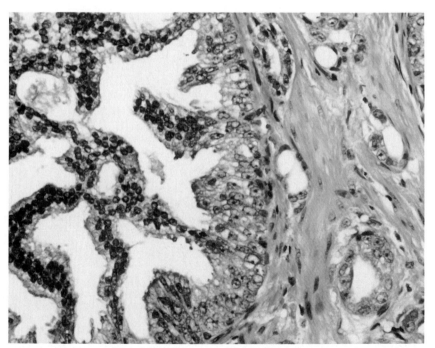

FIG. 7.14. Focus of severe cribriform dysplasia with associated small glands of infiltrating carcinoma found on transurethral resection. Note maturation of nuclei toward the center of the gland; nuclear features of severe dysplasia toward the basement membrane are similar to those of surrounding small glands of infiltrating carcinoma. × 316.

our cases with severe dysplasia on transurethral resection and minimal carcinoma, there was no residual tumor within the corresponding radical prostatectomy specimen. The finding of severe dysplasia on transurethral resection indicates an increased chance of having carcinoma since only approximately 20% of benign glands harbor severe dysplasia (PIN3).[24,47] However, the finding of severe dysplasia on transurethral resection does not indicate, if there is tumor, to what extent it is present. It may vary from more extensive incidental carcinoma to a single focus of low-grade adenocarcinoma. The management of a patient with severe dysplasia on transurethral resection would be in large part determined by other factors, such as the patient's age. For example, in an elderly patient with severe dysplasia on transurethral resection, after ruling out a clinically significant tumor on rectal examination, probably no further management would be instigated (Fig. 7.15). The finding of severe dysplasia on transurethral resection in a younger individual would trigger a more aggressive workup to rule out a clinically significant tumor. This might include, in addition to rectal examination, the performance of a transrectal ultrasound with or without biopsies as well as close follow-up.

The finding of moderate dysplasia on transurethral resection in which there is no palpable mass or peripherally located hypoechoic lesion is probably of lesser significance since between 20 and over 60% of prostate glands without carcinoma may harbor moderate dysplasia. Given the greater amount of tissue sampled on

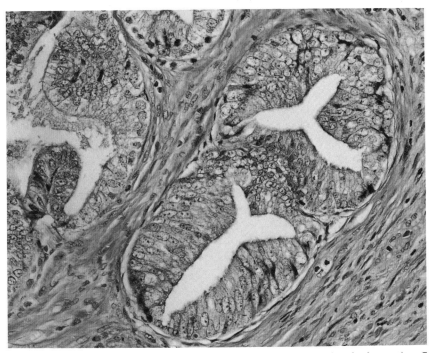

FIG. 7.15. Several glands of severe dysplasia found in a focus on transurethral resection. Small glands of infiltrating adenocarcinoma were not identified. This focus was found incidentally in an elderly man and no further therapy was instigated. × 260.

transurethral resection, as compared to needle biopsy, the finding of moderate dysplasia probably has little significance. Potentially in a younger individual one would tend to work up this finding more thoroughly, such as by the performance of a transrectal ultrasound to look for a peripherally located tumor. If moderate or severe dysplasia is found on transurethral resection specimen and the specimen has not been put through in its entirety, the remainder of the transurethral resection specimen should be processed in order to look for infiltrating carcinoma.

The distinction on biopsy material between glands of high-grade dysplasia versus glands of dysplasia with an infiltrating component may be difficult. It is often the large basophilic dysplastic glands that draws the pathologist's attention. Occasionally, only a few infiltrating malignant glands may be identified in a biopsy composed predominantly of dysplastic glands. One should, therefore, carefully examine the intervening stroma between the dysplastic glands to look for small infiltrating glands with similar cytologic features.

Occasionally, several cribriforming glands will be identified on biopsy material in which the differential diagnosis rests between infiltrating cribriforming carcinoma versus cribriforming high-grade dysplasia. In general, with cribriforming dysplastic glands there is the same maturation of the nuclei toward the center of the gland, as seen in dysplastic glands with micropapillary tufts. Within the center of the cribriforming glands the nuclei will have a bland appearance, resembling that of normal nuclei. Toward the edge of the cribriforming gland up against the basement membrane, the cytology will be more characteristic of high-grade dysplasia with enlarged nuclei and prominent nucleoli. Cribriforming carcinoma tends to have more prominent cytologic atypia throughout the cribriforming gland, although infiltrating cribriforming carcinoma on occasion may share dysplasia's maturation of nuclei toward the center of the gland. The finding of basal cells around the cribriforming gland, whether by light microscopy or more objectively by using basal cell-specific stains such as keratin 903, is diagnostic of dysplasia and rules out infiltrating carcinoma.

When there are cribriforming glands on biopsy material without small glands of infiltrating carcinoma I generally will not diagnose carcinoma (Fig. 7.16). Almost all cases of infiltrating cribriforming carcinoma are accompanied by small glands of infiltrating cancer. Upon finding only cribriforming atypical glands on biopsy material, I prefer to be conservative and diagnose the focus as cribriforming dysplasia and strongly recommend repeat biopsy rather than to overdiagnose infiltrating carcinoma.

DYSPLASIA VERSUS CARCINOMA *In Situ*

When deciding if a given focus on biopsy is severe dysplasia or infiltrating carcinoma, the question might arise as to whether both lesions should be treated in the same aggressive fashion. Answering that question raises the issue of distinguishing between severe dysplasia and carcinoma *in situ*; *i.e.*, if there is no distinction, why not use the term "carcinoma *in situ* of the prostate"? Based on many of the articles already quoted, as well as some newer data that will be presented later in this article, there is a growing body of data suggesting that

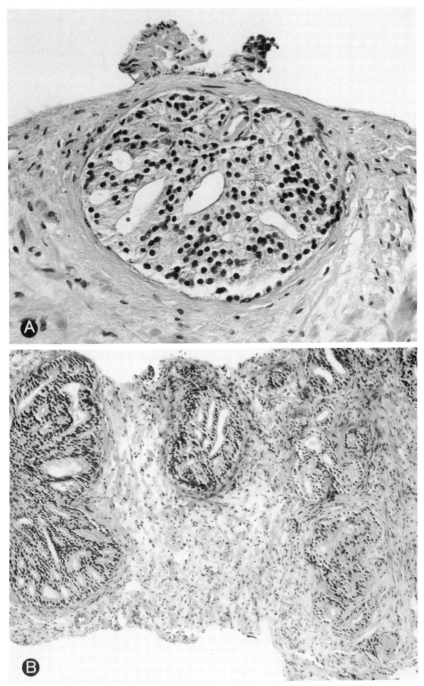

FIG. 7.16. (*A*) Single cribriform gland found on needle biopsy. Although this could represent infiltrating cribriform carcinoma, cribriform dysplasia was diagnosed with the recommendation for repeat biopsy. × 270. (*B*) Repeat biopsy showed several similar cribriform glands (left) as well as smaller glands diagnostic of infiltrating adenocarcinoma (right). × 270.

severe dysplasia (PIN3) is a precursor to some forms of carcinoma of the prostate. For these reasons, some individuals feel that severe dysplasia should be termed carcinoma *in situ*. However, the one piece of evidence that we do have for premalignant lesions in other organs, which is lacking in the prostate, is the natural history of severe dysplasia (PIN3). In the cervix, for example, high-grade dysplastic lesions such as CIN3 have been followed and a higher than expected number of these lesions will, over a period of time, develop into an infiltrating carcinoma at the site of the precursor lesion. In other organs, such as the breast, we have good imaging techniques to follow the site where biopsy of a putative *in situ* lesion has been done to determine whether that area is at increased risk to develop infiltrating carcinoma. Consequently, when we diagnose *in situ* carcinoma of the breast or of the cervix we have a good understanding as to what percentage of patients, if left untreated, will progress to infiltrating carcinoma over a defined period of time. This data can then be factored into the therapeutic decision-making process. With the prostate, there is currently no such capability of monitoring a dysplastic focus to determine whether: (1) there is already infiltrating carcinoma at that site, or (2) when infiltrating carcinoma evolves, has it done so in the immediate vicinity of the dysplastic focus?

There are a few reports of prostatic lesions seen on ultrasound where dysplasia was found on biopsy, and the patient was followed for a relatively short period of time and subsequently shown to have infiltrating carcinoma.[26] Severe dysplasia has also been reported on fine-needle aspiration biopsy where the patient was followed and later demonstrated to have infiltrating carcinoma.[28] Although these cases were interpreted as showing evolution from dysplasia to carcinoma, more likely the infiltrating component was already present at the time of the initial biopsy or aspiration and was not sampled.

Because we do not yet know when severe dysplasia (PIN3) is found on biopsy material what percentage of these patients will develop infiltrating carcinoma over a given follow-up interval, most authorities do not prefer the term carcinoma *in situ*. Carcinoma *in situ* has implications that these dysplastic lesions will develop into infiltrating carcinoma at a sufficiently high frequency that may lead some aggressive clinicians to treat these lesions in a radical fashion. Given that there is still controversy as to whether even infiltrating adenocarcinoma of the prostate should always be treated aggressively, it is doubtful that these potential precursor lesions should be treated by aggressive therapy until their natural history is better understood.

In a parallel system, some gastrointestinal pathologists favor the use of the term "high-grade dysplasia" when assessing a focus of marked epithelial atypia in a tubular adenoma, rather than the term carcinoma *in situ*. While these gastrointestinal pathologists understand that the lesions they prefer to term high-grade dysplasia in a tubular adenoma are morphologically equivalent to carcinoma *in situ* within a tubular adenoma, they prefer the former term in order to prevent overly aggressive therapy of these biologically benign lesions. Whereas some surgeons might perform partial colectomies for the diagnosis of tubular adenoma with carcinoma *in situ*, they would not do so for a lesion termed high-grade dysplasia arising in a tubular adenoma. In the prostate, for both this practical reason to prevent overly aggressive therapy as well as for the theoretical consideration that we lack a more complete understanding of the natural history of these dysplastic lesions, the term severe dysplasia (PIN3) is preferred over carcinoma *in situ.*

FURTHER EVIDENCE RELATING DYSPLASIA TO CARCINOMA

In addition to the light microscopic evidence that intraductal dysplasia is a precursor lesion to some forms of adenocarcinoma of the prostate, newer techniques have demonstrated further evidence of similarities between intraductal dysplasia and carcinoma. Some of these studies have shown that, compared to benign prostatic epithelium, there is an increased expression of various markers and substances within intraductal dysplasia similar to carcinoma, and others have shown a decreased expression of various antigens in dysplasia similar to carcinoma. Many of these studies showing an increase in a specific marker are based on relatively few cases and there are often other studies that show conflicting results. Consequently, until more studies are performed, some of the information provided within this section must be regarded as being preliminary.

Two recent works have analyzed DNA ploidy in PIN versus carcinoma and benign tissue. O'Malley *et al.*[40] analyzed 11 cases of low-grade PIN and 56 cases of high-grade PIN by flow cytometry and compared them to adenocarcinoma of the prostate. All cases of low-grade PIN were diploid and only one case (1.8%) of high-grade PIN was aneuploid. In a few prostates, PIN was compared to adenocarcinoma from the same case; in three cases both the adenocarcinoma and the high-grade PIN were diploid, and in one case the adenocarcinoma was tetraploid and the associated high-grade dysplasia was diploid. The second study, by Amin *et al.*,[1] utilized computerized image analysis to assess ploidy in PIN2 and PIN3 as compared to cancer and benign prostate. In 13 cases, PIN and cancer ploidy patterns matched (59%), whereas 9 cases were discordant. There was a statistically significant difference in the mean optical density between cancer cases and benign prostate tissue, and cancer cases versus PIN; however, the differences between benign tissue and PIN were not statistically significantly different.

Nucleolar organizing regions (AgNOR) have been shown to correlate with growth fraction, and have been shown in other organ systems to be increased in malignant tissues when compared to normal or benign conditions. Several recent studies have analyzed the AgNOR counts in intraductal dysplasia as compared to benign and malignant prostatic epithelium. In the study by Deschenes and Weidner[11] there was a statistically higher AgNOR count for carcinomas with Gleason pattern 4 or 5 as compared to intraductal dysplasia and benign prostatic tissue, although there were significant overlaps among the groups. AgNOR counts for intraductal dysplasia were significantly higher than those for benign prostatic tissue, again with overlaps among the groups. However, there were no statistically significant differences in AgNOR counts between intraductal dysplasia and Gleason pattern 2 or 3 tumor. No significant differences in AgNOR counts between the three grades of PIN were identified. In a conflicting study, Cheville et al.[9] found no difference in AgNOR counts in hyperplasia, PIN, or adenocarcinoma or between grades of PIN. Mostofi et al.[37] cite preliminary studies stating that AgNOR counts were lowest in benign tissue, highest in carcinoma, and intermediate in dysplasia, although the data from this study have not yet been presented.

Other markers have been shown to be increased in dysplasia that are not as directly related to proliferation, but reflect cytoplasmic differentiation. Perlman and Epstein[42] and Nagle et al.[39] have shown enhanced expression of the lectin UEA-1 in both intraductal dysplasia and invasive carcinoma, but not in normal or hyperplastic glands. Conflicting studies on the expression of UEA-1 have come from McNeal et al.[33] Of interest in our study was the finding that the increased UEA-1 staining was seen in dysplasia and intermediate and high-grade carcinoma, and not in low-grade carcinoma[42]; this result supports prior studies suggesting that the close relationship that dysplasia has with peripherally located higher grade carcinomas may not exist with lower grade carcinoma.[15,43] The increased expression of Leu-7, which is a differentiation marker for a lymphocyte subpopulation, has been shown to be increased in dysplasia and carcinoma as compared to benign glands, according to Mostofi et al.[37] Again, conflicting studies on the expression of Leu-7 in dysplasia come from McNeal et al.,[31] who showed a reduction in Leu-7 staining in dysplasia. In a recent study on the expression of various cytokeratins in carcinoma, dysplasia, and benign prostatic tissue, Nagle et al.[39] demonstrated that KΛ4, which detects cytokeratin 14, 15, 16, and 19, was enhanced in dysplasia and carcinoma as compared to benign tissue. This marker, however, was only enhanced in frozen tissue; in formalin-fixed tissue, the distinction between dysplasia, carcinoma, and hyperplasia could not be demonstrated.

In addition to the immunohistochemical evidence of similarities between carcinoma and dysplasia as compared to benign tissue, Humphrey[21] has demonstrated, using histochemical staining, that there was enhanced secretion of acidic mucin in severe dysplasia similar to that seen in carcinoma, as compared to the rare production of acidic mucins in benign or hyperplastic glands.

Studies showing a decrease in various markers similar to carcinoma have also been reported. Bostwick and Brawer[4] have demonsttated the loss of the basal cell layer in dysplasia using basal cell-specific antibodies such as keratin 903. Furthermore, with increasing grades of dysplasia, the discontinuity of the basal cell layer became more pronounced. Although some authors have proposed utilizing keratin 903 in the assessment of dysplastic glands looking for microinvasion, we feel that there is relatively little utility of this antibody for this purpose. Because even normal glands may show a patchy absence of keratin 903 staining, we would be hesitant to diagnose infiltrating carcinoma based on discontinuous keratin 903 staining.[19] Furthermore, we feel that the light microscopic finding of small glands with nuclear atypia in and among larger dysplastic glands is usually readily diagnosable as infiltrating carcinoma.

Other substances shown to be decreased in dysplasia paralleling that seen with carcinoma include blood group antigens A and B,[42] and prostate-specific antigen and prostate-specific acid phosphatase.[31,37] Utilizing frozen sections, Nagle *et al.*[39] have demonstrated a decrease in vimentin expression within dysplasia and carcinoma when compared to benign tissue. However, this result could not be duplicated in formalin-fixed tissue.

Although many of these studies are preliminary and some studies demonstrate conflicting results, the overall trend of these studies show that intraductal dysplasia and carcinoma share diverse histochemical and immunohistochemical similarities in their nuclear and cytoplasmic characteristics.

ANIMAL STUDIES

Finally, there have been several animal studies suggesting that dysplasia may evolve into carcinoma under the appropriate circumstances. Leav *et al.*[25] demonstrated that the simultaneous implant of Noble rats with testosterone and 17 β-estradiol-filled silastic capsules for 16 weeks caused a lesion that they termed dysplasia. Similarly, Drago[12] reported the presence of microscopic carcinomas in 88% of Noble rats treated for over 18 months with testosterone and 17 β-estradiol-filled silastic implants. These studies in combination suggest that dysplasia may progress to adenocarcinoma and raise the question of long-term hormonal stimulation playing a significant role in the genesis of dysplasia and carcinoma of the prostate. Isaacs[22] studied the ACI/Seg rat, which is highly susceptible to spontaneous prostatic carcinoma, and demonstrated lesions that were thought to be dysplastic. In contrast, nonsusceptible strains did not demonstrate these dysplastic foci. It must be recognized, however, that the prostate glands of these animal and their tumors and dysplasia show significant histological differences from that seen in man.

SUMMARY

In recent years we have made great strides in our understanding of various atypical lesions within the prostate. This clarity originated with the recognition that lesions of atypical hyperplasia of the prostate are diverse both in their histology and in their potential relationship to adenocarcinoma. While the possible relationship of adenosis to carcinoma is still somewhat controversial, there has been a growing body of histological, histochemical, and immunohisto-logical evidence demonstrating that intraductal dysplasia (PIN) is closely linked to some forms of adenocarcinoma of the prostate. Whether there are significant differences in the relationship of intraductal dysplasia to clinically detectable peripherally located adenocarcinoma and centrally located incidentally found carcinomas needs additional clarification. Further studies on all forms of atypical hyperplasia are still required to determine their relative risk of developing carcinoma, similar to those that have been recently published on various atypical hyperplastic lesions within the breast. In order for these studies to be successful, better imaging techniques of the prostate must become available to rule out invasive carcinoma already being present when one of the forms of atypical hyperplasia is identified on biopsy. Additional directions of research in the future will also undoubtedly probe the molecular biology of various forms of atypical hyperplasia, in particular intraductal dysplasia and its relationship to carcinoma, although at this time the molecular characteristics of adenocarcinoma of the prostate is still in its infancy.

REFERENCES

1. Amin, M. B., Schultz, D. S., Zarbo, R. P. H., Kubus, J., and Shaheen, C. Computerized static DNA ploidy analysis of prostatic intraepithelial neoplasia. *Mod. Pathol. 4:* 43A, 1991.
2. Blute, M. L., Zincke, H., and Farrow, G. M. Long-term follow-up of young patients with stage A adenocarcinoma of the prostate. *J. Urol. 136:* 840–843, 1986.
3. Bostwick, D. G. Prostatic intra-epithelial neoplasia (PIN). *Urology (Suppl) 34:* 16–22, 1989.
4. Bostwick, D. G., and Brawer, M. K. Prostatic intra-epithelial neoplasia and early invasion in prostate cancer. *Cancer 59:* 788–794, 1987.
5. Brawer, M. K., Nagle, R. B., Pitts, W., Freiha, F. S., and Gamble, S. Keratin immunoreactivity as an aid to the diagnosis of persistent adenocarcinoma following prostatic irradiation. *Cancer 63:* 454–460, 1989.
6. Brawer, M. K., Peehl, D. N., Stamey, T. A., and Bostwick, D. G. Keratin immunoreactivity in the benign and neoplastic human prostate. *Cancer Res. 45:* 3663–3667, 1985.
7. Brawn, P. N. Adenosis of the prostate: A dysplastic lesion that can be confused with prostate adenocarcinoma. *Cancer 49:* 826–833, 1982.
8. Brawn, P. N. *Interpretation of Prostate Biopsies.* New York, Raven Press, 1983, pp. 48–81.
9. Cheville, J. C., Clamon, G. H., and Robinson, R. A. Silver-stained nucleolar organizer regions in the differentiation of prostatic hyperplasia, intra-epithelial neoplasia, and adenocarcinoma. *Mod. Pathol. 3:* 596–598, 1990.
10. Christensen, W. N., Partin, A. W., Walsh, P. C., and Epstein, J. I. Pathologic findings in stage A2 prostate cancer: Relation of tumor volume, grade and location to pathologic stage. *Cancer 65:* 1021–1027, 1990.
11. Deschenes, G., and Weidner, N. Nucleolar organizer region (NOR) in hyperplastic and neoplastic prostate disease. *Am. J. Surg. Pathol. 14:* 1148–1155, 1990.
12. Drago, J. R. The induction of Nb rat prostatic carcinomas. *Anticancer Res. 4:* 255–256, 1984.
13. Eble, J. N., and Epstein, J. I. Stage A carcinoma of the prostate: In *Pathology of the Prostate, Seminal Vesicles, and the Male Urethra*, edited by L. M. Roth; D. G. Bostwick, consultant editor. New York, Churchill Livingstone, 1990
14. Epstein, J. I. *Interpretation of Prostate Biopsies.* New York, Raven Press, 1989.
15. Epstein, J. I., Cho, K. R., and Quinn, B. D. Relationship of severe dysplasia to stage A (incidental) adenocarcinoma of the prostate. *Cancer 65:* 2321–2327, 1990.
16. Epstein, J. I., Paull, G., Eggleston, J. C., and Walsh, P. C. Prognosis of untreated stage A1 prostatic carcinoma: A study of 94 cases with extended follow-up. *J. Urol. 136:* 837–839, 1986.
17. Gown, A. N., and Vogel, A. M. Monoclonal antibodies to human intermediate filament protein: Distribution of filament proteins in normal human tissues. *Am. J. Pathol. 114:* 309–321, 1984.
18. Hamper, U. M., Sheth, S., Walsh, P. C., Holtz, P. N., and Epstein, J. I. Stage B adenocarcinoma of the prostate: Transrectal US and pathologic correlation of non-malignant hypoechoic peripheral zone lesions. *Radiology 180:* 101–104, 1991.
19. Hedrick, L., and Epstein, J. I. Use of keratin 903 as an adjunct in the diagnosis of prostate carcinoma. *Am. J. Surg. Pathol. 13:* 389–396, 1989.
20. Helpap, B. The biological significance of atypical hyperplasia of the prostate. *Virchows Arch. A Pathol. Anat. Histol. 387:* 307–317, 1980.
21. Humphrey, P. A. Mucin in severe dysplasia of the prostate. *Modern Pathol. 4:* 48A, 1991.
22. Isaacs, J. T. The aging ACI/Seg versus Copenhagen male rat as a model system for the study of prostatic carcinogenesis. *Cancer Res. 44:* 5785–5796, 1984.

23. Kastendieck, H. Correlations between atypical primary hyperplasia and carcinoma of the prostate: A histological study of 180 total prostatectomies. *Path. Res. Practice 169:* 366–387, 1980.
24. Kovi, J., Mostofi, F. K., Heshmat, M. Y., and Enterline, J. P. Large acinar atypical hyperplasia and carcinoma of the prostate. *Cancer 61:* 555–561, 1988.
25. Leav, I., Ho, S., Ofner, P., Merk, F. B., Kwan, P. W., and Damassa, D. Biochemical alterations in sex hormone-induced hyperplasia and dysplasia of the dorsal lateral prostates of Noble rats. *J. Natl. Cancer Inst. 80:* 1045–1053, 1988.
26. Lee, F., Torp-Pedersen, S. T., Carroll, J. T., Siders, D. B., Christensen-Day, C., and Mitchell, A. E. Use of transrectal ultrasound and prostate-specific antigen in diagnosis of prostatic intra-epithelial neoplasia. *Urology (Suppl.) 34:* 4–8, 1989.
27. Lepor, H., Gregerman, M., Crosby, R., Mostofi, F. K., and Walsh, P. C. Precise localization of the autonomic nerves from the pelvic plexus to the corpora cavernosa: A detailed anatomical study of the adult male pelvis. *J. Urol. 133:* 207–212, 1985.
28. Markham, C. W. Prostatic intra-epithelial neoplasia: Detection and correlation with invasive cancer and fine-needle biopsy. *Urology (Suppl.) 34:* 57–61, 1989.
29. McNeal, J. E. Morphogenesis of prostatic carcinoma. *Cancer 18:* 1659–1666, 1965.
30. McNeal, J. E. Significance of duct-acinar dysplasia in prostatic carcinogenesis. *Urology (Suppl.) 34:* 9–15, 1989.
31. McNeal, J. E., Alroy, J., Leav, I., Redwine, E. A., Freiha, F. S., and Stamey, T. A. Immunohistochemical evidence of impaired cell differentiation in the pre-malignant phase of prostate carcinogenesis. *Am. J. Clin. Pathol. 90:* 23–32, 1988.
32. McNeal, J. E., and Bostwick, D. G. Intraductal dysplasia: A pre-malignant lesion of the prostate. *Hum. Pathol. 17:* 64–71, 1986.
33. McNeal, J. E., Leav, I., Alroy, J., and Skutelsky, E. Differential lectin staining of central and peripheral zones of the prostate and alterations in dysplasia. *Am. J. Clin. Pathol. 89:* 41–48, 1988.
34. McNeal, J. E., Price, H. N., Redwine, E. A., Freiha, F. S., and Stamey, T. A. Stage A versus stage B adenocarcinoma of the prostate: Morphological comparison and biological significance. *J. Urol. 139:* 61–65, 1988.
35. Miller, A., and Seljelid, R. Cellular atypia in the prostate. *Scand. J. Urol. Nephrol. 5:* 17–21, 1971.
36. Moore, R. A. Benign hypertrophy of the prostate: A morphological study. *J. Urol 50:* 680–710, 1943.
37. Mostofi, F. K., Sesterhenn, I. A., and Davis, C. J., Jr. Malignant change in hyperplastic prostate glands: The AFIP experience. *Urology (Suppl.) 34:* 49–51, 1989.
38. Nagle, R. B., Ahmann, F. R., McDaniel, K. N., Paquin, N. L., Clark, V. A., and Celniker, A. Cytokeratin characterization of human prostatic carcinoma and its derived cell lines. *Cancer Res. 47:* 281–286, 1987.
39. Nagle, R. B., Brawer, N. K., Kittelson, J., and Clark, V. Phenotypic relationships of prostatic intra-epithelial neoplasia to invasive prostatic carcinoma. *Am. J. Pathol. 138:* 119–128, 1991.
40. O'Malley, F., Grignon, D., Keeney, M., Kerkvliet, N., and McLean, C. DNA flow cytometric studies of prostatic intra-epithelial neoplasia. *Mod. Pathol. 4:* 50A, 1991.
41. Oyasu, R., Bahnson, R. R., Nowels, K., and Garnett, J. E. Cytological atypia in the prostate gland: Frequency, distribution, and possible relevance to carcinoma. *J. Urol. 135:* 959–962, 1986.
42. Perlman, E. J., and Epstein, J. E. Blood group antigen expression in dysplasia and adenocarcinoma of the prostate. *Am. J. Surg. Pathol. 14:* 810–818, 1990.
43. Quinn, B. D., Cho, K. R., and Epstein, J. I. Relationship of severe dysplasia to stage B adenocarcinoma of the prostate. *Cancer 65:* 2328–2337, 1990.
44. Tannenbaum, M. Differential diagnosis in uropathology: Carcinoma in situ of prostate gland. *Urology 5:* 143–146, 1975.
45. Thompson, I. M., and Zeidman, E. J. Extensive follow-up of stage A1 carcinoma of prostate. *Urology 33:* 455–458, 1989.

46. Totten, R. S., Heineman, N. W., Hudson, P. B., Sproul, E. E., and Stout, A. P. Microscopic differential diagnosis of latent carcinoma of prostate. *Arch. Pathol. 55:* 131–141, 1953.

47. Troncoso, P., Babaian, R. J., Ro, J. Y., Grignon, D. J., von Eschenbach, A. C., and Ayala, A. G. Prostatic intra-epithelial neoplasia and invasive prostatic adenocarcinoma in cystoprostatectomy specimens. *Urology (Suppl.) 34:* 52–56, 1989.

48. Walsh, P. C. Radical prostatectomy: Preservation of sexual function, Cancer Control: The controversy. *Urol. Clin. North. Am. 14:* 663–673, 1987.

49. Walsh, P. C., and Donker, P. J. Impotence following radical prostatectomy: Insight into etiology and prevention. *J. Urol. 128:* 491–497, 1982.

50. Wernert, N., Seitz, G., and Achtstatter, T. H. Immunohistochemical investigation of different cytokeratins and vimentin in the prostate from the fetal period up to adulthood and in prostate carcinoma. *Pathol. Res. Pract. 182:* 617–626, 1987.

Chapter 8

Diagnostic Correlations with Whole Mounts of Radical Prostatectomy Specimens

GARY J. MILLER AND JAMES M. CYGAN

Prostatic carcinoma has become the most frequently diagnosed malignancy of men in the United States.[3] It is estimated that by the year 2020 approximately 65,000,000 individuals in the United States will become 65 years old.[46] As this graying of our population occurs, it is anticipated that the number of patients with clinically manifest prostatic carcinoma will rise dramatically. Previous data showed that over one-third of patients diagnosed with this disease are found after it has spread outside the prostate, at clinical stages C and D.[41] It is generally accepted that once this disease has become locally invasive or metastatic, available treatment strategies are mainly palliative.[49] Therefore, the last 5 years have been witness to an intensification of efforts to develop the ability to intervene earlier, at clinical stages A and B. During these initial stages, the disease is considered potentially curable both by radical prostatectomy[52,53] and radiotherapy.[2,22] Although it remains to be proven whether earlier intervention will actually increase disease-free survival,[24] the clinical perception is that it will. Consequently, there has been widespread introduction and use of new diagnostic technology such as transrectal ultrasonography and magnetic resonance imaging in an attempt to detect earlier more "curable" lesions. Likewise, there has been extensive evaluation of the more conventional modalities such as digital rectal examination and the serum marker prostate-specific antigen.[7-9] The culmination of such efforts is yet to come with the institution of a nationwide, NIH-sponsored, screening trial to evaluate the efficacy of the available techniques, alone or in combination, at detecting prostatic cancer.[6]

As has previously been the case, the role of diagnostic pathology in the advancement of such knowledge will be pivotal. Any study of the natural history or clinical progression of prostatic cancer could not be considered complete without thorough evaluation of those factors with demonstrated prognostic significance. At present, the list is somewhat short, including only histological grade (for review see Reference 32), tumor volume,[14,28,29,36,45] pathological stage,[5,11,17] and DNA ploidy.[16,33,47] While controversy still exists over the exact value of each of these factors for individual patients (i.e., the precise time and manner of each patient's death cannot be accurately predicted), it is unquestionable that histological grade, for example, is a very powerful tool when large patient cohorts are examined.[18] It has also been recognized for almost 20 years that pathological staging of prostatic carcinomas in clinical stage B disease can be used as a predictor of 5-year survival. Byar and Mostofi[5] demonstrated that when resected prostates were examined using the "whole-mount" technique, penetration of tumors through the prostatic capsule into the surrounding soft tissue markedly decreased survival. Finally, recent studies by McNeal and co-workers[28,29] and others[14] have suggested that tumor volume also may have predictive value with respect to capsular penetration, seminal vesicle invasion, and lymph node metastasis.

In spite of the data that exists regarding the importance of accurate evaluation of the pathological aspects of stage B disease, whole-mount examination of radical prostatectomy specimens is generally considered by practicing pathologists to be a "research" technique. This appraisement is probably justified, at least in part, due to the high cost for material and technical time that whole mounts require. While time consuming and somewhat costly, the use of whole mounts provides a level of information that is difficult to obtain using conventional sections. It is the purpose of the discussion that follows to (1) provide a working description of the process of preparing prostatectomy whole mounts that can be carried out in the routine histology laboratory with little or no modification of existing facilities; (2) review the significant differences encountered in sampling the prostatic capsule using "representative" sections as opposed to whole mounts; (3) provide examples of the types of clinically significant data that can be derived from whole mounts; and (4) give example of the utility of whole-mount preparations in correlating histopathological findings with those obtained using the currently popular methods of diagnostic imaging. In so doing, we hope to foster the use of such methods in pursuing the systematic study of the interrelationships between the pathobiology of early prostatic carcinomas and their clinical management.

PREPARATION OF PROSTATE WHOLE MOUNTS

While considered difficult by many, the preparation of transverse whole-mount sections from radical prostatectomy specimens can be carried out in the routine histology laboratory with the same equipment used for the processing of standard surgical pathology specimens. The procedure described below was developed in our laboratory and has been successfully used to prepare sections of over 300 prostates during the last 3 years. Similar techniques have recently been described in detail elsewhere.[13,23] Following the description of our usual method, some minor modifications are also described to facilitate examination of prostates when whole mounts cannot be prepared.

Following receipt of specimens from surgery, standard measurements of weight and linear dimension are recorded. The volume of prostate is then determined by displacement of water in a graduated cylinder. The specimen should then be fixed for at least 3 days while suspended in a minimum of 9 volumes of 10%

neutral-buffered formaldehyde. While not absolutely necessary, fixation in a suspended state decreases gravity-associated shape artifacts and results in a specimen with a more natural form. The specimen can be suspended using string as is the convention with the brain following autopsy. Alternatively, a short length of alcohol lamp wick can be inserted into the urethra and is then used to tether the specimen to the top of an appropriate container. The latter approach has the advantage that the wick allows fixation to occur from the center of the specimen at an accelerated rate. If possible, it is preferable to renew the formalin solution after 24 hours to assure adequate fixation. The importance of this cannot be overstated since inadequately fixed specimens are subject to several associated artifacts that interfere with histological interpretation. These include (1) retraction of the prostatic capsule after slicing, (2) excessive autolysis that can complicate the diagnosis of well-differentiated lesions, and (3) inadequate further processing, which makes it extremely difficult to cut histological sections. Thorough fixation is, therefore, necessary to the success of the remainder of the technique.

Following fixation, the volume and linear dimensions of the specimen are again determined and recorded. The difference in volume between the unfixed and fixed states can then be used to determine a shrinkage factor. Under our routine conditions, shrinkage is rarely greater than 3–5% of the starting value. More concentrated formalin solutions have been reported to produce greater changes.[28] Shrinkage factors can be used to correct tumor volumes determined from histological sections only if significant spreading or stretching of sections does not occur while transferring paraffin sections to glass slides.

To simplify orientation of the histological sections during microscopic inspection, the left and right sides of the fixed specimens are color coded with Davidson inks (Bradley Products, Inc., Bloomington, MN). The entire outer surface is then painted with India ink to establish the surgical margin of resection. Retention of the inks on the surface of the specimen is enhanced by briefly dipping the inked prostate into 5% acetic acid solution. Five percent acetic acid solution is preferred over Bouin's fixative for this purpose since its use eliminates the problems associated with picric acid. The painted prostates are then sliced at 4-mm intervals in either the transverse or sagittal planes as desired. Numerous means have been devised to assure even, parallel section spacing. Plexiglass "jigs" can be used to both anchor the section and determine the distance between slices. We have used a commercially available rotary meat slicer with good success for many of our cases. The advantage of mechanical over free-hand slicing is that the resulting sections are of more uniform thickness. In addition, the use of a rotating blade seems to eliminate some curling of the slice during subsequent paraffin infiltration and embedding.

Each slice is then labeled and secured within a nylon net envelope. The latter is made by simply folding an appropriately sized rectangle of nylon net (available at retail fabric shops) around each slice and stapling the edge near but not through the tissue. The advantage to this material is that the mesh is of large size, which precludes the trapping of air bubbles that can hamper infiltration. These net envelopes are much less expensive than commercial alternatives such as embedding bags or oversized cassettes. They take up little room in the processing chamber and can be disposed of after use. If excessive room is not left between the tissue and the nylon net, paper labels are retained during processing on the desired side of the slice that will be sectioned. We routinely section the proximal side of each slice, assuring that the resulting histological sections are near 4 mm apart from each other.

Processing can be carried out on existing instruments with little or no modification. Vacuum processing is preferred over simple immersion due to the necessity to infiltrate these large pieces of tissue. If possible, it is also preferred to increase the normal processing times by approximately 20% to permit adequate diffusion of solvents and paraffin. Care should be taken to assure that paraffin infiltration temperatures are not excessive since dried or brittle specimens present a greater challenge to the microtomist.

Following processing, the infiltrated slices are cast into paraffin blocks using L-shaped metal forms to build an appropriately sized rectangular mold. At present we do not attempt to insert specimen rings or blockholders into the backs of the solidifying blocks. Instead, we have obtained an oversized clamp device that can be opened to a width that will accept the smaller dimension of nearly any block commonly encountered. Alternatively, the back of the block can be carved with a sharp knife to produce a "stub" that will directly fit into conventional microtome clamps. Microtomy, transfer of sections to large glass slides (3 × 2 inches) and staining are then finished using standard histotechnique.

As an alternative to preparing whole-mount sections, each transverse slice can be divided into smaller portions (*e.g.*, halves or quarters) such that the resulting pieces will fit into conventional embedding cassettes (*e.g.*, 21). The chief complication encountered using this approach is difficulty in orienting each of the histological sections. One simple remedy to this problem is the use of photocopies as described by Rosai.[39] After the transverse slices are cut, they can be placed on a sheet of transparent acetate and photocopied to produce a quick, inexpensive but accurate map of section shapes and surface features. As the transverse sections are divided, the locations of each piece can be diagrammed on the map. Continuing the process, as each section is examined, the presence of tumor can be recorded on the map along with indication of capsule penetration or margin involvement. Using this method, multifocality, zones of origin, and pathological stage can be readily assessed.

Confusion can result from two potential sources. First, additional cuts perpendicular to the prostatic capsule provide added opportunities for capsule retraction and/or misinterpretation of the pathological stage. Second, embedding more sections increases the probability that the wrong side of a given section might be examined. The latter can be avoided by inking with a unique color, the side of each piece opposite to that which should be cut. One final useful modification is the cutting of the apical slice in a "clockface" fashion, similar to the usual method used for cervical cone biopsies.[1] In this way, more of the apical margin is examined than with a single transverse slice. This can be important since it has been noted that the prostatic apex is a frequent site for capsule penetration.[50]

SAMPLING OF THE PROSTATE USING WHOLE MOUNTS VERSUS REPRESENTATIVE SECTIONS

As previously discussed, one recognized prognostic variable regarding disease recurrence and survival following radical prostatectomy is the presence or absence of capsular penetration. The prostatic capsule is a somewhat vague structure[1] that varies with respect to location around the gland. While it is somewhat well-defined as a compact band of fibromuscular cells along the posterolateral aspects, the demarcation of the anterior fibromuscular structures from the surrounding connective tissue elements is less obvious. Nonetheless, when penetration of malignant cells into the surrounding soft tissue occurs, 5-year survival decreases.[5,11,17] At present, it remains unestablished precisely how much capsule must be penetrated to have clinical consequences. But over one-half of patients believed to have disease confined within the prostate before surgery can be shown to have capsular penetration following thorough inspection.[40,53] Current trends in the clinical management of pathological stage C-patients are still evolving, but it seems prudent to be as accurate as possible in any assessment of tumor stage.

While the question of sampling error in pathological inspection of transurethrally resected prostates has been addressed,[35,51] no formal discussion of the sampling of radical prostatectomy specimens is available. Our inspection of over 100 prostates has revealed an average volume of 38 cc measured by displacement. Assuming a spherical shape, the surface of an average prostate can be calculated to be approximately 55 cm^2. The amount of capsule that can be examined using representative sections is severely constrained by the size of routine embedding cassettes. Even if each section was maximized for the amount of capsule included, it is unlikely that each section would examine more than 1.25 cm^2. Examination of eight representative cassettes from a radical prostatectomy specimen would, therefore, sample only 20% of the prostate surface. Although an experienced pathologist can select suspicious areas and improve the chance of finding capsule penetration,[13] this approach is unreliable. While it is true that some prostatic carcinomas are yellow in color and grossly apparent, many are not. Furthermore, as clinical diagnostic techniques become more sensitive, the size of tumors present in resected prostates will decrease making them less likely to be seen on gross inspection.

CLINICAL VERSUS PATHOLOGICAL STAGING

As the search for more sensitive clinical diagnostic tools progresses, larger numbers of early stage prostatic cancers will be found. The resultant increase in the number of radical prostatectomy specimens that will become available for pathological review provides a unique opportunity to study the tumor biology of these neoplasms. Early studies by Moore[34] using whole-mount sections revealed that nearly three-fourths of carcinomas arise in the peripheral prostate. Furthermore, Moore concluded that the occurrence of prostatic carcinoma is not infrequently multicentric. In 52 cases, he found 68 separate malignant foci. McNeal and co-workers[28,29,45,50] have reported on several recent series of studies in which autopsy and surgical specimens were examined using the whole-mount technique. Besides confirming the findings of Moore regarding multifocality, McNeal and co-workers have also developed a new hypothesis regarding the natural history of early stage tumors. They have concluded that as tumors increase in volume, their degree of differentiation decreases.[28] Using this relationship, they suggest that, at a critical volume of 3.8 cc, tumors frequently develop the ability to become metastatic.[29] The combination of histological grade (Gleason score sum) and tumor volume appears, therefore, to be a powerful predictor of malignant potential.

Our own studies on such specimens have confirmed some previous findings, but have revealed significant differences regarding the interrelationships of stage and grade. The data from our first 50 cases have, for example, documented the multicentric nature of prostatic carcinoma (Fig. 8.1). Using three-dimensional reconstruction,[31] we have found that approximately 50% of patients have more than one focus of cancer in their prostatectomy specimen. In fact, this probably represents an underestimation since we cannot rule out the possibility that some large "single" tumors arose from the collision of two smaller lesions. The significance of multifocality is most apparent when one considers the diagnostic importance of an original biopsy in directing clinical management. It has recently been suggested that expectant therapy cannot be reliably recommended for patients with low-grade cancers diagnosed by needle biopsy since these patients may have multifocal tumors with more aggressive malignant potentials.[15]

Regarding the relationship of histological grade to tumor volume, the data from our first 50 cases are seen in Figure 8.2. While there is a modest correlation between the two variables ($r_s = 0.4175$), it appears that volume and grade are not uniformly related in these specimens. This lack of correlation is just as apparent ($r_s = 0.3563$) when the index tumor for each case (*i.e.*, the largest tumor per prostate) is identified according to the criteria of McNeal and co-workers[28] and compared to its Gleason sum (Fig. 8.3). While several lower grade tumors were

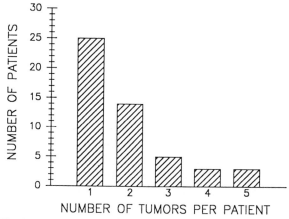

FIG. 8.1. Multifocality of prostatic carcinoma. Only 25 of the 50 patients studied had a single prostatic carcinoma. The other 25 have multifocal disease ranging from 2 to 5 carcinomas per prostate.

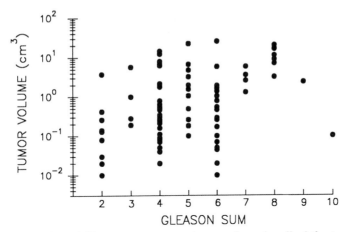

FIG. 8.2. Relationship of Gleason score sum to tumor volume for all of the tumors ($n = 98$) detected in 50 radical prostatectomy specimens.

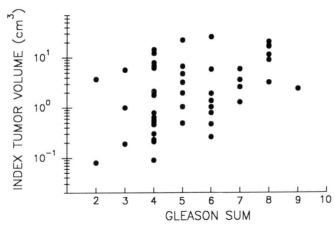

FIG. 8.3. Relationship of Gleason score sum to the tumor volume of the index tumor ($n = 50$) for each prostate. The index tumor was defined as the largest volume tumor in each radical prostatectomy specimen.

found to be of low volume, the highest grade tumors are not the largest. Tumors with highest volume are found in intermediate grade lesions, such as those with Gleason score sums of 5 to 8.

Gleason sum was also found to lack direct correlation with the surface area of prostatic capsule that had been penetrated (Fig. 8.4). Again, the largest amounts of capsule penetration occur over a range of Gleason sums from 4 to 8. However, Gleason sum was found to be related to the simple presence or absence of penetration. Most tumors with Gleason score sums of 2 were confined to the prostate, whereas the majority of tumors with Gleason score sums of 7 or greater demonstrated focal penetration. From our results it can be concluded that neither the volume nor the surface area of capsule penetration can be predicted prior to

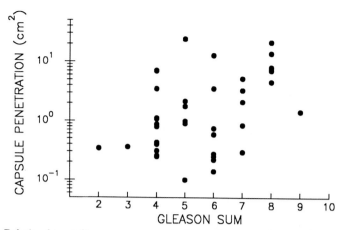

FIG. 8.4.   Relationship of Gleason score sum to the surface area of prostatic capsule penetrated by tumor cells. Penetration was defined by the presence of malignant cells invading into periprostatic tissue. Those cases in which penetration did not occur (*i.e.,* penetration = 0) are not shown.

surgery based on Gleason sum alone. The extremes of Gleason scores do, however, provide an indication of whether or not any capsule penetration might be present.

In agreement with Stamey and co-workers,[45] we have found a clear relationship between tumor volume and the amount of capsule penetration, as seen in Figure 8.5. Here it is apparent that these two variables are directly correlated ($r =$ 0.8883). These data clearly show that as a tumor becomes larger, it is likely to penetrate more of the prostatic capsule. To summarize, the higher the histological grade and the larger the tumor volume, the more likely that a given tumor will be found to be of higher pathological stage than was clinically suspect.

Lastly, Epstein[13] has recently examined the significance of radical prostatectomy surgical margins designated as positive or negative in a series of 40 patients. These patients first underwent nerve-sparing prostatectomy and subsequently had their neurovascular bundle removed following the diagnosis of stage C disease by gross inspection. This study provided a relatively unique opportunity to compare the findings from the prostate with those from surrounding soft tissue obtained during a single surgical procedure. All of the 20 cases that were found to have negative margins on histological inspection of the prostate specimen also failed to contain malignant cells in the neurovascular bundle. Tumor was present in 6 of 10 neurovascular bundles when the prostate margins were unequivocally positive. However, tumor cells could not be found in the neurovascular bundles of 11 cases that had tumor extending near to or at the inked margin. While this study suggests that a conservative approach should be taken regarding the interpretation of positive margins, this area remains controversial. Since the residual postprostatectomy soft tissue surrounding the prostate can not be histologically examined with the same scrutiny as the prostate itself, local recurrence must serve as the ultimate measure of the failure to completely excise such tumors.

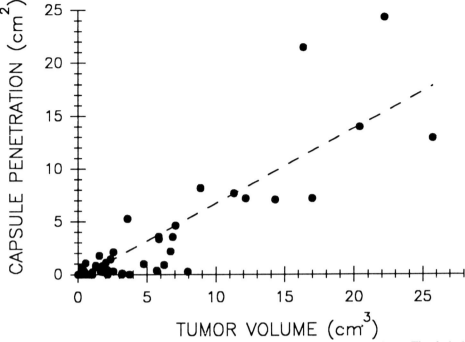

FIG. 8.5. Relationship of the surface area of capsule penetration to tumor volume. The *dashed line* represents a first-order regression line plotted through the data points.

CORRELATION WITH IMAGING TECHNIQUES

One of the great advantages in preserving the prostatic anatomy with whole mounts is the ability to correlate histopathological findings directly with imaging results. The prostate is a dynamic organ subject to several common disease processes including benign hyperplasia, acute prostatitis, chronic prostatitis, and cystic atrophy, in addition to carcinoma. It is not at all uncommon to find several of these entities occurring concurrently. In fact, it is likely that several benign diseases represent a disease complex that is part of a pathogenetic cascade beginning with benign hyperplasia. Confusion regarding the meaning of various imaging findings can result from the intimacy of unrelated disease to the one of interest. For example, carcinomas invade through the prostatic stroma and are frequently found admixed with atrophic acini or hyperplastic epithelium. Inflammatory infiltrates that accompany acute prostatitis often extend away from their origins and involve focal carcinomas. The juxtaposition of these disparate processes makes it imperative that correlative studies of diagnostic imaging and histopathology should be carried out with all the precision that is possible. This necessity has led to the suggestion that whole-mount sections of radical prostatectomy specimens should be used as a "gold standard" against which diagnostic findings should be compared.[37] In spite of this, many current studies have attempted to analyze such complex problems using biopsy techniques. For example some studies correlating transrectal ultrasonographic (TRUS) findings to various clinical findings use whole mounts,[19–21,42,43] yet many others have been interpreted using comparison to needle biopsy results.[4,7,9,10,25,26]

The power of direct correlation with whole mounts is well illustrated in the recent studies of Shinohara *et al.*[43] For example, these authors found that in 98 patients the principal tumor was seen as a hypoechoic area in only 66 cases. In 31 patients, the region of the prostate known to contain a tumor by histological analysis appeared similar to normal prostate by ultrasonography (isoechoic). One patient was found to have a tumor with hyperechogenicity. In view of the importance of tumor volume cited above, the accuracy of sonographic estimation of tumor size was also examined. Comparing the maximum diameter for each of the 66 tumors that were visible by ultrasound with their diameter determined from whole-mount sections revealed that ultrasonography consistently underestimated tumor size by approximately 4 mm. Finally, the relationship of tumor grade to echogenic appearance was examined. These authors found that hypoechoic tumors were more likely to be moderate to poorly differentiated. Isoechoic tumors were more often well or moderately differentiated.

We have also examined prostates from 30 patients who underwent transrectal ultrasonography prior to radical prostatectomy.[30] A total of 61 tumors were identified in the whole-mount sections from these specimens. Correlations with ultrasonography revealed that 32 tumors were correctly identified prior to surgery, 29 were missed, and 11 patients' sonographic "lesions" were false-positives (Fig. 8.6). Seventy-one percent of the false-negatives were located in the anterior prostate. This is particularly relevant since about one-third of all unifocal tumors in our series have been confined to the anterior half of the prostate. In part, the inability to image tumors in the anterior prostate is probably due to the presence of calcified corpora amylacea near the prostatic urethra which cast acoustic shadows. False-positives were attributed to cystic atrophy (seven cases), simple atrophy (two cases), acute prostatitis (one case), benign hyperplasia (one case), and granulomatous prostatitis (one case). All of these benign conditions are extremely common in the aged prostate and have been shown to contribute to the poor specificity of TRUS by others.[42]

The finding of granulomatous prostatitis presenting as a hypoechoic lesion suggests that this iatrogenic inflammatory process (typically a sequela of transurethral prostatectomy[44]) would hamper our ability to accurately assess the presence of residual stage A cancers.[30,42] Sixteen of the 21 tumors identified by ultrasound were hypoechoic. These were predominantly (14 of 16) Gleason sums of 7 or less and 7 of 16 had Gleason sums of 2–4. A larger fraction of the isoechoic tumors (16 of 22) were well-differentiated (Gleason 2, 3, or 4). However, considerable overlap existed between grades. This has prompted us to examine the epithelial/stromal (E/S) ratio of tumors in an attempt to directly explain their echogenic characteristics. Preliminary studies have indicated that tumors that appear hypoechoic have E/S ratios greater than 1, whereas isoechoic lesions have E/S ratios of 1 or less. Five tumors in our series were hyperechoic. Two of these mucinous carcinomas had focal calcifications. The other three were high-grade "comedocarcinomas," which contained central necrosis.[27] Similar findings by

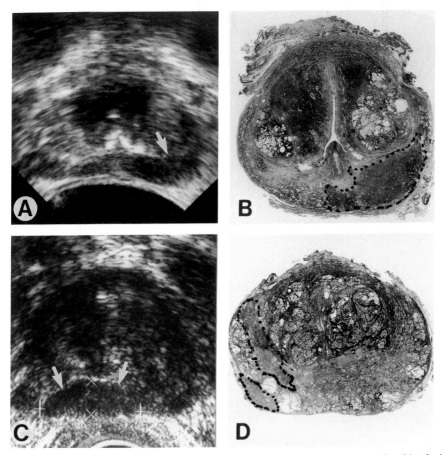

FIG. 8.6. Comparison of TRUS images of prostatic carcinoma to their corresponding histological whole mounts. Note the close correlation between the position of the hypoechoic lesion (*white arrow*) in A with the carcinoma (*dotted*) seen in B. The comparison of C and D reveals almost no direct correlation. The hypoechoic lesion in C (*white arrows*) corresponds to a field of cystic atrophy.

others[19] have confirmed this observation. The presence of mixed or hyperechogenicity may, therefore, indicate the presence of highly aggressive tumors. Lastly, the ability of TRUS to detect capsular invasion has been studied by Hamper *et al.*[21] using hemisectioned prostatectomy specimens. These authors found that of the 250 half-prostates that were examined, 86 contained areas of capsular penetration. TRUS correctly identified pericapsular tumor invasion in 59 halves. In 15 halves, false-positive results were obtained. It appears, therefore, that TRUS may be somewhat effective at detecting relatively large amounts of capsular penetration.

As new imaging modalities are further developed, additional opportunities occur for correlation with histopathology. Magnetic resonance imaging (MRI) is an example of such a technique. Using whole-mount sections, we have examined the ability of 0.35 Tesla MRI to detect and estimate the volume of prostate carcinomas.[48] MRI correctly identified 82% of carcinomas greater than 5 mm in maximum diameter. These lesions were best identified when they involved the midposterior prostate. Individual tumor volumes, however, were poorly estimated. It was concluded that while MRI can identify prostatic carcinomas, the technique may have limitations as a screening modality and in accurately assessing the amount of a given prostate that is involved by cancer. Finally, the results of a multi-institutional cooperative trial of MRI and TRUS in the imaging and staging of early prostatic cancer have recently been reported.[38] Although, as stated above, these techniques are capable of detecting some tumors, it was concluded by the authors that the available equipment is not highly accurate, mainly because of an inability to identify microscopic spread of disease.

SUMMARY

While probably not necessary in routine diagnosis, whole-mount sections of radical prostatectomy specimens can provide valuable information that is difficult to obtain by other means. Contrary to popular belief, the technique can be carried out in the routine histology laboratory with only minor modifications of existing methods. The use of this technique has provided valuable insight into the tumor biology of early stage prostatic cancer pointing to a multifocal origin for this disease. Likewise, the study of tumor volume, histological grade, and capsular penetration has provided a basis for the use of such prognostic markers in clinical management. The continuing development of new screening tools such as TRUS and MRI requires careful correlation with histopathology to assure a fundamental understanding of their abilities and limitations to detect and stage early-stage tumors. Only with such continued effort will diagnosis and clinical intervention allow us to make a meaningful impact on the natural history of this common malignancy.

ACKNOWLEDGMENTS

This work was supported in part by the University of Colorado Cancer Center, USPHS grant CA-46934, through the Histopathology Core Laboratory. James Cygan was supported in part by the American Cancer Society Brooks Trust and by NIH grant R25 CA-49981 through the University of Colorado Summer Cancer Student Fellowship program. The authors would like to thank Nancy J. Dunscomb for preparing whole-mount sections, Robert McCullough for photography, and Nancy Hart and Clairene Mraz for preparing the manuscript.

REFERENCES

1. Ayala, A. G., Ro, J. Y., Babaian, R., Troncoso, P., and Grignon, D. J. The prostatic capsule: Does it exist? Its importance in the staging and treatment of prostatic carcinoma. *Am. J. Surg. Pathol. 13:* 21–27, 1989.
2. Bagshaw, M. A., Ray, G. R., and Cox, R. S. Selecting initial therapy for prostate cancer: Radiation therapy perspective. *Cancer 60:* 521–525, 1987.
3. Boring, C. C., Squires, T. S., and Tong, T. Cancer statistics, 1991. *CA 41:* 19–36, 1991.
4. Burks, D. D., Drolshagen, L. F., Fleischer, A. C., Liddell, H. T., McDougal, W. S., Karl, E. M., and James, A. E. Jr. Transrectal sonography of benign and malignant prostatic lesions. *AJR 146:* 1187–1191, 1986.

5. Byar, D. P., and Mostofi, F. K. Carcinoma of the prostate: Prognostic evaluation of certain pathologic features in 208 radical prostatectomies. *Cancer 30:* 5–13, 1972.
6. The Cancer Letter. Advisors OK 16 year, $60 million trial of cancer screening methods. *17 (7),* Feb. 15, 1991, pp. 4–6.
7. Chodak, G. W., Wald, V., Parmer, E., Watanabe, H., Ohe, H., and Saitoh, M. Comparison of digital examination and transrectal ultrasonography for the diagnosis of prostatic cancer. *J. Urol. 135:* 951–954, 1986.
8. Cooner, W., Mosley, B. R., Rutherford, C. L. Jr., Beard, J. G., Bond, H. S., Terry, W. J., Igel, T. C., and Kidd, D. D. Prostate cancer detection in a clinical urological practice by ultrasonography, digital rectal examination and prostate specific antigen. *J. Urol. 143:* 1146–1154, 1990.
9. Devonec, M., Chapelon, J. Y., and Cathignol, D. Comparison of the diagnostic value of sonography and rectal examination in cancer of the prostate. *Eur. Urol. 14:* 189–195, 1988.
10. Devonec, M., Fendler, J. P., Monsallier, M., Mouriquand, P., Maquet, J. H., Mestas, J. L., Dutrieux-Berger, N., and Perrin, P. The significance of the prostatic hypoechoic area: Results in 226 ultrasonically guided prostatic biopsies. *J. Urol. 143:* 316–319, 1990.
11. Elder, J. S., Jewett, H. J., and Walsh, P. C. Radical perineal prostatectomy for clinical Stage B2 carcinoma of the prostate. *J. Urol. 127:* 704–706, 1982.
12. Epstein, J. I. Evaluation of radical prostatectomy capsular margins of resection: The significance of margins designated as negative, closely approaching and positive. *Am. J. Surg. Pathol. 14:* 626–632, 1990.
13. Epstein, J. I. The evaluation of radical prostatectomy specimens. Therapeutic and prognostic implications. In *Pathology Annual: Nineteen Ninety-One*, edited by P. R. Rosen and R. E. Fechner, East Norwalk, Conn., Appleton & Lange, 1991, pp. 159–210.
14. Epstein, J. I., Oesterling, J. E., and Walsh, P. C. Tumor volume versus percentage of specimen involved by tumor correlated with progression in Stage A prostatic cancer. *J. Urol. 139:* 980–984, 1988.
15. Epstein, J. I., and Steinberg, G. D. The significance of low-grade prostate cancer on needle biopsy. *Cancer 66:* 1927–1932, 1990.
16. Fordham, M. V. P., Burdge, A. H., Matthews, J., Williams, G., and Cooke, T. Prostatic carcinoma cell DNA content measured by flow cytometry and its relationship to clinical outcome. *Br. J. Surg. 73:* 400–403, 1986.
17. Fowler, J. E., and Mills, S. E. Operable prostatic carcinoma: Correlations among clinical stage, pathological stage, Gleason histological score and early disease-free survival. *J. Urol. 133:* 49–52, 1985.
18. Gleason, D. F., and the Veterans Administration Cooperative Urologic Research Group. Histologic grading and clinical staging of prostatic carcinoma. In *Urologic Pathology: The Prostate*, edited by M. Tannenbaum, Philadelphia, Lea & Febiger, 1977, pp. 171–198.
19. Hamper, U. M., Sheth, S., Walsh, P. C., and Epstein, J. I. Bright echogenic foci in early prostatic carcinoma: Sonographic and pathologic correlation. *Radiology 176:* 339–343, 1990.
20. Hamper, U. M., Sheth, S., Walsh, P. C., Holtz, P. M., and Epstein, J. I. Carcinoma of the prostate: Value of transrectal sonography in detecting extension into the neurovascular bundle. *AJR 155:* 1015–1019, 1990.
21. Hamper, U. M., Sheth, S., Walsh, P. C., Holtz, P. M., and Epstein, J. I. Capsular transgression of prostatic carcinoma: Evaluation with transrectal US with pathologic correlation. *Radiology 178:* 791–795, 1991.
22. Hanks, G. E. Radical prostatectomy or radiation therapy for early prostate cancer. Two roads to the same end. *Cancer 61:* 2153–2160, 1988.
23. Hostetter, A. L., Pedersen, K. V., Gustafsson, B. L., Månson, J.-C., and Boeryd, B. R. G. Diagnosis and localization of prostate carcinoma by fine-needle aspiration cytology and correlation with histologic whole-organ sections after radical prostatectomy. *Am. J. Clin. Pathol. 94:* 693–697, 1990.
24. Johansson, J. E., Adami, H. O., Anderson, S. O., Bergstrom, R., Krusemo, U. B., and Kraaz, W. Natural history of localised prostatic cancer: A population-based study in 223 untreated patients. *Lancet I:* 799–803, 1989.

25. Lee, F., Littrup, P. J., Torp-Pedersen, S. T., Mettlin, C., McHugh, T. A., Gray, J. M., Kumaska, G. H., and McLeary, R. D. Prostate cancer: Comparison of transrectal US and digital rectal examination for screening. *Radiology 168:* 389–394, 1988.
26. Lee, R., Gray, J. M., McLeary, R. D., Meadows, T. R., Kumasaka, G. H., Borlaza, G. S., Straub, W. H., Lee, F., Jr., Solomon, M. H., McHugh, T. A., and Wolf, R. M. Transrectal ultrasound in the diagnosis of prostate cancer: Location, echogenicity, histopathology, and staging. *Prostate 7:* 117–129, 1985.
27. Lile, R., Thickman, D., and Miller, G. J. Prostatic comedocarcinoma: Correlation of sonograms with pathologic specimens in three cases. *AJR 155:* 303–306, 1990.
28. McNeal, J. E., Bostwick, D. G., Kindrachuk, R. A., Redwine, E. A., Freiha, F. S., and Stamey, T. A. Patterns of progression in prostate cancer. *Lancet I:* 60–63, 1986.
29. McNeal, J. E., Villers, A. A., Redwine, E. A., Freiha, F. S., and Stamey, T. A. Histologic differentiation, cancer volume, and pelvic lymph node metastasis in adenocarcinoma of the prostate. *Cancer 66:* 1225–1233, 1990.
30. Miller, G. J. Histopathologic correlates with sonographic findings. In *Clinical Aspects of Prostate Cancer: Assessment of New Diagnostic and Management Procedures*, edited by W. J. Catalona, D. S. Coffey, and J. P. Karr. New York, Elsevier, 1989, pp. 73–78.
31. Miller, G. J. Histopathology of prostate cancer: Prediction of malignant behavior and correlations with ultrasonography. *Urology 33:* 18–26, 1989.
32. Miller, G. J. New developments in grading prostate cancer. *Semin. Urol. 8:* 9–18, 1990.
33. Montgomery, B. T., Nativ, O., Blute, M. L., Farrow, G. M., Meyers, R. P., Zincke, H., Therneau, T. M., and Lieber, M. M. Stage B prostate adenocarcinoma: Flow cytometric nuclear DNA ploidy analysis. *Arch. Surg. 125:* 327–331, 1990.
34. Moore, R. A. The morphology of small prostatic carcinoma. *J. Urol. 33:* 224–234, 1935.
35. Murphy, W. M., Dean, P. J., Brasfield, J. A., and Tatum, L. Incidental carcinoma of the prostate: How much sampling is adequate? *Am. J. Surg. Pathol. 10:* 170–174, 1986.
36. Paulson, D. F., Stone, A. R., Walther, P. J., Tucker, J. A., and Cox, E. B. Radical prostatectomy: Anatomical predictors of success or failure. *J. Urol. 136:* 1041–1043, 1986.
37. Rifkin, M. D. Prostate cancer: Sonographic characteristics. In *Ultrasound of the Prostate*, edited by M. D. Rifkin. New York, Raven Press, 1988, pp. 157–184.
38. Rifkin, M. D., Zeerhouni, E. A., Gatsonis, C. A., Quint, L. E., Paushter, D. M., Epstein, J. I., Hamper, U., Walsh, P. C., and McNeil, B. J. Comparison of magnetic resonance imaging and ultrasonography in staging early prostatic cancer. *N. Engl. J. Med. 323:* 621–626, 1990.
39. Rosai, J. Gross techniques in surgical pathology. In *Ackermans Surgical Pathology. Vol. I*, edited by J. Rosai. St. Louis, C. V. Mosby Co., 1989, pp. 13–29.
40. Scardino, P. T., Shinohara, K., Wheeler, T. M., and Carter, S. St. C. Staging of prostate cancer: Value of ultrasonography. *Urol. Clin. N. Am. 16:* 713–734, 1989.
41. Schmidt, J. D., Mettlin, C. J., Natarajan, N., Peace, B. B., Beart, R. W. Jr., Winchester, D. P., and Murphy, G. P. Trends in patterns of care for prostatic cancer, 1974–1983. Results of surveys by the American College of Surgeons. *J. Urol. 136:* 416–421, 1986.
42. Sheth, S., Hamper, U. M., Walsh, P. C., Holtz, P. M., and Epstein, J. I. Stage A adenocarcinoma of the prostate: Transrectal US and sonographic-pathologic correlation. *Radiology 179:* 35–39, 1991.
43. Shinohara, K., Scardino, P. T., Carter, S. St. C., and Wheeler, T. M. Pathologic basis of the sonographic appearance of the normal and malignant prostate. *Urol. Clin. N. A. 16:* 675–691, 1989.
44. Sorenson, F. B., and Marcussen, N. Iatrogenic granulomas of the prostate and urinary bladder. *Pathol. Res. Pract. 182:* 822–830, 1987.
45. Stamey, T. A., McNeal, J. E., Freiha, F. S., and Redwine, E. Morphometric and clinical studies on 68 consecutive radical prostatectomies. *J. Urol. 139:* 1235–1241, 1988.
46. *Statistical Abstract of the United States: 1987.* 107th edition. Washington, D. C., U.S. Bureau of the Census. 1987.
47. Stephenson, R. A. Flow cytometry in genitourinary malignancies using paraffin-embedded material. *Semin. Urol. 6:* 45–52, 1988.

48. Thickman, D., Miller, G. J., Hopper, K. D., and Raife, M. Prostate cancer: Comparison of pre-operative 0.35T MRI with whole-mount histopathology. *Mag. Res. Imaging 8:* 205–211, 1990.

49. Venner, P. M. Therapeutic options in treatment of advanced carcinoma of the prostate. *Semin. Oncol. 17:* 73–77, 1990.

50. Villers, A., McNeal, J. E., Redwine, E. A., Freiha, F. S., and Stamey, T. A. The role of perineural space invasion in the local spread of prostatic adenocarcinoma. *J. Urol. 142:* 763–768, 1989.

51. Vollmer, R. T. Prostate cancer and chip specimens: Complete versus partial sampling. *Hum. Pathol. 17:* 285–290, 1986.

52. Walsh, P. C. Radical retropubic prostatectomy with reduced morbidity: An anatomic approach. *NCI Monogr. 7:* 133–137, 1988.

53. Walsh, P. C., and Lepor, H. The role of radical prostatectomy in the management of prostatic cancer. *Cancer 60:* 526–537, 1987.

Chapter 9

The Biology of Prostate Cancer: New and Future Directions in Predicting Tumor Behavior

ALAN W. PARTIN, H. BALLENTINE CARTER,
JONATHAN I. EPSTEIN, AND DONALD S. COFFEY

Both the incidence and mortality from prostate cancer in the United States have risen markedly in the past 13 years.[42] The life-time risk of developing prostate cancer in the United States is 1 in 11.5, which is presently equal to the risk of developing lung cancer.[58] The risk of developing prostate cancer has risen 42.6% since 1975, as compared to an increase of only 26% in the risk of developing lung cancer for that same time period. In addition, approximately 10 million United States males harbor histological prostate cancer, the majority of which will never manifest clinically. Approximately 400,000 operations are performed each year in the United States for benign prostatic hyperplasia (BPH), of which 10% will display incidental cancer (*i.e.*, stage A). Currently there are no accurate methods of predicting which of these cancers will become clinically manifest.

There has been little progress in terms of new effective therapy with regard to prostate cancer and at present only pathologically localized prostate cancer is considered potentially curable. It has been estimated that approximately 40% of the new cases of prostate cancer this year will represent disease confined to the organ.[3] Within this population of potentially curable patients, the relative risk of progression during the next 10–15 years approaches 25% even after definitive surgery.[20,29,40,53,54,56,65] These observations mandate new and better methods for determining the biological potential of prostate cancers in order to: (1) evaluate better which patients have tumors that need treatment, and (2) determine the prognosis of patients with prostate cancer pathologically localized to the gland, after surgery, so that treatment of those patients with a high probability of disease progression might begin earlier in the natural course of the disease. This Chapter is devoted to describing new methods developed to predict accurately tumor behavior in patients with prostate cancer.

TUMOR GRADE, STAGE, AND SERUM MARKERS

While widely accepted and utilized for evaluation of an individual patient's prognosis, the current methods for predicting tumor behavior [graded as Gleason score, stage, serum prostate-specific antigen (PSA), and serum prostatic acid phosphatase (PAP)] have been unreliable for prediction of prognosis of the individual patient with prostate cancer.

The most commonly used grading system, Gleason, has been shown to predict accurately prognosis for patients with low grade (Gleason score 2–4) and high grade (Gleason score 8–10). However, the majority of patients (more than 75%) have tumors of intermediate grade (Gleason score 5–7) where the Gleason system has shown limited prognostic ability for individual patients. Figure 9.1 represents graphically the generalized problem in assessing the prognosis of patients with prostate cancer using the Gleason score as a prognostic factor. When prognosis is plotted as a function of prognostic factors (*e.g.*, grade, stage, serum PSA value or serum PAP value) there is little correlation ($r = -0.15$, $p = 0.42$) for those patients within the intermediate zone (Gleason 5–7, $n = 75$; squares on Fig. 9.1). However, the patients lying at the extremes (Gleason 2–4 and 8–10, $n = 25$; triangles on Fig. 9.1) yield a much better correlation ($r = -0.78$, $p < 0.00001$) and elevate the overall correlation coefficient ($r = -0.42$, $p = 0.001$) for the entire group. A goal of future efforts in predicting prognosis is to resolve the grades of

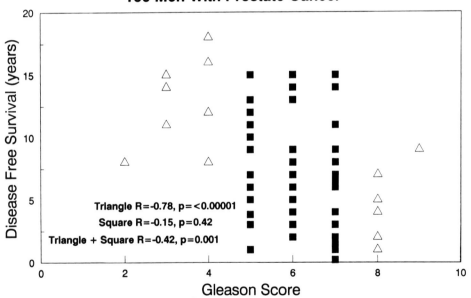

**Correlation of Gleason Score
With Disease Free Survival For
100 Men With Prostate Cancer**

Triangle R=-0.78, p=<0.00001

Square R=-0.15, p=0.42

Triangle + Square R=-0.42, p=0.001

FIG. 9.1.   Correlation of Gleason score with prognosis. Graphic representation of the generalized problem in assessing the prognosis of patients with prostate cancer. The graph illustrates the present limitations in prognosis determination when using the Gleason score. Patients with Gleason score (5–7) have a correlation of $r = -0.15$, while those on the extremes (2–4 and 8–10) correlate with $r = -0.78$. Unfortunately 75% of the 100 patients fall within the middle range, yet the overall correlation is $r = -0.42$ and significant at $p < 0.001$. The goal is to resolve the middle range.

these patients within the middle zone and provide a more accurate prognosis for this disease.

The Jewett-Whitmore[24,66] staging system for prostate cancer, plus recent advances of serum PSA measurements and transrectal ultrasound imaging of prostate cancer, are currently used by most urologists and pathologists to predict which patients harbor potentially curable prostate cancer. As many as 60% of patients diagnosed with prostate cancer each year in the United States have what is defined as clinically localized disease, yet unfortunately, as many as 40% of this group of patients will prove to have nonorgan-confined disease when examined histopathologically.[3] Both tumor volume and percent of the gland involved with tumor have been shown to be predictive of tumor behavior.[28,48] A more precise staging of incidentally found (stage A) prostate cancer was introduced by Cantrell *et al.*[2] and has been expounded upon in more recent works[2,13,17,28,48] in which tumor volume and percent are used to describe better tumor aggressiveness.

Figure 9.2 demonstrates the relationship between both tumor volume and the percent of gland involved with tumor for a group of 56 step-sectioned radical prostatectomy specimens. While both volume and percent show an increased trend with advancing stage, due to the great overlap between stages neither is

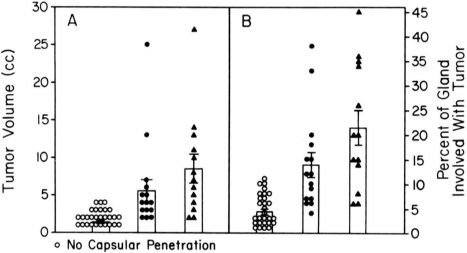

○ No Capsular Penetration
● Positive Capsular Penetration
▲ Seminal Vesicle Involvement

FIG. 9.2.   Correlation of tumor volume and percent of gland involved with tumor with pathological stage. Correlation distribution of 56 step-sectioned radical prostatectomy specimens by tumor volume (*A*) and percent of gland involved with tumor (*B*) versus pathological stage. *Open circles* represent patients with localized tumor and no prostatic capsular penetration. *Closed circles* represent patients with positive capsular penetration only. *Closed triangles* are those patients with seminal vesicle involvement. *Bars* represent mean plus or minus standard deviation of mean for the groups. From Partin, A. W., Epstein, J. I., Cho, K. R., Gittelsohn, A. M., and Walsh, P. C. Morphometric measurement of tumor volume and percent of gland involvement as predictors of pathologic stage in clinical stage B prostate cancer. *J. Urol. 141:* 341–345, 1989.

useful for prediction of stage for an individual patient with prostate cancer. This relationship between tumor volume/percent and tumor aggressiveness is predicted from what is known about solid tumor heterogeneity in general.[43] As the tumor grows, increased genetic instability within the tumor occurs, resulting in a growth advantage for subpopulations of cells.[16,18,44] These changes eventually result in populations of cells with varied phenotypes capable of growth in the absence of androgens, and with differing metastatic ability and resistance to chemotherapeutic agents. Unfortunately, at present there is no precise method to quantify accurately tumor volume prior to definitive therapy. Although recent improvements in transrectal imaging of the prostate via both magnetic resonance and ultrasound may improve local tumor staging by volume determinations, the accurate quantitation of small volume (<1 cc) remains beyond the resolution of current instruments.

The currently used serum markers for prostate cancer (PSA and PAP) have shown little value in the prediction of tumor behavior for an individual patient with prostate cancer localized to the gland. An elevation of PAP, while indicative of metastatic disease, is a late finding in the natural course of prostate cancer and, when elevated, is specific only for advanced disease.[25] Serum prostate-specific antigen, on the other hand, is a very sensitive marker for secretion from the prostatic epithelium,[61] but because of its relative nonspecificity, a single PSA level does not differentiate between normal, inflamed, hyperplastic, and cancerous epithelium. It is thus not useful alone as a marker of prostate cancer or a predictor of tumor behavior.[7,15,25,47,60,61] Figure 9.3 demonstrates the marked overlap in serum PSA levels among different pathological stages for individual men with prostate cancer and BPH. There is evidence that serial measurements of PSA with evaluation of rate of change in PSA may accurately differentiate between men with BPH and those with malignancy.[6] The organ specificity of PSA makes serum PSA measurements a valuable tool for surveillance of patients after radical prostatectomy. For example, an elevated PSA prior to therapy, which does not return to normal or subnormal values after therapy, or a subsequent elevation in serum PSA after therapy is the best marker of residual disease. In summary, while not shown to be a specific marker for prostate cancer prior to therapy, elevation in serum PSA levels postoperatively may help in selecting patients who harbor more aggressive tumors and might benefit from additional forms of therapy.

FUTURE PROGNOSTIC FACTORS

It is well accepted that the transformation of a normal prostatic epithelial cell to a cancer cell with progression to a metastatic phenotype requires multiple steps.[16] This progression, from normal to cancer to aggressive cancer is accompanied by changes in the individual cells, as depicted in Figure 9.4. The development of methods to quantify accurately these changes in order to predict better tumor behavior has been the subject of much experimental work in prostate cancer.

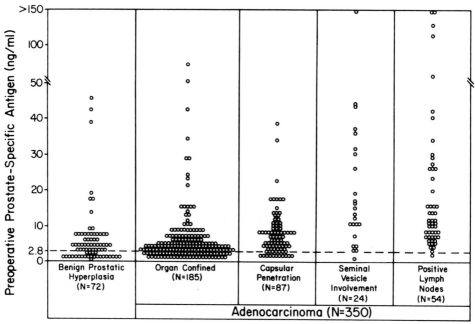

FIG. 9.3.   Serum prostate-specific antigen versus pathological stage. Plot of individual preoperative serum PSA values (nanograms per milliliter) for 350 men with prostate cancer and 72 men with histologically confirmed BPH only with respect to pathological stage. *Dashed line* represents upper limit of normal for men (range, 0–2.8 ng/ml). From Partin, A. W., Carter, H. B., Chan, D. W., Epstein, J. I., Oesterling, J. E., Rock, R. C., Weber, J. P., and Walsh, P. C. Prostate specific antigen in the staging of localized prostate cancer: Influence of tumor differentiation, tumor volume and benign hyperplasia. *J. Urol. 143:* 747–752, 1990.

NUCLEAR SHAPE

As early as 1851, pathologists recognized that cancer cells had very pleomorphic and irregularly shaped nuclei and that the more abnormal the shape of the nuclei, the worse the prognosis for the patient harboring that tumor.[64] Now, more than a century later, the diagnosis of cancer and the determination of prognosis still depends heavily on the appreciation of these cytological abnormalities. Several grading systems have evaluated the degree of nuclear anaplasia[21,37,38] to assess prognosis for patients with prostate cancer. The inaccuracies and poor reproducibility in these grading systems have led many investigators to search for more objective and quantitative methods for grading prostate cancer. Morphometry has permitted a more careful quantification of these nuclear characteristics.

Diamond and associates[9,10] were the first to employ a simple nuclear shape factor (nuclear roundness) to describe the shape of cancerous nuclei for patients with stage B1 and B2 prostate cancer and accurately predicted outcome for these patients. Since then, several investigators have used this method to predict prognosis for patients with various stages of prostate cancer.[8,12,13,30,33,36,41,46,52] More recently, we have used a multivariate analysis of the variance of nuclear roundness, clinical stage, Gleason score, and the patient's age to predict disease-

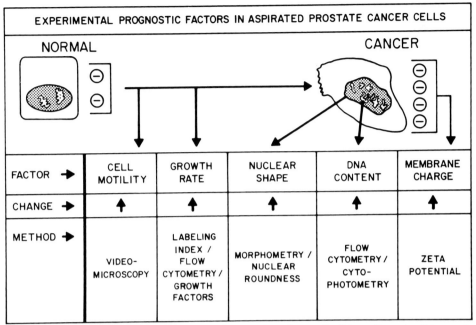

FIG. 9.4. Experimental prognostic factors. Progression of normal cell to malignant cell is associated with changes in the nucleus (shape, DNA content), cell membrane (membrane charge), and alterations in cell motility and growth rate. These changes can be used to help predict tumor behavior in prostate cancer. From Carter, H. B., and Coffey, D. S. Prediction of tumor behavior in prostate cancer. In *Prostate Cancer: The Second Tokyo Symposium*, edited by James P. Karr and Hidetoshi Yamanaka. New York, Elsevier Science Publishing Co., Inc., 1989, pp. 19–27.

free survival among a group of 100 postoperative patients with prostate cancer.[50] Figure 9.5 demonstrates the Kaplan-Meier survival curve for the variance of nuclear roundness as predictor of disease-free survival time for a group of 100 men with prostate cancer. These exciting new techniques have recently been applied to other urological malignancies including Wilms' tumor,[19,51] rhabdomyosarcoma,[27] and renal cell carcinoma.[39] In addition, recent advances in computer and image analysis technologies have made this quantitative modality available for routine analysis of patient samples in clinical practice.

CELL MOTILITY

Many grading systems, both architectural and cytological, have been developed to assess the metastatic potential of prostate cancers. These quantitative techniques have been applied to the prediction of prognosis based on the study of fixed, *i.e.*, *dead* cancer cells. Until recently, methods did not exist for study of the dynamic biological properties of *live* cancer cells. Time-lapse videomicroscopy of living cancer cells has revealed that some cancer cells demonstrate dynamic forms of cell motility. Cancer, often termed a disease of cell structure, has been recognized histologically by pathologists for over 100 years by its altered morphology. The diversity of cell shape and size among cancer cells is described by

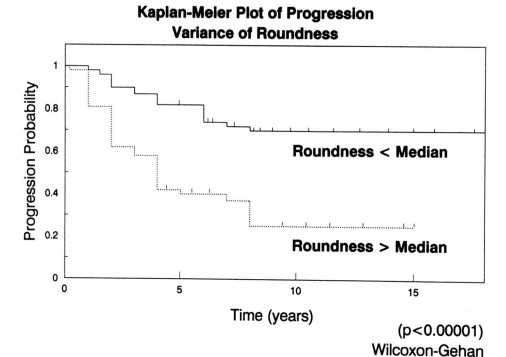

FIG. 9.5. Nuclear morphometry as a predictor of disease-free survival on prostate cancer. Kaplan-Meier actuarial time to progression survival curve for morphometric variance of nuclear roundness. *Solid line* = < median; *dotted line* = > median.

pathologists through the static analysis of fixed, *dead* cells and only represents a "freeze-frame" of the dynamic motility events occurring within *living* cancer cells.

Preliminary time-lapse studies of cancer cells taken from the Dunning R3327 rat model of prostatic adenocarcinoma demonstrated various distinct types of cell motility including cell membrane ruffing, pseudopodal extension, undulation, and cell translation. The development and testing of a visual motility grading system of these types of cancer cell motility[31,34,35] proved an accurate method for predicting prognosis among the Dunning model of prostate cancer[11,23] and established the feasibility for the development of a more quantitative approach. This technique, based on a combined temporal-spatial Fourier analysis of cell motility,[49] allowed accurate simultaneous measurement of these types of cell motility that correlated well with metastatic potential in this animal model of prostate cancer.

We studied the motility of live cancer cells aspirated directly from 55 human radical prostatectomy specimens[32] with clinically localized prostate cancer. Preliminary investigation of the motility of these live human cancer cells has demonstrated the feasibility and limitations of these methods for grading human prostate cancer.

A time-lapse videomicroscopy system was developed[34] with which we studied the motility of live cells from five Dunning tumors with varying metastatic potential. Visual grading of three parameters of cell motility, cell membrane ruffling, pseudopodal extension, and translation (Fig. 9.6) contained the information necessary for optimal identification of cells from the various cell lines. Membrane ruffling represents rapid rhythmic movement of short segments of cell membrane. Pseudopodal extension represents extension and retraction of short segments of cell membrane over long distances. Translation represents movement of the entire cell. This method of grading cell motility proved accurate and reproducible with intra-assay, intraobserver, and interobserver reproducibility of 75, 80, and 75%, respectively.

We then tested whether this visual grading system of cell motility could be used to predict the metastatic potential among various Dunning sublines.[31] Time-lapse films were made and visually graded using isolated cells taken from seven (four low metastatic and three highly metastatic) of the Dunning variants. Figure 9.7 demonstrates the marked differences found between cells taken from the highly metastatic cell lines and those from the low metastatic lines. Measurement of cell translation allowed correct categorization of 26 of 28 specimens, whereas the combination of translation and pseudopodal extension allowed correct categorization of 27 of the 28 tumors studied.

Our time-lapse videomicroscopy studies and subjective visual motility grading system demonstrated the ability of the human eye to recognize, classify, and categorize various types of cell motility that correlate well with metastatic potential in cells from the Dunning model of prostate cancer. Cell motility measurements from zero to five were too subjective and lack descriptive labels such as microns, degrees, and seconds. With this in mind, we combined the use of time-lapse videomicroscopy, image analysis techniques, and a new spatial-temporal two-dimensional Fourier analysis of cell motility to correlate metastatic potential with measurements of cell motility within the Dunning model.[49]

We used DynaCELL (JAW Associates Inc., Annapolis, MD), Motility Morphometry Measurement Workstation (Fig. 9.8) and a two-dimensional Fourier

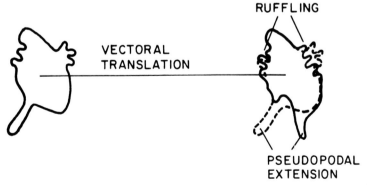

FIG. 9.6.   Visual cell motility grading system. Each parameter of cell motility was graded from 0, none observed, to 5, excessive amounts of motility. From Mohler, J. L., Partin, A. W., Isaacs, W. I., and Coffey, D. S. Time-lapse videomicroscopic identification of Dunning R3327 adenocarcinoma and normal rat prostate cells. *J. Urol. 137:* 544–547, 1987.

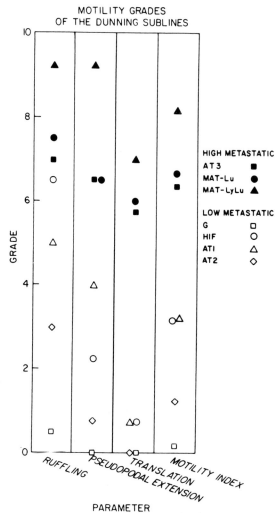

FIG. 9.7.   The motility grades for the three motility parameters, ruffling, pseudopodal extension, and translation as well as the motility index are depicted for seven of the Dunning sublines. Solid figures represent cell lines with ≥90% of subcutaneously inoculated animals developing metastases and open figures represent sublines, in which ≤20% of animals develop metastases. From Mohler, J. L., Partin, A. W., Isaacs, J. T., and Coffey, D. S. Metastatic potential prediction by a visual grading system of cell motility: Prospective validation in the Dunning R3327 prostatic adenocarcinoma model. *Cancer Res. 48:* 4312–4317, 1988.

analysis of cell motility to quantitate cell motility among the Dunning cell lines. Figure 9.9 is a flow diagram depicting the quantitative measurement of cell motility of single cells with a spatial-temporal Fourier analysis of cell motility by this method. We then measured the motility with this method for 26 cells from each of 6 of the Dunning tumor cell lines with varying metastatic potential. Figure 9.10 demonstrates the mean and distribution of the various Dunning cell lines as well as their metastatic potential. The motility coefficients for translation

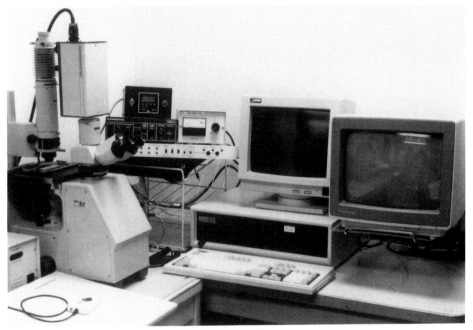

FIG. 9.8. Equipment used for Fourier analysis of cell motility. Photograph depicts the equipment used for this new Fourier method of analyzing cell motility. The equipment consists of a computer, frame grabber, VGA monitor, multisync color video monitor, digitizer tablet, Nomarski optics, heated stage, time-date generator, and time controller box.

and pseudopodal extension were higher for cells from tumor sublines with higher metastatic potential. Fourier motility coefficients yielded correlation coefficients of 0.63 for pseudopodal extension ($p < 0001$), 0.59 for undulation ($p < 0.001$), 0.50 for translation ($p < 0.001$), and 0.50 for ruffling ($p < 0.001$). This new spatial-temporal Fourier analysis accurately quantified the different types of cell motility and should aid in the study of the motility of individual cells in many areas of cell and tumor biology.

We studied the motility of cancer cells from 55 radical prostatectomy specimens from patients with clinically localized prostatic carcinoma.[32] Forty-five of these yielded adequate attachment to culture plates to allow analysis by time-lapse videomicroscopy for visual grading of the various types of cell motility. This group consisted of B1N ($N = 6$), B1 ($N = 28$), B2 ($N = 10$), and C1 ($N = 1$). The average motility index (sum of the three visual motility parameters) varied markedly within the patients, not only between histopathological grades, but within a single histopathological grade as well. This separation of patients within and between pathological grade and stage provides hope that a motility grading system similar to this may add to the limited ability of stage and grade to predict the prognosis of individual patients with prostatic carcinoma. These early results with human prostatic carcinomas are too preliminary to ascertain the usefulness as a predictor of progression due to the long natural history of this disease (1 of 45 patients to date has progressed). Nonetheless, these data did demonstrate an

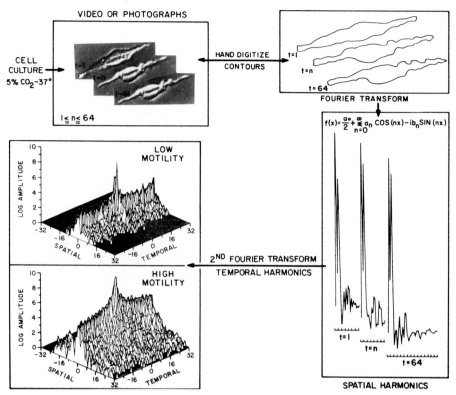

FIG. 9.9. Quantitative measurement of the motility of individual cells with a spatial-temporal Fourier analysis of time-lapse images. Cells were inoculated at low density on glass. Individual cells were viewed at ×400 with an inverted Nomarski optics microscope. Images were collected at 60-second intervals for 64 minutes. Cell contours were manually traced with a digitizer tablet in succession. The X-Y coordinates of each successive cell contour were then subject to a spatial complex fast Fourier transform (FFT) to determine the spatial Fourier motility coefficients describing the cell shape. The spatial Fourier coefficients for each of the 64 cell contours were then combined into a matrix and subject to a second FFT to determine the temporal changes in the spatial Fourier coefficients. The root sum of the square of the coefficient produces the Fourier motility coefficients. This is graphically depicted in a three-dimensional plot. The results of a highly motile cell are compared with that of a low motile cell. From Partin, A. W., Schoeniger, J. S., Mohler, J. L., and Coffey, D. S. Fourier analysis of cell motility: Correlation of motility with metastatic potential. *Proc. Natl. Acad. Sci. USA 86:* 1254–1258, 1989.

increased heterogeneity (coefficient of variation average of 68%) not seen among the cells studied in the Dunning model (coefficient of variations averaging 33%).

In summary, we feel that it is too early to assess the usefulness of cell motility in the evaluation of human prostate cancer. We are optimistic, however, with further research and the use of the quantitative methods previously described that this valuable method of studying the dynamic nature of *live* cancer cells will undoubtedly aid in the study of prostate cancer and other forms of cancer.

GROWTH RATE

Tumor growth rate often correlates directly with tumor aggressiveness, and increased growth rate, as measured by estimating the percentage of cells repli-

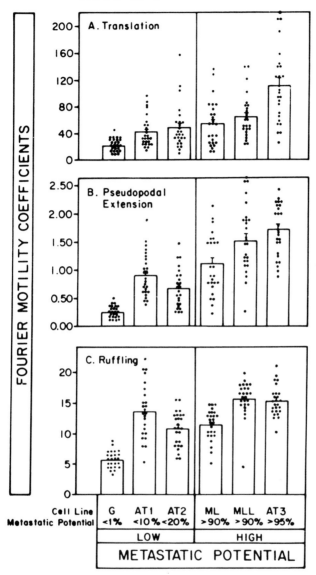

FIG. 9.10. Comparison of the Fourier motility coefficients for translation (*A*), pseudopodal extension (*B*), and ruffling (*C*) for six Dunning cell sublines with varying metastatic potential. Twenty-six cells from each of six Dunning cell lines were analyzed with the spatial-temporal Fourier method described in Figures 9.3 and 9.4. The metastatic potential of each cell line is expressed as the percent of animals that develop distant metastases following subcutaneous injection of 10^5 cells found at the time of death or at autopsy 42 days postinjection. Metastatic potential is arbitrarily defined as low metastatic when <20% of rats develop distant metastases and high when >90% develop distant metastases. *Bars* represent the mean ± SEM for 26 cells from each cell line. *ML* and *MLL* represent MAT-Lu and MAT-LyLu, respectively. From Partin, A. W., Schoeniger, J. S., Mohler, J. L., and Coffey, D. S. Fourier analysis of cell motility: Correlation of motility with metastatic potential. *Proc. Natl. Acad. Sci. USA* 86: 1254–1258, 1989.

cating their DNA (labeling index), has been correlated with aggressiveness in prostate cancer.[26,59,63] Classically, tumor proliferation rate has been estimated by incubation of cells with tritiated thymidine, which is taken up by cells in the S-phase of the cell cycle (DNA replication phase). Subsequent production of an autoradiogram then allows quantitation of the number of cell in S-phase, and thus a method of estimating tumor proliferation rate. Newer methods of estimating the growth fraction of tumors utilize flow cytometric quantification of the number of cells with DNA content between diploid and tetraploid (S-phase fraction). Specific fluorescent labeling of DNA precursors taken up by cells synthesizing DNA can also be detected using flow cytometry.[22] In addition, cell cycle markers have recently been described which allow the quantification of not only the cells in S-phase but all cells in the cell cycle (G1,S, G2,M).[67] These antigens appear to be present in the nucleus of cells, and monoclonal antibodies to these antigens (*e.g.*, Ki-67, Fig. 9.11) allow quantification of cells expressing the antigens. Newly characterized growth factors which are thought to play a roll in the loss of growth control in tumor cells may add further to the evaluation of tumor growth rate, and thus help predict tumor behavior.[67]

DNA CONTENT

There are both quantitative as well as qualitative changes in the DNA content of cells as they undergo progression from normal to cancer cells. These changes

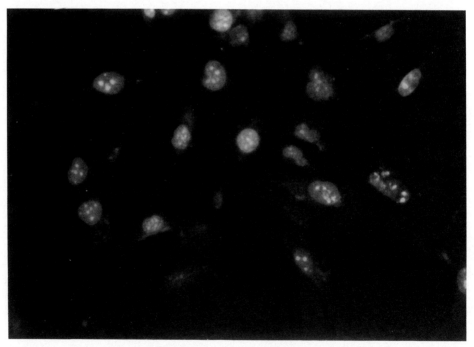

FIG. 9.11.   Ki-67 staining of Dunning rat prostate cancer cells. Immunofluorescent staining of highly metastatic Dunning R-3327 rat prostate cancer cells at ×2240 magnification. Note the intense staining of the nuclear border and nucleolar region.

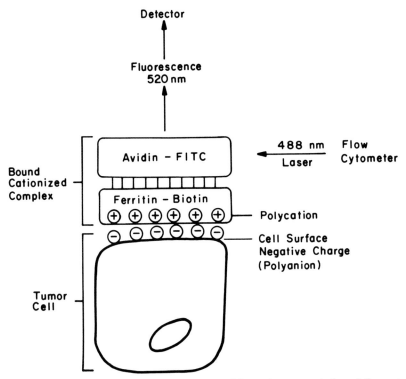

FIG. 9.12. Cell surface charge and flow cytometry. Schematic representation of flow cytometric method for quantification of cell surface charge. Cationized ferritin-biotin is bound to tumor cell surface prior to addition of fluoresceinated avidin (*avidin-FITC*). Measurement of fluorescent emission and cell size for each tumor cell using flow cytometry allows calculation of a relative surface charge. From Carter, H. B., Partin, A. W., and Coffey, D. S. Prediction of metastatic potential in an animal model of prostate cancer: Flow cytometric quantification of cell surface charge. *J. Urol. 142:* 1338–1341, 1989.

are associated with the changes in nuclear shape mentioned above. Indirect quantification of DNA content (ploidy) has been possible using light microscopy (cytophotometry) and laser-induced fluorescence (flow cytometry). Using fluorescent dyes capable of specifically staining DNA allows ploidy measurements on thousands of cells within minutes when flow cytometry is used to quantitate fluorescence. The measurement of tumor cell DNA content may add to the ability to predict tumor behavior in prostate cancer[62]; however, because not all potentially aggressive tumors have abnormal DNA content that can be detected by fluorescence measurements, additional parameters will probably be required to accurately predict a patient's prognosis. This topic is dealt with in detail in Chapter 5 within this text.

MEMBRANE CHARGE

It would appear that changes at the surface of the cell are important in the metastatic process.[57] For example, all eukaryotic cells have a net negative surface

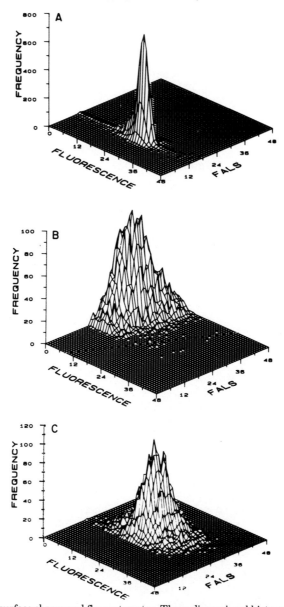

FIG. 9.13.   Cell surface charge and flow cytometry. Three-dimensional histogram plots of standard microspheres (*A*), AT-1 (low metastatic) Dunning tumor (*B*), and MAT-LyLu (high metastatic) Dunning tumor (*C*). X-axis, log forward angle light scatter (FALS); Y-axis, log green fluorescent intensity of sample minus control; Z-axis, frequency of events. From Carter, H. B., Partin, A. W., and Coffey, D. S. Prediction of metastatic potential in an animal model of prostate cancer: Flow cytometric quantification of cell surface charge. *J. Urol. 142:* 1338–1341, 1989.

Measurement Of Cell Surface Charge
By Electrophoresis And Flow Cytometry
Dunning Prostate Tumor Model

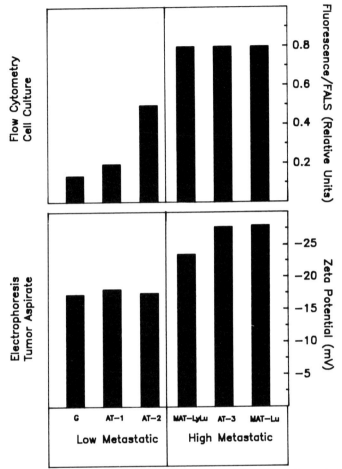

FIG. 9.14. Comparison of electrophoretic and flow cytometric surface charge techniques. Flow cytometric measurement of cell surface charge (top graph) and electrophoretic measurement of cell charge (bottom graph) on low (G, AT-1, and AT-2) and high (MAT-LyLu, AT-3, and MAT-Lu) metastatic sublines of the Dunning R-3327 rat prostatic animal model. Y-axis of top graph represents relative units of log mean fluorescent intensity/log mean FALS. Y-axis of bottom graph represents zeta potential in millivolts calculated from electrophoretic mobility. From Carter, H. B., and Coffey, D. S. Prediction of tumor behavior in prostate cancer. In *Prostate Cancer: The Second Tokyo Symposium*, edited by James P. Karr and Hidetoshi Yamanaka. New York, Elsevier Science Publishing Co., Inc., 1989, pp. 19–27.

charge, and an increase in this negative charge has been associated with both transformation from a normal cell to a cancer cell, and from nonmetastatic to metastatic cells.[1,55] The Dunning R-3327 animal model previously described[11,23] has been used widely in the study of prostate cancer because of its similarities with human prostate cancer. Using six different sublines of the Dunning model (G, AT1, AT2—low metastatic; AT3, MAT-Lu, MAT-LyLu—high metastatic) growing subcutaneously in rats, the relationship between cell surface charge and metastatic potential was studied.[4]

Cells were aspirated in a similar fashion to fine-needle aspiration when the tumors were palpable. Tumor cell movement in an electric field was measured in microns per second per volt per centimeter (electrophoretic mobility). A simple equation (Helmholtz equation) was then used to calculate a zeta potential (surface charge) from the electrophoretic mobility. On 100 cells from each of the six Dunning sublines studied, a zeta potential in millivolts was calculated. There was a significant difference in cell surface charge noted between the low and high metastatic tumor cells. We noticed more negativity at the cell surface associated with a greater metastatic potential.

Because this method of measuring cell surface charge is time consuming and requires large numbers of cells for each assay, a flow cytometric method for measuring cell surface charge was investigated for the same Dunning sublines. A chemical complex between cationized ferritin and biotin was made and used to tag the regions of apparent negativity on the cell membrane. In a second step, fluoresceinated avidin was used to label the positively charged ferritin-biotin complex.[5] In this manner, the fluorescent intensity as measured by flow cytometry was used as an indirect measure of cell surface negativity. Figure 9.12 demonstrates a schematic representation of this flow cytometric method for quantification of cell surface charge. In addition, the forward angle light scatter (FALS) was measured for each cell line as an indirect measure of surface area, and thus the ratio of fluorescent intensity and the FALS represented an indirect measure of net charge per surface area. Figure 9.13 demonstrates the three-dimensional representations of the flow cytometric data comparing the surface charge and FALS for a standard microsphere of known size and charge with those of a population of low versus highly metastatic Dunning cells. Figure 9.14 shows the results of the flow cytometric and electrophoretic measurements of surface charge on the low and high metastatic sublines of the Dunning tumor. Using either method to measure cell surface charge, an increase in negativity at the cell surface was associated with a greater metastatic potential.

SUMMARY

Because the present ability to treat and cure patients with prostate cancer is limited to those patients with pathologically organ-confined disease, it has become increasingly important to diagnose this disease at an early stage when cure is most likely. Recent advances in imaging may allow the urologist and pathologist to make the diagnosis of prostate cancer much earlier in the natural course of the disease. It therefore becomes imperative to have methods available to predict which patients have a high probability of progressing so that treatment can be assigned logically and appropriately. Our current methods of prognosis determination (stage and grade) do not allow accurate assessment of tumor behavior in the majority of individual patients with prostate cancer. Therefore, more accurate quantification of nuclear and cellular changes that take place as a tumor progresses to take on the aggressive (metastatic) phenotype are urgently needed. Experimental techniques have proven useful in answering these questions in animal models and now seem ready for large-scale testing in clinical studies.

ACKNOWLEDGMENTS

The authors wish to thank Ms. Ruth Middleton for her expert assistance in the preparation of this manuscript. This work was supported by a grant (CA 15416) from the National Cancer Institute.

REFERENCES

1. Ambrose, E. J., James, A. M., and Lowick, J. H. B. Differences in the electrical charge carried out by normal and homologous tumor cells. *Nature (Lond.) 177:* 576, 1956.
2. Cantrell, B. B., deKlerk, D. P., Eggleston, J. C., Boitnott, J. K., and Walsh, P. C. Pathological factors that influence prognosis in stage A prostatic cancer: The influence of extent versus grade. *J. Urol. 125:* 516, 1981.
3. Carter, H. B., and Coffey, D. S. Prostate cancer: The magnitude of the problem in the United States. In *A Multidisciplinary Analysis of Controversies in the Management of Prostate Cancer*, edited by D. S. Coffey, M. I. Resnick, F. A. Dorr, and J. P. Karr. New York, Plenum Press, 1988, pp. 1–7.
4. Carter, H. B., and Coffey, D. S. Cell surface charge in predicting metastatic potential of aspirated cells from the Dunning rat prostatic adenocarcinoma model. *J. Urol. 140:* 173, 1988.
5. Carter, H. B., Partin, A. W., and Coffey, D. S. Prediction of metastatic potential in an animal model of prostate cancer: Flow cytometric quantification of cell surface charge. *J. Urol. 142:* 1338, 1989.
6. Carter, H. B., Pearson, J. D., Metter, J. E., Brant, L., Chan, D. W., Andres, R. E., Fozard, J., and Walsh, P. C. Longitudinal evaluation of prostate specific antigen in men with and without prostate disease. *J.A.M.A.* (In Press).
7. Chan, D. W., Bruzek, D. J., Oesterling, J. E., Rock, R. C., and Walsh, P. C. Prostate-specific antigen as a marker for prostate cancer: A monoclonal and a polyclonal immunoassay compared. *Clin. Chem. 33:* 1916, 1987.
8. Clark, T. D., Askin, F. B., and Bagnell, C. F. Nuclear roundness factor: A quantitative approach to grading in prostatic carcinoma, reliability of needle biopsy tissue, and the effect of tumor stage on usefulness. *Prostate 10:* 199, 1987.
9. Diamond, D. A., Berry, D. S., Jewett, H. J., Eggleston, J. C., and Coffey, D. S. A new method to assess metastatic potential of human prostate cancer: Relative nuclear roundness. *J. Urol. 128:* 729, 1982.
10. Diamond, D. A., Berry, S. J., Umbricht, C., Jewett, H. J., and Coffey, D. S. Computerized image analysis of nuclear shape as a prognostic factor for prostatic cancer. *Prostate 3:* 321, 1982.
11. Dunning, W. F. Prostate cancer in the rat. *NCI Monograph 12:* 351, 1963.
12. Eichenberger, T., Mihatsch, M. J., Oberholzer, M., Gschwind, R., and Rutishauser, G. *Prostate Cancer. Part A: Research, Endocrine Treatment, and Histopathology.* New York, Alan R. Liss, Inc., 1987, pp. 533–537.
13. Epstein, J. I., Berry, S. J., and Eggleston, J. C. Nuclear roundness factor: A predictor of prognosis in untreated stage A2 prostate cancer. *Cancer 54:* 1666, 1984.
14. Epstein, J. I., Oesterling, J. E., and Walsh, P. C. Tumor volume versus percentage involved by tumor correlated with progression in stage A prostatic cancer. *J. Urol. 139:* 980, 1988.
15. Ercole, C. J., Lange, P. H., Mathiesen, M., Chiou, R. K., Reddy, P. K., and Vessella, R. L.

Prostatic specific antigen and prostatic acid phosphatase in the monitoring and staging of patients with prostatic cancer. *J. Urol. 138:* 1181, 1987.

16. Farber, E. The multistep nature of cancer development. *Cancer Res. 44:* 4217, 1984.

17. Freiha, F. S. Selection criteria for radical prostatectomy based on morphometric studies. In *Consensus Development Conference on Management of Clinically Localized Prostate Cancer, National Institutes of Health, Bethesda, Md., Program and Abstracts,* June 15–17, 1987, p. 73.

18. Frost, J. E., editor. *The Cell in Health and Disease.* New York, Karger, 1986, p. 1.

19. Gearhart, J. P., Partin, A. W., Leventhal, B., Beckwith, J. B., and Epstein, J. I. The use of nuclear morphometry to predict response to therapy in Wilms' tumor. *Cancer 69:* 804–808, 1992.

20. Gibbons, R. P., Correa, R. J., Jr., Brannen, G. E., and Mason, J. T. Total prostatectomy for localized prostatic cancer. *J. Urol. 131:* 73, 1984.

21. Gleason, D. F., Mellinger, G. T., and the Veterans Administrative Cooperative Urological Research Group. Prediction of prognosis for prostatic adenocarcinoma by combined histological grading and clinical staging. *J. Urol. 111:* 58, 1974.

22. Gray, J. W., and Mayall, B. H., editors. *Monoclonal Antibodies Against Bromodeoxyuridine.* New York, Alan R. Liss, Inc., 1985.

23. Isaacs, J. T., Isaacs, W. B., Feitz, W. F. J., and Scheres, J. Establishment and characterization of seven Dunning rat prostatic cancer cell lines and their use in developing methods for predicting metastatic abilities of prostatic cancers. *Prostate 9:* 261, 1986.

24. Jewett, H. J. The present status of radical prostatectomy for stages A and B prostatic cancer. *Urol. Clin. North Am. 2:* 105, 1975.

25. Lange, P. H., and Winfield, H. N. Biological markers in urologic cancer. *Cancer 60:* 464, 1987.

26. Lelle, J. J., Heidenreich, W., Stauch, G., and Gerdes, J. The correlation of growth fractions with histologic grading and lymph node status in human mammary carcinoma. *Cancer 59:* 83, 1987.

27. Leonard, M. P., Partin, A. W., Epstein, J. I., Jeffs, R. D., and Gearhart, J. P. Nuclear morphometry as a prognostic index for pediatric genitourinary Rhabdomyosarcoma. *J. Urol. 144:* 1222, 1990.

28. McNeal, J. E., Kindrachuk, R. A., Freiha, F. S., Bostwick, D. G., Redwine, E. A., and Stamey, T. A. Patterns of progression in prostate cancer. *Lancet 1:* 60, 1986.

29. Middleton, R. G., Smith, J. A., Jr., Metzer, R. B., and Hamilton, P. E. Patient survival and local recurrence rate following radical prostatectomy for prostatic carcinoma. *J. Urol. 136:* 422, 1986.

30. Miller, G. J., and Shikes, J. L. Nuclear roundness as a predictor of response to hormonal therapy of patients with stage D2 prostatic carcinoma. In *Prognostic Cytometry and Cytopathology of Prostate Cancer,* edited by J. P. Karr, D. S. Coffey, and W. Gardner. New York, Elsevier Science Publishing Co., Inc., 1988, pp. 349–354.

31. Mohler, J. L., Partin, A. W., and Coffey, D. S. Prediction of metastatic potential by a new grading system of cell motility: Validation in the Dunning R3327 prostatic adenocarcinoma model. *J. Urol. 138:* 168–170, 1987.

32. Mohler, J. L., Partin, A. W., and Coffey, D. S. Cancer cell motility: A visual grading system for assessment of prognosis in prostatic cancer. In *Prognostic Cytometry and Cytopathology of Prostate Cancer,* edited by J. P. Karr, D. S. Coffey, and W. Gardner, Jr., New York, Elsevier Science Publishing, Co., 1988, pp. 337–348.

33. Mohler, J. L., Partin, A. W., Epstein, J. I., Lohr, D. W., and Coffey, D. S. Nuclear roundness factor measurement for assessment of prognosis of patients with prostatic carcinoma. II. Standardization of methodology for histologic sections. *J. Urol. 139:* 1085–1090, 1988.

34. Mohler, J. L., Partin, A. W., Isaacs, W. I., and Coffey, D. S. Time-lapse videomicroscopic identification of Dunning R3327 adenocarcinoma and normal rat prostate cells. *J. Urol. 137:* 544–547, 1987.

35. Mohler, J. L., Partin, A. W., Isaacs, J. T., and Coffey, D. S. Metastatic potential prediction by a visual grading system of cell motility: Prospective validation in the Dunning R3327 prostatic adenocarcinoma model. *Cancer Res. 48:* 4312–4317, 1988.

36. Mohler, J. L., Partin, A. W., Lohr, D. W., and Coffey, D. S. Nuclear roundness factor measurement for assessment of prognosis of patients with prostatic carcinoma. I. Testing of a digitization system. *J. Urol. 139:* 1080, 1988.

37. Mostofi, F. K. Grading of prostatic carcinoma. *Cancer Chem. Rep. 59:* 111, 1975.
38. Murphy, G. P., Gaeta, J. F., Pickren, J., and Wajsman, Z. Current status of classification and staging of prostate cancer. *Cancer 45:* 1889, 1980.
39. Murphy, G. F., Partin, A. W., Maygarden, S. J., and Mohler, J. L. Nuclear shape analysis for assessment of prognosis in renal cell carcinoma. *J. Urol. 143:* 1103, 1990.
40. Myers, R. P., and Fleming, T. R. Course of localized adenocarcinoma of the prostate treated by radical prostatectomy. *Prostate 4:* 461, 1983.
41. Narayan, P., Michael, M., Jajodia, P., Stein, R., Gonzalez, J., Ljung, B., Chu, K., and Myall, B. Automated image analysis—a new technique to predict metastatic potential of prostate carcinomas? (Abstract.) *J. Urol. 141* (4 part 2): 183, 1989.
42. National Cancer Institute Division of Cancer Prevention and Control. *Annual Cancer Statistics Review.* NIH Publication No. 88-2789, 1987.
43. Nowell, P. C. Genetic instability in cancer cells: Relationship to tumor cell heterogeneity. In *Tumor Cell Heterogeneity: Origins and Implications*, edited by A. H., Jr., Owens, D. S. Coffey, and S. B. Baylin. New York, Academic Press, 1982, pp. 351–364.
44. Nowell, P. C. Mechanisms of tumor progression. *Cancer Res. 46:* 2203, 1986.
45. Oesterling, J. E., Chan, D. W., Epstein, J. I., Kimball, A. W., Jr., Bruzek, D. J., Rock, R. C., Brendler, C. B., and Walsh, P. C. Prostate specific antigen in the preoperative and postoperative evaluation of localized prostatic cancer treated with radical prostatectomy. *J. Urol. 139:* 766, 1988.
46. Partin, A. W. The development of a system for the quantitative analysis of tumor cell motility: Application to prostate cancer. Baltimore, The Johns Hopkins University, 1988. Thesis.
47. Partin, A. W., Carter, H. B., Chan, D. W., Epstein, J. I., Oesterling, J. E., Rock, R. C., Weber, J. P., and Walsh, P. C. Prostate specific antigen in the staging of localized prostate cancer: Influence of tumor differentiation, tumor volume and benign hyperplasia. *J. Urol. 143:* 747–752, 1990.
48. Partin, A. W., Epstein, J. I., Cho, K. R., Gittelsohn, A. M., and Walsh, P. C. Morphometric measurement of tumor volume and percent of gland involvement as predictors of pathologic stage in clinical stage B prostate cancer. *J. Urol. 141:* 341–345, 1989.
49. Partin, A. W., Schoeniger, J. S., Mohler, J. L., and Coffey, D. S. Fourier analysis of cell motility: Correlation of motility with metastatic potential. *Proc. Natl. Acad. Sci. USA 86:* 1254–1258, 1989.
50. Partin, A. W., Steinberg, G. D., Pitcock, R. V., Wu, L., Piantadosi, S., Coffey, D. S., and Epstein, J. I. Use of nuclear morphometry, Gleason histologic scoring, clinical stage and age to predict disease free survival among patients with prostate cancer. *Cancer* (In Press).
51. Partin, A. W., Walsh, A. C., Epstein, J. I., Leventhal, B. G., and Gearhart, J. P. Nuclear morphometry as a predictor of response to therapy in Wilms' tumor: A preliminary report. *J. Urol. 144:* 952, 1990.
52. Partin, A. W., Walsh, A. C., Pitcock, R. V., Mohler, J. L., Epstein, J. I., and Coffey, D. S. A comparison of nuclear morphometry and Gleason grade as a predictor of prognosis in stage A2 prostate cancer: A critical analysis. *J. Urol. 142:* 1254, 1989.
53. Paulson, D. F. Radiotherapy versus surgery for localized prostatic cancer. *Urol. Clin. North Am. 14:* 675, 1987.
54. Paulson, D. F., Stone, A. R., Walther, P. J., Tucker, J. A., and Cox, E. G. Radical prostatectomy: Anatomical predictors of success or failure. *J. Urol. 136:* 1041–1045, 1986.
55. Purdom, A., Ambrose, E. J., and Klein, G. A correlation between electrical surface charge and some biological characteristics during the stepwise progression of a mouse sarcoma. *Nature (Lond.) 181:* 1586, 1958.
56. Robey, E. L., and Schellhammer, P. F. Local failure after definitive therapy for prostatic cancer. *J. Urol. 137:* 613, 1987.
57. Robbins, J. C., and Nicolson, G. L. Surfaces of normal and transformed cells. In *Cancer: A Comprehensive Treatise*, edited by F. F. Becker. New York, Plenum Press, 1975, pp. 12–42.
58. Seidman, H., Mushinski, M. H., Gelb, S. K., and Silverberg, E. Probabilities of eventually developing or dying of cancer: United States, 1985. *CA 35:* 36, 1985.

59. Sledge, G. W., Jr., Eble, J. N., Roth, B. J., Wihrman, B. P., Fineberg, N., and Einhorn, L. H. Relation of proliferative activity to survival in patients with advanced germ cell cancer. *Cancer Res. 48:* 3864–3868, 1988.

60. Stamey, T. A., Kabalin, J. N., McNeal, J. E., Jr., Johnstone, I. M., Frieha, F., Redwine, E. A., and Yang, N. Prostate specific antigen in the diagnosis and treatment of adenocarcinoma of the prostate. II. Radical prostatectomy treated patients. *J. Urol. 141:* 1076, 1989.

61. Stamey, T. A., Yang, N., Hay, A. R., McNeal, J. E., Freiha, F. S., and Redwine, E. A. Prostate-specific antigen as a serum marker for adenocarcinoma of the prostate. *New Engl. J. Med. 317:* 909, 1987.

62. Tribukait, B. Flow cytometry in assessing the clinical aggressiveness of genitourinary neoplasms. *World J. Urol. 5:* 108, 1987.

63. Uchida, K., Hattomi, K., Kawai, K., Nishijima, Y., and Nemoto, R. A cell kinetics study of prostate cancer with bromodeoxyuridine—microscopic growth pattern and S-phase fraction. Presented at 83rd Annual Meeting of the American Urological Association, Boston, June, 1988.

64. Virchow, R. Ueber bewegliche thierische zellen. *Arch. Pathol. Anat. Physiol. Klin. Med. 28:* 237, 1863.

65. Walsh, P. C., and Jewett, H. J. Radical surgery for prostatic cancer. *Cancer 45:* 1906, 1980.

66. Whitmore, W. F., Jr. Hormone therapy in prostatic cancer. *Am. J. Med. 21:* 697, 1956.

67. Wilson, E. M., and Smith, E. P. Growth factors in the prostate. *Prog. Clin. Biol. Res. 239:* 205, 1987.

Index

Page numbers followed by italic "t" denote tables; those followed by italic "f" denote figures.